# THE PROMOTION OF WELLNESS IN CHILDREN AND ADOLESCENTS

Edited by
Dante Cicchetti, Julian Rappaport,
Irwin Sandler, Roger P. Weissberg

CWLA Press ■ Washington, D.C.

CWLA Press is an imprint of the Child Welfare League of America. The Child Welfare League of America (CWLA), the nation's oldest and largest membership-based child welfare organization, is committed to engaging all Americans in promoting the well-being of children and protecting every child from harm.

CHILD WELFARE LEAGUE OF AMERICA, INC.
440 First Street, NW, Third Floor, Washington, DC 20001-2085
E-mail: books@cwla.org

CURRENT PRINTING (last digit)
10 9 8 7 6 5 4 3 2 1

Cover design by James D. Melvin
Text design by Peggy Porter Tierney

Printed in the United States of America
ISBN # 0–87868–791–2

*Library of Congress Cataloging-in-Publication Data*
The promotion of wellness in children and adolescents / edited by Dante Cicchetti ... [et al.].
    p. cm.
  Includes bibliographical references.
  ISBN 0-87868-791-2
  1. Health promotion--United States. 2. Mental health promotion--United States. 3. Children--Health and hygiene--United States. 4. Children--Mental health--United States. 5. Teenagers--Health and hygiene--United States. 6. Teenagers--Mental health--United States. 7. Child mental health--United States. 8. Developmental psychology--United States. 9. Medical policy--United States. I. Cicchetti, Dante.

RJ102.P76 2000
613'.0432'0973--dc21

00-030364

# Issues in Children's and Families' Lives
## An Annual Book Series

### Senior Series Editor
Thomas P. Gullotta, *Child and Family Agency of Southeastern Connecticut*

### Editors, The University of Chicago At Illinois Series on Children and Youth
Arthur J. Reynolds, *University of Wisconsin-Madison*
Herbert J. Walberg, *University of Illinois at Chicago*
Roger P. Weissberg, *University of Illinois at Chicago*

Drawing upon the resources of the Child and Family Agency of Southeastern Connecticut, one of the nation's leading family service agencies, **Issues in Children's and Families' Lives** is designed to focus attention on the pressing social problems facing children and their families today. Each volume in this series will analyze, integrate, and critique the clinical and research literature on children and their families as it relates to a particular theme. Believing that integrated multidisciplinary approaches offer greater opportunities for program success, volume contributors will reflect the research and clinical knowledge base of the many different disciplines that are committed to enhancing the physical, social, and emotional health of children and their families. Intended for graduate and professional audiences, chapters will be written by scholars and practitioners who will encourage readers to apply their practice skills and intellect to reducing the suffering of children and their families in the society in which they live and work.

*Thomas P. Gullotta*
Chief Executive Officer
Child and Family Agency of
Southeastern Connecticut

# Contents

# Foreword

I have long felt a strong kinship with Emory Cowen, but I was not fully aware of some subtle connections between us until I was able to pry some biographical details from him. These data were difficult to obtain because he urged me to err in the direction of brevity—"the briefer and less ostentatious the better," he wrote. But in the interest of history, there are some things the record should show.

Emory grew up on "the streets of Brooklyn," the city of his birth, during the Great Depression. I am about four years older, and I also was deeply affected by that same depression. In my small town in rural Pennsylvania, food was hard to come by, with the exception of venison and brook trout, which were free for the taking.

Emory went to Brooklyn College, unsure of his vocational goals. My late first wife, eldest daughter of Sicilian immigrant parents, moved with her family to Brooklyn from Manhattan's Lower East Side, and she attended Brooklyn College at the same time as Emory. Indeed, it is probable that they sat together in the same psychology classes because both were strongly influenced by Abraham Maslow. Emory went into the new field of clinical psychology that Maslow found promising, especially the development called "nondirective therapy." In 1946, he entered graduate school at Syracuse University to study with Arthur W. Cooms, a former student of Carl Rogers. (My late wife went into graduate school to study social group work and social change.) In 1946, I enrolled in clinical psychology at the University of Pittsburgh to study with Victor Raimy, another former student of Carl Rogers. I was also able to take courses with Thomas Gordon and Virginia Axline, both Rogerians. Our early publications included articles on psychotherapy. My late first wife was so entranced by Maslow that when he and I were both on the APA presidential ballot, she campaigned for him! (I was elected two years later with her support.) Unfortunately, Maslow was too ill to serve actively as APA President, so George Miller and I substituted for him during part of his term as president and past president.

In those early years, when clinical psychology was young, when there were few of us in universities and when fewer still were doing meaningful research, I wrote a letter to Emory. Because neither my memory nor my organizational skills allow me to pinpoint the exact date, I must approximate it—probably the mid-1960s. Anyway, the date is not important; it was Emory's response that is forever fixed in my head. I was on the Editorial Board of the *Annual Review of Psychology*, and it was the task of board members to recommend and enlist people to be writers of chapters reviewing research on a specific topic. My letter to Emory was a request that he do a review of research on psychotherapy. I was familiar with his reputation as a solid scientist and gifted researcher. His publications included articles on group therapy and others on psychotherapy research. His response to my invitation was direct and clear. No, he replied, I am moving into work in the schools and community. He went on to explain that one-to-one psychotherapy was not going to solve the mental health problems of the nation, and that a better strategy was to work with young children in the schools to prevent early problems from growing into big problems later. The letter had an impact on me. I was already convinced from my work with the Eisenhower Commission (Joint Commission on Mental Illness and Health) that our nation would never have enough therapists to deal effectively with the vast number of people with problems. Emory's approach, his reprints enclosed, was a ray of light. While the growing field of clinical psychology was hell-bent to do one-on-one psychotherapy, Emory already saw a more important and effective way. I shared his view: mental disorders could not be treated out of existence.

I wish I had preserved his letter. (Later I learned that every letter from Emory is a jewel, carefully crafted and original, and I began to keep them in a special file.) When I retired from the University of Vermont in 1993 and was forced, finally, to attack and sort endless boxes of papers stored in the basement of my farm house, I arranged to ship those of historical significance to the new library of the American Psychological Association. An archivist, I was told, would put things in order and preserve these historical treasures. Of course I included my collection of letters from Emory, so future historians of psychology will find these critical data.

In doing honor to Emory, his generous sharing of time with his graduate students must be noted, a great many of whom have gone on to important positions of influence in community psychology. Emory has supervised more than 70 doctoral students and has influenced many more in educational institutions around the world. (One of the things I learned in studying his history was his NIMH Special Senior Research Fellowship at the University of Paris in the early 1960s, and his subsequent visits to France and publications in French in several French psychological journals.)

Ten years or so after our first exchange of correspondence, Emory did a review of social and community interventions for the 1973 *Annual Review of Psychology* [Cowen 1973] and I, with Marc Kessler, did a review of the field of primary prevention in the 1975 volume [Kessler 1975].

It had become clear to both of us that to work in the community, and especially in primary prevention, was the only effective way to reduce the rate of mental/emotional disorders in the population. Cowen focused his attention on enhancing wellness and the prevention of human ineffectiveness and suffering by programs aimed at reducing or preventing the early problems of children in the schools. His writings include seven books, 50 chapters and monographs, and more than 200 articles in the scientific and professional literature. Probably the most important of his many contributions is the Primary Mental Health Project involving the early detection and prevention of children's impending maladjustment in the schools. This clearly defined and well-researched intervention is now being used in 500 school systems throughout the world. These programs have a major emphasis on fostering children's competencies "known to subserve wellness," changing classroom practices "to enhance children's adaptation," and "to help children at risk cope with stressful life events" [see American Psychologist, April 1990, pp. 477-478]. Cowen, with several colleagues, published *School-based prevention for children at risk: The primary Mental Health Project* [1996], a detailed review of this major effective program.

During the mid-1970s, Emory and I served as members of the Task Panel on Prevention of the President's (Carter) Commission on Mental Health [1978]. There were twelve members on this Panel representing diverse fields including psychiatry, social work, consumers, etc. We reviewed much of the literature on primary prevention, and our report had a strong impact on the Commission and especially its honorary chair Rosalynn Carter. She, along with Commission member Beverly Long (President of the National Mental Health Association and, more recently, President of the World Federation for Mental Health), pushed hard for increasing emphasis on prevention at the National Institute for Mental Health in the final Commission report.

The final report of our Task Panel on Prevention was written largely by Emory and me (with significant input from the other members). One of the issues we wrestled with was the setting of priorities for federally funded primary prevention efforts. We noted the following in our report:

## Priorities

Our Task Panel was asked by the Commission to order our priorities among a range of prevention interventions and among the variety of target groups for whom primary prevention efforts are possible. It is not easy to set such priorities; indeed, decisions about them could well vary as a function of the weights given to social value judgments versus scientific criteria.

We illustrated the kinds of choices we considered in setting priorities among the large variety of primary prevention programs the Task Panel reviewed. We found ourselves considering:

1. Programs with high potential for success that affect relatively few people,

2. Programs with significant research effectiveness demonstrated on small samples but with good prospects for reaching large numbers,

3. Programs with strong theoretical promise for success affecting potentially large numbers of people.

Priority setting may be premature, we thought. One rational, possible approach would be to base priorities on three sources of judgment:

1. Epidemiological information on prevalence of distress;

2. Value judgments solicited from affected groups, e.g., minorities, the aged, the impoverished—all at high risk; and

3. Research and demonstrations of effectiveness.

The last year of the Carter presidency was a high point for the field of primary prevention. The Mental Health Systems Act was passed, and NIMH was urged to set up prevention programs as a high priority. With the Reagan victory, much of these new interactives collapsed. This is not the place to detail the changes that occurred in the prevention agenda. But it is important to note that for nearly two decades now, the NIMH models have emphasized genetic and biological causation of mental disorders. The 1990s is designated the "Decade of the Brain." NIMH has developed a new, narrow, safe prevention model that insists on research using only experimental-control intervention trials seeking to reduce risk for specific psychiatric disorders. There has also been a clear rejection of mental health promotion efforts, particularly those seeking to promote wellness. (The reason is not difficult to determine. If wellness reduces the overall rate of emotional distress, then the myth of discrete, separate mental illnesses is destroyed.)

Cowen's work has long focused on the importance of fostering wellness. His work is a rock-solid bulwark against the limitations of the new "scientific prevention." In his 1991 address, "In Pursuit of Wellness," following his receipt of the award for Distinguished Contributions to Psychology in the Public Interest, he stressed four approaches to the promotion of wellness: competence, resilience, social system modification, and empowerment [Cowen 1991; see also his longer paper on wellness, Cowen 1994]. His clear thinking, his inspiring research and writing, and his unswerving allegiance to careful science will remain a strong beacon in a field replete with false prophets.

Cowen's writings keep up my spirits at a time when the outlook often seems gloomy for those of us concerned with the need for social changes to achieve a more just and equitable society, one that is more child friendly and less stressful. Elsewhere I have described Emory Cowen as the tallest oak in the forest of prevention—sturdy, productive, deeply-rooted, and a guide to those unsure of their way. When the history of prevention is written a hundred years hence, Cowen's ideas, achievements, and influence will lead all the rest.

*George W. Albee*
Professor-Emeritus, University of Vermont
Courtesy Professor, Florida Mental Health Institute

# References

American Psychologist. (1990). Awards for Distinguished Contributions to Psychology in the Public Interest: 1989—Emory L. Cowen. *American Psychologist, 45,* 477–479.

Cowen, E. L. (1973). Social and community interventions. *Annual Review of Psychology, 24,* 423–472.

Cowen, E. L. (1991). In pursuit of wellness. *American Psychologist, 46,* 4, 404–408.

Cowen, E. L. (1994). The enhancement of psychological wellness; Challenges and opportunities. *American Journal of Community Psychology, 22,* 149–179.

Cowen, E. L., Hightower, A. D., Work, W. C., Pedro-Carroll, J. L., Wyman, P. A. & Haffey, W. G. (1996). *School-based prevention for children at risk: The Primary Mental Health Project.* Washington, DC: American Psychological Association.

Kessler, M. & Albee, G. W. (1975). Primary prevention. *Annual Review of Psychology, 26,* 557–591.

President's Commission on Mental Health, Task Panel on Prevention. (1978). *Report to the President.* Washington, DC: U.S. Government Printing Office, Vol. IV.

# Preface

## A Tribute to Emory L. Cowen: "Social Criticism, a Belief in Ordinary People, and the Creation of Contexts"

This volume, entitled "The Promotion of Wellness in Children and Adolescents," is a tribute to Emory L. Cowen, a leading researcher, mentor *par excellence*, and tireless policy advocate for populations that lack the power and voices to influence others. Accordingly, the volume strives to unify several subfields of psychology. Specifically, we believe that concepts central to the wellness perspective, including: "the enhancement of competence through the provision of programs for primary prevention of individual and social disorder," "the creative use of community resources," and "the importance of resilient adaptation in the face of adversity," can best be understood and elucidated by drawing upon the ways in which community psychology, developmental psychopathology, and an ecological perspective on development intersect. The integrative perspective that Emory Cowen has so willingly shared with others, and his ability to communicate complex concepts in both professional contexts and to society more broadly, has revolutionized the provision of mental health services to children.

In his eminent career that has now spanned half a century, Emory Cowen has received numerous awards, with accompanying verbal praise and vignettes provided to illustrate his professional accomplishments, as well as his extensive personal attributes. An overarching theme evident throughout the bestowal of such honors has been Emory's modesty and discomfort with being singled out for accolades. Thus, it was with considerable trepidation that we decided to organize a Festschrift to highlight Emory's career achievements and to present him with a planned scholarly volume devoted to the construct of wellness, an approach that strives to maximize the likelihood that children will develop in wholesome ways. Rappaport, Sandler, and Weissberg were graduate students with Emory during the 60s and 70s, while Cicchetti has been a colleague of Emory's at the University of

Rochester since 1985. The longevity of these relationships with Emory is no small coincidence, as Emory exerts long-term intellectual, professional, and personal influences on those with whom his path has crossed. Similarly, a lasting commitment and loyalty is consistent among those fortunate enough to know Emory.

Being cognizant of Emory's aversion to the limelight, in this preface we have opted to draw from the sentiments of others, communicated throughout the span of Emory's career, as well as from his own writings. We chose the former to convey the magnitude of personal respect and admiration that he engenders, and the latter to communicate directly the clarity and passion embodied in his work.

Before turning to Emory's own words, we summarize the sentiments represented in the eloquent tribute given upon Emory's receipt of the APA Psychology in the Public Interest award. Emory's work has changed public schools throughout the United States and in distant countries. His ideas and his research, his model programs, program evaluations, and workshops, all have inspired others—including psychologists, educators, administrators, teachers, and volunteer lay people—to generate new programs that have provided affordable human services to thousands of children who otherwise would not have received help. He has improved the lives of countless individuals, ranging from school-aged children through the elderly. He pioneered early detection and secondary prevention research, and his clear thinking has fostered the study of primary prevention and wellness in mental health. In essence, we, among others too numerous to name, believe that Emory has revolutionized how we, as a society, view mental health.

In the presentation that accompanied Emory Cowen's 1991 APA award for Distinguished Contributions to Psychology in the Public Interest, he seized upon the opportunity to introduce the concept of psychological wellness. In this presentation and the subsequent article published in *American Psychologist* [Cowen, 1991], Emory emphasized the need for an alternative to the emphasis on the diagnosis and repair of established disorders. According to Cowen [1991], "This analysis suggests that a comprehensive approach to the promotion of wellness requires active pursuit of complex and divergent strategies. Four concepts, each with a promising, established research base that holds the potential for advancing a richer psychology of wellness are identified. These concepts are competence, resilience, social system modification, and empowerment." [p. 404]. In concluding, Emory [1991] states, "Wellness remains an idyllic, abstract concept. However absorbing and socially significant, it will not be pursued easily. ... Advancing the early formation of wellness will depend heavily on inputs from child development specialists, educators, experts in policy and planning for children, systems analysts, as well as psychologists. Similarly, healthy development and application of empowerment notions call for major inputs beyond psychology, from political scientists, economists, and urban planners, and from the criminal justice, legal, and welfare systems." [p. 408]. Such an ambitious and, to most individuals, overwhelming agenda might dissuade mere mortals from the pursuit and promotion of psychological wellness. Not so for Emory! In fact, challenges such as this have been the "stuff" of which his career has been made. Emory battles with tradition valiantly and, more often than not, succeeds in redefining established practices and initiating broad social movements.

Thus, it is not surprising that the concept of psychological wellness, as evident in the current volume, has achieved increased visibility and generated research and practice initiatives in the decade since Emory first emphasized its importance. In a recent volume that describes the Primary Mental Health Project, Emory and his colleagues [Cowen, Hightower, Pedro-Carroll, Work, & Wyman, 1996] raise the question, "What can be done from the start and throughout to maximize the likelihood that children will develop in wholesome ways?" [p. 292]. The authors go on to state, "A multipronged search for pathways to wellness is an objective that must increasingly capture our imagination, challenge our ingenuity, and guide our effort in the decades to come." [p. 292] It is no coincidence that Emory has and will continue to capture our imaginations, challenge our ingenuity, and guide our efforts in the decades ahead.

In the current volume, we have invited scientists in the fields of developmental psychopathology, developmental psychology, and community psychology, all unified by their admiration and affection for Emory Cowen, to contribute chapters to this volume. They all have been influenced in personal and/or professional ways by Emory, not only as a renowned scholar, but just as importantly, for the values that characterize Emory as a human being. We have no doubt that the lives that Emory has touched could fill many volumes. Thus, this book serves as but a small example of the influence that Emory has exerted.

The volume opens with a foreword by George W. Albee, a pioneer in the field of primary prevention, a longtime colleague of Emory's, and, along with Emory, a major founder of community psychology. Lorion then provides a comparative and historical perspective on the study of wellness, in which he urges us to consider possible iatrogenic effects of categorizing people as "less than well." He calls for conceptualizing wellness from the perspective of individuals actively adapting to the demands of their environment, rather than from the perspective of state or trait characteristics of individuals. Luthar and Burack then examine the concept of adolescent wellness, proffering the perspective that definitions of successful adaptation among adolescents vary greatly as a function of who is determining the presence or absence of competence. Specifically, discrepancies emanating from conceptualizations drawn from mainstream Western society versus those resulting from subcultures present in contemporary inner cities are highlighted. With a similar emphasis on the importance of considering varied contexts, Wiley and Rappaport ask if it is useful to mix metaphors like wellness (a bio-medical construct) with empowerment (a sociopolitical construct). They argue that if developmental psychology is to be central to a wellness perspective, then we are obligated to explore the range of normative but distinct paths of development that exist in different communities, especially those outside the mainstream. Accordingly, issues of methods, values, interpretation, and advocacy will become more transparent.

In moving toward applications of wellness, Wyman, Sandler, Wolchik, and Nelson engage in the ambitious undertaking of understanding processes that foster resilience (framed within the broader concept of wellness), with the development of programs designed to promote resilience in children and adolescents. They integrate studies of multiple risk factors and resilience with studies focusing on processes of stress and coping in the context of specific life stressors. Emphasizing neighborhood structures and processes, Aber and Nieto take up Cowen's charge to identify features of influential social environments that support the development of psychological wellness. They examine how the influential community theories of the Chicago School Sociologists have influenced the direction and assumptions of past and contemporary neighborhood research. They argue that a wellness agenda focused on neighborhoods, in which the intention is to build on prior neighborhood and community theory and research, must grapple with thorny definitional issues, and must appreciate and move beyond the limitations posed by assumptions inherent in much of this work. Durlak next presents a model of adjustment that incorporates healthy functioning and serves as a context for understanding prevention through health promotion. He then summarizes outcome data on the success of health promotion prevention programs, focusing on programs for children and adolescents. In the next chapter, Elias and Weissberg provide an overview of school-based prevention programs to enhance children's wellness, using a unique format: an imaginary dialogue between Emory Cowen and his grandchild! They describe a diverse array of research-based preventive efforts and conclude by describing a growing international movement in social and emotional education and the efforts of a new national organization devoted to turning "good science into widespread helping." Continuing with an emphasis on schools as a context for the promotion of wellness, Felner advocates deep and widespread systemic, systematic educational reform based on knowledge of the ecological contexts in which schooling takes place. He discusses the Project on High Performance Learning Communities, a program that has, for the last two decades, been developing a model and knowledge base to guide the creation of contexts in which students are enabled to reach the high levels of achievement and adjustment necessary for success in today's society. Barrera and Prelow review a wide range of efforts to promote wellness by improving children's social support, including interventions that provide mentoring and support groups, and change the supportiveness of settings. Their review indicates that although many promising support enhancement intervention models have been developed, there is a critical need for evaluation designs that systematically test the effects of the intervention to increase support and the effects of improving support on improving wellness outcomes. Fantuzzo and Mohr then address the limitations inherent in an "illness, deficiency-based" system of care in child psychology and psychiatry and argue for an alternative "pursuit of wellness" model based on individual and community strengths. The utilization of this model in assessment, intervention, and training in Head Start programs is discussed. Trickett and Birman discuss the importance of utilizing wellness constructs for conceptualizing, developing, and evaluating interventions with culturally diverse groups. Their chapter elucidates a concept seen throughout much of this volume, namely, the centrality and importance of attending to issues of culture and context in the study of the promotion of wellness. In the next chapter, Cicchetti, Toth, and Rogosch bring the principles of psychological wellness to bear on the body of research on the sequelae of child maltreatment. Maltreatment represents one of the greatest failures of the environment to offer opportunities for fostering psychological wellness and, as such, knowledge of the factors that may erode the development of psychological wellness, as well as those that promote resilience, provides insight into how best to promote wellness in these vulnerable children.

Sarason next creatively integrates historical reactions to George Gershwin's *Porgy and Bess*, issues in the classification of human behavior, possible roles for "wellness psychologists," and struggles the field faces in defining the complex concept of wellness. Recognizing the limitations of a DSM-IV psychopathology orientation, wellness advocates offer an alternative perspective for enhancing human development by identifying characteristics and capacities that enable people to deal with obstacles in order to achieve their goals and fulfill social responsibilities. While applauding this direction, Sarason challenges wellness researchers to recognize the broader conceptualization that "wellness is not a feature in or of an individual. Rather, it refers to interpersonal phenomena suffused with the imprint of time and era, a viewpoint that possesses implications for definition, assessment, intervention, and evaluation. In the penultimate chapter of the volume, Schneider provides both a vision and a roadmap for training professionals to enhance psychological wellness. Schneider contends that behavioral and social science research must go beyond a focus on understanding, treating, and preventing mental illness to an emphasis on promoting psychological wellness in order to enhance their growth. As part of his analysis, he highlights four areas of multidisciplinary training relevant to psychological wellness: developmental neurobiology and genetics, the development of age-related emotional competence, practical knowledge of health economics and policy, and understanding the cultural context of wellness and illness. In a fitting, and perhaps the only possible ending to the volume, Cowen puts forth his hopes for what he would like to see occur with respect to a wellness enhancement approach in the future. Cowen highlights a number of areas necessary to foster the continued development of the construct of wellness, including: the importance of distinguishing between "risk-driven, disease-prevention" models of primary prevention and the enhancement of psychological wellness; the need to develop further a wellness enhancement approach; and the necessity of elucidating a life-span wellness-enhancement approach that can coexist with less proactive strategies. Although Cowen acknowledges that systematic wellness enhancement may never *fully* be realized, his chapter provides a much needed framework for guiding evolving conceptualizations and for promoting program development and research.

## ELC: An Appreciation

On October 26, 1996, colleagues, friends, and family gathered in Rochester, New York, to honor Emory L. Cowen and to recognize his extensive contributions. The assembled group included individuals spanning each decade of Emory's career.

In preparing to speak at the Festschrift for Emory, we prepared some notes, among them the following: "Emory's influence has been in large measure a function of the ability to reframe practical problems as conceptual/scholarly thought problems that, once reconceptualized, lead to fairly simple interventions and straightforward empirical studies. He uncomplicates difficult problems. When he does so, three fairly specific concepts emerge: Social Criticism, Belief in Ordinary People, and the Creation of Contexts. These concepts are evident, to varying degrees, throughout Emory's research, theoretical writings, and approach to education.

The impact of Emory's graduate mentorship was summarized as follows: "Emory's Community Practicum was an extraordinary training experience that may have laid the foundation for future career directions. It taught everyone the difference between direct service versus conceptualizing and designing a program and then consulting to others that would implement it. In my case, I designed my first social problem-solving project and trained three teachers to implement it. My work has built from that modest—but very demanding and ambitious at the time—start."

Unlike those who have benefited from his mentorship, the collegiality provided by Emory to colleagues at the University of Rochester was also highlighted. In directing an off-campus Center for disadvantaged children and families, Emory has freely shared his collective wisdom with others, imparting his knowledge and giving his support and loyalty to help his less experienced colleagues build successful research, clinical, and training facilities. Emory's openness, integrity, and compassion, as well as his ongoing strivings to grow as a psychologist, have been frequently noted. Emory has never been one to rest on his laurels.

Moving back in time a decade, to a nomination letter for the American Psychological Association's Distinguished Scientific Award for the Applications of Psychology (which, not surprisingly, Emory won), Roger Weissberg sought to address the question "What difference would it make if Dr. Cowen's research and writings disappeared?" Roger writes as follows, "First, ... without Dr. Cowen's research, none of the 100,000 high-risk youngsters participating in the Primary Mental Health Project would have received preventive services, especially in view of the extremely limited mental health resources available for children. Second, the quality of research and theory in community psychology and mental health prevention would be significantly poorer and less respected without Dr. Cowen's insightful contributions on the ways to improve the definitional and methodological shortcomings of work in these areas. And last, Professor Cowen is a master teacher and a dedicated mentor. No other scholar in the country has trained more scientist-practitioners who have positively influenced research and practice in preventive mental health and community psychology. The intellectual legacy of Dr. Cowen in community psychology and prevention will live on. ..."

Whether as a critic, conceptualizer, exemplar, or mentor, it is clear that Emory has and continues to exert a giant influence on the field. He has been a constant critic of current thinking, whether of the structure of clinical mental health services in favor of services with greater population impact, of fuzzy definitions of primary prevention, or of the neglect of the promotion of positive mental health as part of the prevention agenda. His telling critiques have consistently led to important conceptual advances. His belief that the steps toward primary prevention lead through a clearer understanding of the influence of social environments and the development of human competencies; that prevention research needs to develop through complementary generative and executive studies; and his insistence on rigorous hard-nosed evaluations of prevention programs presage the best of current thinking in the field. His research on theoretical issues (e.g., resilience) and interventions (e.g., the Primary Mental Health Project; interventions with children of divorce) exemplifies the payoff from his ideas. Through his ideas and his attention he has personally brought out the best in several generations of students who follow in his footsteps.

In efforts to draw upon Emory's extraordinary memory, we asked him to provide us with the number of doctoral students that he has advised. Emory has mentored approximately 80 doctoral students from 1950 through the present, an average of almost 2 students produced each year for a period of 50 years!" In view of his prodigious record in mentoring, it is fitting that the Society for Community Research and Action (Division 27 of APA) established the Emory L. Cowen dissertation award for the Promotion of Wellness. This award will honor the best dissertation of the year on a range of topics within Emory's conceptualization of wellness, including the promotion of positive well-being and the prevention of dysfunction. This honor demonstrates yet another lasting legacy of Emory's.

In a continued quest to provide a window into Emory's own perspective on his body of work, we requested that he list what he considered to be his most important publications. The list he provided reflects the breadth of Emory's interest in at-risk children. Emory's 1967 book, *Emergent approaches to mental health problems: An overview and directions for future work*, lays the foundation for 30 years of identifying and fostering alternative ways to extend mental health research, prevent psychopathology, and promote wellness. Two of Emory's collaborative books, *New ways in school mental health* [1975] and *School-based prevention for children at risk* [1996], provide conceptual, programmatic, and research information about the Primary Mental Health Project, one of the most extensively evaluated school-based preventive mental health models. Emory's publications from the late 1950s through the late 1990s also elucidate the historical evolution of his work. From the 1950s through the present, early secondary prevention in the form of the Primary Mental Health Project is apparent. During the late 1970s and 1980s a focus on the primary prevention of mental health problems emerges. Competence promotion and wellness enhancement is ascendant during the 1980s and 1990s. This list follows:

Cowen, E. L., Underberg, R. P., Verrillo, R .T., & Benham, F. G. (1961). *Adjustment to visual disability in adolescence*. New York: American Foundation for the Blind.

Cowen, E. L., Gardner, E. A., & Zax, M. (Eds.). (1967). *Emergent approaches to mental health problems: An overview and directions for future work*. New York: Appleton-Century-Crofts.

Rappaport, J., Chinsky, J. M., & Cowen, E. L. (Eds.). (1971). *Innovations in helping chronic patients: College students in a mental hospital*. New York: Academic Press.

Cowen, E. L. (1973). Social and community interventions. *Annual Review of Psychology, 24,* 423–472.

Cowen, E. L., Pedersen, A., Babigian, H., Izzo, L. D., & Trost, M. A. (1973). Long-term follow-up of early detected vulnerable children. *Journal of Consulting and Clinical Psychology, 41,* 438–446.

Cowen, E. L., Trost, M. A., Lorion, R. P., Dorr, D., Izzo, L. D., & Isaacson, R. V. (1975). *New ways in school mental health: Early detection and prevention of school maladaptation*. New York: Human Sciences Press.

Zax, M. & Cowen, E. L. (1976). *Abnormal psychology: Changing conceptions*. (2nd ed.). New York: Holt, Rinehart, & Winston.

Cowen, E. L. (1977). Baby-steps toward primary prevention. *American Journal of Community Psychology, 5,* 1–22.

Cowen, E. L. (1980). The wooing of primary prevention. *American Journal of Community Psychology, 8,* 258–284.

Cowen, E. L. (1982). Help is where you find it: Four informal help-giving groups. *American Psychologist, 37,* 385–395.

Cowen, E. L. (1982). Research in primary prevention in mental health. *American Journal of Community Psychology, 10*, 239–367.

Cowen, E. L. (1984). A general structural model for primary prevention program development in mental health. *Personnel and Guidance Journal, 62*, 485–490.

Cowen, E. L. (1985). Person centered approaches to primary prevention in mental health: Situation-focused and competence enhancement. *American Journal of Community Psychology, 13*, 31–48.

Cowen, E. L. (1986). Primary prevention in mental health: Ten years of retrospect and ten years of prospect. In M. Kessler & S. E. Goldston (Eds.), *A decade of progress in primary prevention* (pp. 3–45). Hanover, NH: University Press of New England.

Cowen, E. L. & Work, W. C. (1988). Resilient children, psychological wellness and primary prevention. *American Journal of Community Psychology, 16*, 591–607.

Price, R. H., Cowen, E. L., Lorion, R. P., & Ramos-McKay, J. (1988). *Fourteen ounces of prevention.* Washington, DC: American Psychological Association.

Cowen, E. L. (1994). The enhancement of psychological wellness: Challenges and opportunities. *American Journal of Community Psychology, 22*, 149–179.

Cowen, E. L., Hightower, A. D., Pedro-Carroll, J. L., Work, W. C., Wyman, P. A., & Haffey, W. G. (1996). *School based prevention for children at risk.* Washington, DC: American Psychological Association.

Cowen, E. L. (1999). In sickness and in health: Primary prevention's vows revisited. In D. Cicchetti & S. L. Toth (Eds.), *Rochester Symposium on Developmental Psychopathology, Vol. IX: Developmental approaches to prevention and intervention.* (pp. 1–24). Rochester, NY: University of Rochester Press.

Cowen, E. L. (2000). Psychological wellness: Some hopes for the future. In D. Cicchetti, J. Rappaport, I. Sandler, & R. P. Weissberg (Eds.), *The promotion of wellness in children and adolescents* (pp. 477–504). Washington, DC: CWLA Press.

The magnitude of Emory's influence also is noted in a vignette included in the Introduction to the Distinguished Contributions Award that he received from Division 27 of the American Psychological Association. Chinsky and Rappaport [1980] write:

Emory, having been justifiably identified as a past reviewer of psychotherapy literature, was asked by the editors of the *Annual Review of Psychology* to do a review of psychotherapy. In essence, what Emory told them was more than 'no.' What he did was suggest that there were now a variety of other forms of human services called collectively 'social and community interventions,' and that perhaps the series editors needed to consider expanding their topics. He modestly filed that letter away and forgot about it until several months later when he was asked to write such a chapter. The rest is history. ... He reshaped the thinking for the field collectively, as he had done for so many of us individually, and he brought the problem of social and community interventions to a place of wider visibility in psychology. [p. 257]

In closing, Emory, on behalf of your many colleagues, your past, current, and future students, and the countless children and families whose lives you have improved, we dedicate this volume to you. Although technically a "Festschrift," we know that your vitality, scholarly productivity, and extensive influence in the field will continue to blossom and astound us all!

*Dante Cicchetti*
*Julian Rappaport*
*Irwin Sandler*
*Roger P. Weissberg*

.

# 1

## Theoretical and Evaluation Issues in the Promotion of Wellness and the Protection of "Well Enough"

*Raymond P. Lorion*

The concept of psychological "wellness" represents an important challenge for the mental *health* disciplines which, to this day, remain far more conversant with mental *illness* than with mental *health*. A quarter century ago, as today, most doctoral programs prepare their graduates to apply interviewing, observational, and assessment skills to diagnose *dis*tress, *dis*order, *mal*adaptation, *mal*adjustment and, generally, emotional and behavioral *problems*. Emphasis on the negative is both dominant and assumed to be appropriate. Not unlike carpenters with hammers for whom everything appears as nails, mental health service providers are equipped to detect symptoms, diagnose their formation into syndromes, select an appropriate label from the accepted nosology [American Psychiatric Association 1994], and administer appropriate treatment. These clinical emphases, in turn, have defined the priorities of mental health scientists for nearly half a century.

Unavailable still, although beginning to be recognized as missing, is access to a similar nosology and science of adaptation and behavioral health. Absent is a parallel sequence of steps to nurture emotional growth, to enrich cognitive development, and to foster satisfying interpersonal exchanges. Contact with clients occurs when problems appear in individuals or relationships, but not when the individuals or the relationships are doing well. Metaphorically, mental health providers are like carpenters equipped to repair damage yet with neither the blueprints nor tools required to craft raw materials into a solid, unique, and satisfying structure.

## Moving Toward Prevention

The effectiveness of psychotherapeutic services was and is measured, case by case, in terms of the reduction or elimination of emotional distress and behavioral problems. Traditionally, the service system assumes that the provider will wait for the patient to seek treatment. Long ago, Dumont [1968] described as absurd the fact that clinical effectiveness was evidenced *not* by an empty waiting room, but rather by one which remained filled with changing clients. Then, as now, the flow of clients rarely stopped! That it was not expected to stop led some [e.g., Albee 1982; Caplan 1964; Cowen 1973] to realize that the nation's burden of emotional and behavioral problems could never be relieved one person, one relationship, or one problem at a time. Among these, Cowen [1973] urged the mental health disciplines to expand beyond reliance on treatment strategies to the development and application of ways to prevent emotional and behavior disorders. His appeal echoed Caplan's [1964] earlier calls for these disciplines to validate the public health maxim that significant threats to health were controlled not by treatment of disorders, but rather by their avoidance.

Over three decades, the field has learned that developing effective interventions to prevent emotional and behavioral disorders requires a "theory of the problem," i.e., an understanding of the mechanisms and processes defining the etiological path by which disorder evolves, and a "theory of the solution," i.e., a conceptually and empirically supported (or supportable) intervention that alters those mechanisms and processes in ways which normalize the underlying developmental trajectory. Ideally, prevention efforts remove pathogens or neutralize their negative effects entirely or early enough that a "primary" preventive outcome can be achieved, i.e., the incidence level is reduced in the targeted population. If diagnosable levels of dysfunction cannot be avoided, they might be mitigated through "secondary" efforts, i.e., early detection and effective early treatment that reduces the duration of illness and initiates healing and recuperation. Adoption of one or both preventive strategies lowers prevalence levels of disorders in targeted populations, as fewer new cases arise and existing cases are resolved [Lorion et al. 1989; Mrazek & Haggerty 1994].

As reflected in meta-analytic studies of preventive intervention effectiveness, substantial evidence exists for optimism concerning the prevention of some child and adolescent disorders [Durlak & Wells 1997, 1998]. Continued progress in these areas is the defining goal of "prevention science." According to Coie, Watt, West, Hawkins, Asarnow, Markam, Ramey, Shure, and Long [1993]:

> [This new research discipline] explicitly addresses the complex biomedical and social processes believed to influence the incidence and prevalence of mental illness. Preventive interventions aim to counteract risk factors and reinforce protective factors in order to disrupt processes that contribute to human dysfunction. [p. 1013]

Coie et al. [1993] outline a series of principles and promising directions for accelerating the development of preventive science, including the design and application of strategies which reduce risk factors (i.e., "variables associated with a high probability of onset, greater severity and longer duration of major mental health problems" [p.1013]) and reinforce protective factors (i.e., "conditions that improve people's resistance to risk factors and disorders" [p.1013]).

Recognition and pursuit of primary and secondary strategies reflected important shifts in the mental health disciplines' targets and procedures. No longer was their involvement restricted simply to established pathology; it now extended to its etiological processes and antecedent conditions. At the outset, this shift was frequently depicted using the metaphor of a river. Treatment strategies such as psychotherapy, medication, or hospitalization were portrayed as attempts to retrieve and resuscitate those who had fallen into a raging river and been tossed about in its rapids. For some, rescue was of no avail. The underlying pathology was unresponsive to known interventions, or the pathology's cumulative effects (i.e., its negative consequences on physical health, intimate relationships, or career) were insurmountable. For others (e.g., members of low-income and minority segments of the population), treatment efforts were frequently inadequate or superficial, the victim and/or rescuer were skeptical of their value, and efforts at rescue were superficial. For yet others, the resuscitation was slow, painful, and uncertain. Even those who responded positively were assumed to sustain a lasting reduction in resistance to subsequent problems.

Contrast this pessimistic scenario with the hopeful image attached to those pioneers who sought to design preventive interventions. These early explorers headed upriver looking for opportunities to extricate the water's victims earlier (i.e., secondary prevention) or to keep them from falling into the river (i.e., primary prevention). Long ago, when I related the river metaphor to my psychoanalytic supervisor, he listened intently and then simply asked, "And how do they learn to swim?"

## Moving Toward Wellness

For more than 25 years, I have thought about that question. The field has long assumed that health defines one's functioning on the shore; perhaps, it should have looked at what occurs in the water. By focusing on those who were drowning (or were feared to be), mental health professionals may have paid too little attention to: a) the majority swimming in the river; b) those who were tossed about but keeping their head above water; and c) those who went under but recovered by themselves or with the assistance of someone nearby. Maintaining the metaphor, if life occurs in the river, wellness is defined as responding to the ebbs and flows within that changing, unpredictable, and challenging environment. If so, pathology represents an incapacity to remain afloat, and treatment and prevention represent intervention strategies designed to enhance this capacity in those who have difficulty in doing so (i.e., treatment cases) or those deemed at risk for such difficulty (i.e., preventive targets). In either case, the focus is on the inability to stay afloat.

This volume seeks to encourage a further shift in the mental health (indeed all of health!) disciplines' perspective, from treatment to and beyond prevention to consideration of issues related to the nature and maintenance of health and wellness. This trend clearly and directly places the focus on the *ability* to remain afloat. More than two decades ago, Kelly [1974] noted the potential for such a shift in the intent of mental health services:

> The work of psychologists is moving from an emphasis upon the troubles, the anxieties, the sickness of people, to an interest in how we develop, how we acquire positive qualities, and how social influences contribute to perceptions of well-being, personal effectiveness, and even joy. There are signs that in the future, psychologists less and less will be viewing us as having diseases. Instead the psychological view will be one of persons in process over time and as participants in social settings. [p. 1]

To get to Kelly's destination, however, required new concepts and methods unavailable at the time of his comments. As noted earlier, traditional training gave most of us hammers (i.e., psychotherapeutic strategies) and a bias toward seeing nail-like qualities (i.e., psychopathology) in those seeking our services. Cowen [1991, 1994, 1996] has provided a glimpse beyond those biases in his presentation of psychological wellness as a logical step in the pursuit of effective prevention programs:

> The term wellness, as used here, is intended to anchor one end of a hypothetical continuum, anchored at the other end by an opposing term such as pathology (sickness). The preceding sentence seeks to highlight two points: (a) wellness should indeed be seen as an extreme point on a continuum, not as a category in a binary classification system; and (b) wellness is something more than/other than the absence of disease, that is, it is defined by the "extent of presence" of positive marker characteristics. ... And, for that reason, many people who fall well short of being glaring psychological casualties also fail to approach a predominant state of wellness. The two preceding points suggest that the ideal of wellness, and the goal of wellness enhancement, pertain to all people, not just to a limited or select portion of the population. [Cowen 1994, p. 153]

As reflected in Cowen's comments, debate can be expected about its nature (e.g., is it continuous or categorical, dynamic or static?), malleability, consistency across time, place, and circumstance, and so forth. The topic is both extraordinarily important and understudied. We are, indeed, in the very early phases of the work that will need to be completed before wellness becomes a substantive and recognized focus of the human services. The intent of this chapter is to bring to the forefront conceptual and methodological issues relevant to this nascent field. As these issues are discussed and its investigatory plan is organized and pursued, the shift envisioned by Kelly and the promise glimpsed by Cowen will add to the mental health disciplines' craft. Many others have advocated for such a shift.

Two decades ago, for example, Surgeon General Richmond [Public Health Service 1979] argued for consideration of health promotion in national health care planning. His groundbreaking report, *Healthy People*, clearly articulated the complementarity among treatment, prevention, and health promotion. In his analysis of the state of the nation's health, Richmond explained:

> The linked concepts of disease prevention and health promotion are certainly not novel. Ancient Chinese texts discussed ways of life to maintain good health—and in classical Greece, the followers of the gods of medicine associated the healing arts not only with the god Aesculapius but also with his two daughters, Panacea and Hygeia. While Panacea was involved with medication of the sick, her sister Hygeia was concerned with living wisely and preserving health. [Public Health Service 1979, p.6]

Further in the report, Richmond explains the interconnections among these elements of health care:

> Medical care begins with the sick and seeks to keep them alive, make them well, or minimize disability.

> Disease prevention begins with a threat to health—a disease or environmental hazard—and seeks to protect as many people as possible from the harmful consequences of that threat.

Health promotion begins with people who are basically healthy and seeks the development of community and individual measures, which can help them to develop lifestyles that can maintain and enhance the state of well being.

Clearly, the three are complementary, and any effective national health strategy must encompass and give due emphasis to all of them. [Public Health Service 1979, p. 119]

Additional endorsement of a focal shift to health and wellness is provided by a recent call for psychology to pursue "positive social science." Seligman [1998a] noted that 50 years ago, psychologists sought to achieve three distinct but overlapping goals: a) finding a cure for mental illness; b) enhancing the lives of people; and c) nurturing individual talent. For a variety of reasons, the discipline focused on the first to the virtual exclusion of the remaining two:

We became a victimology. Human beings were seen as passive foci: Stimuli came on and elicited "responses", or external "reinforcements" weakened or strengthened "responses," or conflicts from childhood pushed human beings around. Viewing the human being as essentially passive, psychologists treated mental illness within a theoretical framework of repairing damaged habits, damaged drives, damaged childhoods and damaged brains. [p. 2]

If people are passive victims of pathology, then they need to be protected from life's ebbs and flows; once in the river's current, they are assumed to have little control over their destinies. *Difficulty* with keeping afloat is equated with an *inability* to do so. For those individuals for whom that is not the case—i.e., they could overcome their difficulty—the application of intervention obscures, both to them and to others, their potential for handling life's currents and for gaining benefit from that struggle. The alternative to saving them is for mental health to design ways to enhance their recognition of that potential as well as their courage, optimism, interpersonal skills, work ethics, hope, honesty, and perseverance—each of which has been associated with resistance to pathology [Cowen 1994] and, analogously, with remaining afloat.

Thus, attention to issues of wellness represents a significant shift for the mental health disciplines toward mental health. The value of this shift seems apparent, yet it moves us in directions that are relatively unfamiliar and, presumably, linked to theories and methods that, at best, are in their nascent stages. Seligman does not underestimate the challenge of this shift:

> Fifty years of working in a medical model on personal weakness and on the damaged brain has left the mental health professions ill-equipped to do effective prevention. We need massive research on human strength and virtue. We need practitioners to recognize that much of the best work they do is amplifying the strengths rather than repairing their patients' weaknesses. [1998a, p. 2]

In addition:

> How has it happened that the social sciences view the human strengths and virtues—altruism, courage, honesty, duty, joy, health, responsibility and good cheer—as derivative, defensive or downright illusions while weakness and negative motivations—anxiety, lust, selfishness, paranoia, anger, disorder and sadness—are viewed as authentic?" [1998b, p.2]

## Should We Go There?

The potential impact of successfully moving beyond prevention to involvement with nurturing health and wellness seems limitless. All in the river may benefit from our efforts. Some gain directly from programs that increase their resistance, their stamina, and their skill in handling the ebbs and flows. Most experiencing difficulty, however, benefit indirectly through the assistance provided by the example and occasional helping hands of those around them. A few will *need rescuing* (the uncertainty of their number and of the extent of their need should be acknowledged!); the challenge for the mental health disciplines is to limit the application of rescue procedures so they appear both *as* needed and *when* needed.

Seligman's [1998a; 1998b] call for development of a "positive social science" certainly encourages movement in that direction. That step must, however, be taken with some caution lest long-standing clinical biases and pathology-oriented perspectives be applied whole-sale. The *social* quality of a positive science must be reflected in the selection of methods of investigation and in considerations of the *social* implications of that work [Sarason 1984]. Typically, such consideration occurs as the work nears or reaches fruition. As noted in a recent paper on the challenges associated with studying inner-city violence [Lorion & Saltzman 1994], the significant personal and economic implications of work on that issue (i.e., urban violence) made evident after the fact that we should have considered such implications *prior to* conducting our studies in targeted communities. I believe that wellness represents such an issue! I also believe that the field needs to engage in thoughtful discussion of the potential implications of our movement into that area of study. Sarason's [1984] attention to the social nature of our science leads inevitably to the question:

> Can science and technology continue to ignore the possibil-ity that what they give to society is frequently a very mixed blessing, that like all other institutions they suffer from the passion of partisanship and the self-serving stance? [p. 480]

and to the assertion that:

> Because something can be studied or developed is in itself an insufficient base for doing it however wondrous it appears to be in regard to understanding and controlling our world. [p. 480]

Applied to wellness, Sarason's admonitions call not for a moratorium on the development of research and programs, but for a considered review of that work to identify potential undesirable detours or unintended consequences it might have.

Society's right to expect such consideration is not without prece-dent. Proposals to modify wetlands or to harvest timber within old growth forests need to be justified in terms of their potential impact on the environment. Should not incursions into admittedly little understood areas of human functioning such as strength and virtue be similarly examined for their iatrogenic potential? Sarason [1984] suggests that the informed consent procedures and Institutional Review Boards procedurally required for federal research funding represent a "people's impact report" [p. 481]. Given the importance attached to the pursuit of preventive interventions and wellness by community psychologists, it is reasonable to expect similar safeguards for such work. As Levine and Perkins [1997] note:

> Most psychologists following the community perspective accept the broader society as it is and see it as their mission to help create or change service organizations or other institutions. They work to achieve the goals of providing humane, effective care and less stigmatizing services to those in need while enhancing human psychological growth and development. [pp. 4–5]

Thus, an initial conceptual and methodological question about the study of wellness becomes "should we go there?" If Sarason's [1984] words are to be heeded, a cautious preview of what could go wrong is a reasonable early step. Long-standing concerns about understanding emotional and behavioral problems from an illness perspective [Levine & Perkins 1997], about the iatrogenic effects of diagnostic labels [e.g., Rappaport 1977] and about the social rather than physical bases of such problems [e.g., Albee 1982] are relevant factors to consider in this early review. Relatedly, we need to ascertain that identified limitations in the reliability and validity of available diagnostic systems [e.g., Dawes 1994] can be overcome as we develop methods to assess the presence and degree of wellness within individuals.

As noted earlier, debate is expected about the nature of wellness. Specifically, is it, as Cowen [1994] implies, an end-state or is it a continuum? Is it even a state characteristic? Might it refer instead to the dynamic process of responding to the positive and negative events of everyday life, i.e., swimming? Defining wellness as a level of functioning attained only by an unknown, but tiny, fraction of the population raises significant conceptual problems. What of those (to some presumably measurable extent) who are "less-than-well" and occupy intermediate states between the "wellness" end and its diag-nostic-state counterpart? Might we label that broad intermediate state as "well enough" and accept its literal meaning?

Thus, the systematic study of wellness must avoid having the "less-than-well" acquire some of the negative labeling characteristics heretofore associated with illness [Scheff 1984; Levine & Perkins 1997]. Otherwise, well intended efforts can be expected, which are designed to improve the "less-than-well." Such efforts to enhance the lives of the "less-than-well" would inevitably confront another of Sarason's [1978] maxims concerning the nature of social problems. To the extent that wellness, like poverty, intelligence, and academic readiness, represents a relative rather than absolute state, such interventions may only have temporary effects that evaporate as the bar defining "wellness" shifts with improvements in the functioning of the reference segments of a population.

In a very real sense, whether conceptualized categorically, stati-cally, or dynamically, wellness has the potential to become yet another parameter by which people are categorized and differentiated. If that were to occur, levels of wellness other than the idealized end-state could be interpreted as another index of relative deficiency. Inevita-bly, then, the "less-than-well" could be deemed in need of repair. Ironically, an intended positive characteristic, i.e., documentation of wellness, assignment to the category of well-enough, and evidence of healthy adaptation, could gain a negative connotation. Staying afloat in spite of a river's strong current and debris may be devalued if emphasis is placed instead on the form and relative efficacy of one's strokes.

To avoid this unintended outcome, initial work on wellness should include critical reflection on the conceptual and methodologi-cal tools available to the mental health disciplines for understanding and describing human conditions. Psychometrics, i.e., the science of measurement, is very clear about its purpose, i.e., the *differentiation* of individuals [Helmstader 1964]. Methodologically, the *sine qua non* of scale development is reliable and valid identification of individual differences. Items that reflect similarity and explain limited or no variability are excluded as non-informative. This focus on difference is also reflected in the intent of the diagnostic interview, i.e., to understand the nature and basis of idiosyncrasies [Dawes 1994], and in the purpose of clinical services, to reduce those differences.

Should these same perspectives be applied as we shift to wellness and examine the merits of well-enough? Without significant change in our basic assumptions and methods, can we measure wellness without creating artificial levels of relative functioning that justify interventions to increase relative wellness? Without a significant shift in our assumptive bases concerning the nature of individual differences, do we risk effectively pathologizing other than endpoint levels of wellness. To avoid this, we may need to examine wellness differently than how we think about and study diagnostic states. To do so, we will need to develop concepts and measurement techniques that do not readily lead us to long-established tendencies to clinical interpretation.

Potentially, wellness might be conceptualized as a *common* characteristic widely shared across individuals, settings, and circumstances. Rather than be measured as a individual status relative to some normative value, being well-enough may represent the "default condition", i.e., that broad band of functioning defining how most people handle most things that confront them. Effectively, it means that recognition will be paid to the variety of ways that one can stay afloat. Particularly complicated is how to balance understandable and socially valuable efforts to optimize health and wellness in each individual with the danger that eligibility for such interventions is interpreted as evidence of deficiency, impairment, or pathology. The very term "intervention" may be so inherently linked to concepts of treatment and problem-solving that health and wellness programs may be more widely accepted and minimally stigmatizing if incorporated within education rather than health or mental health services. As Cowen [1994] notes in his review of promising health promotive strategies, many of those with the best evidence of enhancing normative functioning occur not only within school settings, but are integrated within the curriculum. Simply stated, programs to improve normal functioning need to be delivered and conceptualized as elements of normal settings and processes.

As described below, research to clarify the nature of wellness should begin with the application of qualitative studies of the diversity of its expression across individual, cultural, setting, and temporal characteristics. Barker's [Barker & Wright 1951, 1986] path-breaking forays into the systematic and comprehensive observation of normal children in their daily life offers one example of how such research might be conducted. Such preliminary work is likely to reveal the diversity of individual creativity and adjustment for coping with life's demands in ways that are functional and effective, albeit imperfect. If we observe such processes systematically and longitudinally, we may learn the manner in which later adaptive skills and problem-solving methods evolve cumulatively through experience and feedback. The mechanisms identified by Piaget [1952] for cognitive adaptation, i.e., assimilation and accommodation, are likely to be highly relevant to understanding how individuals cope within seemingly demanding and risky settings and circumstances.

## Development of Wellness

Psychopathology is generally conceptualized as the consequence of a developmental process gone awry due to some combination of individual diathesis (e.g., genetic vulnerability) and experiential or environmental stress [Bronfenbrenner 1979; Sameroff & Fiese 1989; Sroufe 1997]. Earlier explanations of psychoses attributed the resulting disorder to influences ranging from demonic possession to humoral imbalances to biochemical distortions [Zax & Cowen 1972]. Psychoanalysts attributed neurotic processes to defenses against experienced anxiety consequent to a failure in the control of personally and socially unacceptable impulses [Brenner 1974; Freud 1956]. Behaviorists [e.g., Wolpe & Lazarus 1966] examined reinforcement contingencies to understand the establishment and maintenance of maladaptive actions or cognitions [Ellis 1973]. Erikson [1963] explained psychopathology as a by-product of the inadequate resolution of one or more psychosocial crises characteristic of stages in life span development.

These frameworks distinguish normative and pathological pathways. As noted, current views of pathology attribute cognitive, emotional or behavioral dysfunction to some combination of inherited vulnerability and biochemical aberration that directly or indirectly inhibits the individual from effectively responding to situational demands. Across these conceptual models of pathogenesis, the underlying assumption is that normative processes have been disrupted and that something has gone awry in developmental or adaptive processes. By implication, it seems reasonable to view wellness as representing the outcome of normative developmental processes, in programming terms, as the default option. In the absence of that relatively rare combination of individual and situational circumstances, individual development appears to proceed within socially expected and appropriate boundaries reflecting the general capacity to adapt to situational demands and to cope with stressful events. Just as canalization accounts for the limits within which genetic processes emerge within species [Gottlieb 1992], an analogous process may account for the human capacity to adapt to a multitude of settings and circumstances and to cope with seemingly debilitating and pathogenic stressors.

Evidence in support of this position may be found in epidemiological estimates of psychopathology in the general population and segments thereof including the economically disadvantaged, adult survivors of childhood physical and sexual abuse, children of separated and divorced parents, and youth who experiment with alcohol and other drugs. Across these and other known risk conditions, one consistently discovers that the majority of those exposed cope with the risk and ultimately achieve a reasonable state of functioning. In effect, they stay afloat even when the current is strong! , [1999] thoughtful analysis of "adolescent storm and stress" exemplifies the breadth of perspective necessary to appreciate linkages between biological and situational demands and adaptation. By disentangling biological, cultural, situational and generational contributions to the perception and experience of adolescent conflict, Arnett provides a balanced understanding of how seemingly pathogenic situations produce highly different outcomes. Without minimizing the pain or distress suffered by some adolescents and their parents as the former struggle with resolving issues of identity, independence, and biological maturation, Arnett concludes that:

> Finally, to view adolescence as a time of storm and stress is not to say that adolescence is characterized only by storm

and stress. Most adolescents take pleasure in many aspects of their lives, are satisfied with most of their relationships most of the time, and are hopeful about the future. [p. 324]

## Wellness as Process

As noted above, Richmond [Public Health Service 1979] explained that, "Hygeia was concerned with living wisely and preserving health" [p. 6]. Health or wellness, thus, represents an active quality of individuals. Continuing the analogy begun earlier, wellness refers not simply to an individual's being afloat at a particular time, but rather to an individual's capacity to swim, i.e., to remain afloat in spite of turbulence and obstructions in the path. As suggested above, wellness must be studied from a developmental rather than a pathological perspective. In his 1974 address, Kelly cites Audy [1971] as follows: "Health is a continuing property, potentially measurable by the individual's ability to rally from insults, whether chemical, physical, infectious, psychological, or social" [Audy 1971, p. 142]. To this perspective, Kelly adds that "a psychology of healthiness emphasizes that knowledge derives from varied expressions of real life conditions" [Kelly 1974, p. 3]. In effect, wellness refers to the psychological capacity to cope with the demands arising across time, circumstance, and setting.

Echoing this perspective is Erikson's [1963] characterization of individual developmental as a succession of encounters between the growing individual and age-determined aspects of the social environment. These encounters, which define Erikson's classic "eight ages of man," represent opportunities for the incremental development of adaptive capabilities. Importantly, successful early experience represented the building blocks of attitudes, skills, and psychological capacities to deal with subsequent developmental demands. Within his framework, effective coping defined both the process and anticipated outcome of growth. Importantly, Erikson's model seems quite consistent with Seligman's [1998a] call for a positive social science. Psychosocial demands unresolved at their optimal developmental opportunity can be revisited and resolved subsequently. Thus, there is always the hope and assumption that additional experience, skills, and insights can be applied successfully to lingering issues. Erikson's schematic representation of the eight ages reflected, in his view, two primary assumptions:

> (1) that the human personality in principle develops according to steps predetermined in the growing person's readiness to be driven toward, to be aware of, and to interact with a widening social radius; and (2) that society, in principle, tends to be so constituted as to meet and invite this succession of potentialities for interaction and attempts to safeguard and to encourage the proper rate and the proper sequence of their enfolding. This is the "maintenance of the human world." [Erikson 1963, p. 270]

The first assumption argues that inherent within people is a drive toward functional adaptation to environmental demands. Whether conceptualized as the psychological equivalent of the genetic process of canalization, of the philosophical explanation of teleology, or of the Piagetian principles of organization and adaptation (involving the complementary processes of assimilation and accommodation), to achieve equilibrium with the environment, the view that people actively engage with their environment reflects a defining quality of wellness as an inherent human characteristic. As noted before, were the existence of that characteristic and of its positive consequence for adjustment taken as a given, wellness would be viewed as the expected quality or default conditions of individuals.

Implicit within Erikson's second assumption is the expectation that individuals have within themselves the capacity to adapt, to face adversity, and to succeed in that confrontation. This same optimistic and dynamic perspective on the process of growth and adjustment to the demands encountered in the environment is found in Piaget's theory of cognitive development [Ginsburg & Opper 1969], Sroufe's [1997] view of the coherence of human development, Bronfenbrenner's [1979] conception of bio-psycho-social development, Sameroff's transactional view of development [Sameroff & Chandler 1975; Sameroff & Fiese 1989] and Kellam's Life Course/Social Fields theory [Kellam et al. 1975]. In their respective ways, these developmental theorists assume that growth reflects the operation of biological and psychological imperatives toward coping, adaptation, and health. Through a series of active encounters with the physical and social environment, individuals are inherently moving toward adjustment and survival.

Across these theoretical models, wellness as a characteristic of individuals across the life span represents the norm rather than the exception across varying situational demands. Insofar as pathological states are both qualitatively and quantitatively distinct from normative functioning, their avoidance, reduction, or resolution should **not** be the defining markers for wellness. Wellness represents a positive state in and of itself rather than merely serving as an index that dysfunction has been avoided. Thus, understanding wellness depends on an appreciation of the salience of an expanded, ecologically-based developmental psychology for obtaining the scientific base for the design, implementation, and evaluation of interventions to promote health and support wellness. Studies of successful children [Matsen & Coatsworth 1998] and families [Brodsky 1996] living in challenging settings, confirm that processes referred to as "resilience," "invulnerability," or "spontaneous prevention" appear at far greater rates than pathology in their inhabitants.

## Pursuing Wellness

In this chapter, wellness is described as representing a broad expanse of human functioning, distinct from both the pathological conditions defined within existing nosological systems and the earlier cited exceptional state described by Cowen [1994]. As discussed above, Cowen's perception of wellness as the anchor point along a functional continuum raises a series of conceptual, ethical, and methodological challenges. These challenges can be avoided by viewing wellness or well-enough as the normative state involving the active pursuit of equilibrium and adaptation characteristic of most individuals under most circumstances. Insofar as nonreflexive human functioning can be understood as involving some form of cognitive process, Piagetian theory offers insights into thinking about how one would develop a psychology of wellness:

As the individual progresses through the life span, the functions {organization and adaptation (assimilation and accommodation)} will remain the same, but the structures will vary and appear in a fairly regular sequence. Another way of saying this is that intellectual development proceeds through a series of *stages* with each stage characterized by a different kind of psychological structure. An individual of any age must adapt to the environment and must organize his responses continually, but the instruments by which he accomplishes this—the psychological structures—will change from one age level to another. ...

Piaget further proposes that organisms tend toward equilibrium with the environment. The organism—whether a human being or some other form of life—tends to organize structures into coherent and stable patterns. His ways of dealing with the world tend toward a certain balance. He tries to develop structures which are effective in his interaction with reality. This means that when a new event occurs he can apply to it the lessons of the past (or assimilate the events into already existing structures), and he will easily modify his current patterns of behavior to respond of the new situation. With increasing experience he acquires more and more structures and therefore adapts more readily to an increasing number of situations. [Ginsburg & Opper 1969, pp. 23-24]

The above conveys the sense of active interaction between the individual and the environment which defines wellness and is consistent with its metaphoric depiction as the capacity to swim in life's calm, as well as turbulent waters. If this depiction has validity, the methodological task is not to develop a psychological measure of wellness as either a state or trait. Rather the critical work needed at this time is to portray the nature, efficiency, and efficacy of the process of adaptation and adjustment. Strategies for doing so are reflected in Piaget's observational analyses of cognitive development [1952], Barker and Wright's study of a day in the life of a child [1951] and descriptions of the lives of children in the Midwest [Barker & Wright 1955] and emergent ethnographic [e.g., Agar 1986; Fetterman 1989], qualitative [e.g., Crabtree & Miller 1992; Kirk & Miller 1986] and interview [Mishler 1986; Weiss 1994] studies. This need was also recognized by Cowen [1994]:

> At the same time, additional generative information about the ontogenesis of wellness is needed in several areas, including: (a) the *in vivo* study of conditions and processes that nourish the early, spontaneous development of wellness; (b) clarifying understandings of the self-views, skills and competencies, and familial contexts and pathways that operate to advance and maintain wellness; (c) identifying settings, community structures, and policies that further support the development of wellness. [p. 173]

The above suggests that understanding wellness will require an integration of investigatory methods from the developmental sciences, epidemiology, anthropology, and ethnography with protocols characteristic of environmental and ecological psychology. The essential generative task will be to capture the dynamic exchange between individual and environmental characteristics and thereby understand how equilibrium is achieved for a specific individual within a specific situation or context.

Our lack of attention to and understanding of states of health or wellness relative to our focus on disorder and dysfunction appears to parallel our attention to quantitative methods and controlled experimentation relative to qualitative methods. As Trickett [1996] notes:

> The relative neglect of qualitative methods, however, has resulted in an enormous loss in our understanding of context. The instinct behind most qualitative work is the interest in social complexity, in nuance, in understanding how different levels of the ecological environment impinge on the way individuals and communities develop a rhythm, order their priorities, and create resources to cope with stressful life events. Such work is more likely to illuminate how lives are led locally and in context. [p. 217]

Awareness of lives in context seems an essential ingredient to understanding wellness as an active state of grappling with the demands encountered in daily life. Given our current state of knowledge concerning the complexity and predictability of emotional or behavioral outcomes, it seems reasonable that initial attention be given to the creation of taxonomies of situations, of relevant individual characteristics, and of individual-situational transactions. The latter represents a significant challenge but may be simply understood within the Piagetian framework of adaptation, i.e., the related functions of assimilation and accommodation. In this case, adaptation refers to the active experimentation of the individual attempting to understand and respond to environmental demands. To appreciate the nature, variability, and evolution of such experimentation, it seems essential that Piaget's example be followed. Specifically, we must observe how normal people deal with the typical events that define their particular settings and circumstances, i.e., the rhythm described by Trickett above.

A psychology of wellness requires the development of a psychology of everyday life and, by implication, of mental *health*. Understanding wellness requires the accumulation of a knowledge base acquired through the systematic examination of human behavior under naturalistic circumstances, i.e., *in vivo* and with minimal (if any) manipulation of the situation. It will involve far more passive observation than active control if a valid developmental model of the phenomena of interest is to be acquired [Lorion 1990]. In essence, it will reflect an ecological paradigm. Kringy-Westergard and Kelly [1990] explain that paradigm as follows:

> The Ecological approach emphasizes a sequence of activities in which the researcher understands, learns, and becomes informed about phenomena in context ... Research activity according to the Ecological approach is inductive, exploratory, improvisational, and requires constant testing and feedback; testing of ideas occurs by going back and forth between the concepts and the experience of the researcher and the participants. These activities must all take place before the official, public, or "real" research or intervention(s) can begin.
>
> The Ecological approach adapts research styles to incorporate initial uncertainty and ambiguity as the collaborative

enterprise is initiated. In this sense, research becomes an "open" process, because there is tolerance for checking the validity of assumptions, the efficacy of actions, and the very definition and meaning of research. The Ecological approach is empiricist, exploratory, collaborative, and contextual in its theoretical and methodological assumptions. [p. 30]

Consideration of context and of situations cannot be limited to their physical properties or to representation of the observable behaviors of those observed. Attitudes, beliefs and other sociopolitical characteristics of the environment that define parameters of human diversity must be recognized as part of the ecological perspective. Trickett [1993] explains this link as follows:

First, it [the ecological perspective] would attend to the *cultural* context in assessing individual behavior. This may include such issues as how group identification affects the meaning of situations to varied individuals and how behavior adaptive in a monocultural setting may differ from that expressed in a more bicultural one. Yet, this cultural perspective on individuals would be expressly linked to their interaction with their larger social context. Thus, an ecologically grounded community psychology attends to how social values, reflected in social structures and policies, differentially affect the experience of different groups. It investigates how differing cultural contexts define and distribute power and other social resources, and it strives to be explicit in its vision of society and whose interests the field was serving. [p. 273]

As the above suggests, determining the adaptive salience of a behavior or condition requires far more than simply noting the presence or absence of signs, symptoms, and syndromes. Wakefield [1997] addresses this relativism directly in his argument that disorder, regardless of where in the life span it occurs, be conceptualized as: "'harmful dysfunction,' where 'harm' is judged according to social values and a 'dysfunction' is the failure of an internal mental or physical mechanism to perform a function for which it was naturally selected" [p. 269]. This same appreciation of relevance is reflected in Kellam et al.'s [1975] consideration of both developmental stage *and* social field in the theoretical foundation of their work on the assessment of functional status and on the design and assessment of preventive interventions.

## Conclusion

All of the above complicates tremendously the task of studying wellness with the goal of designing conditions for its optimal occurrence. The challenge may be equal to that being undertaken in the human genome project. The latter has required the systematic mapping of the human genetic code as an antecedent to creating strategies for genetic alteration and reducing disease, disorder, and dysfunction. Wellness, as conceptualized as an emotional and behavioral characteristic, appears to represent an equal challenge. In this case, what needs to be mapped are the individual, environmental, and transactional characteristics of human development across time, setting, culture, and circumstance. Such mapping must produce not merely insights into selective slices of life, but somehow model its rhythm and continuity. Does that exceed our methodological capacity?

Beyond traditional qualitative methods known to community psychology, Lerner [1998] builds on Kellam & Rebok [1992] and Lorion's [1990] long-standing advocacy of preventive trials as effective strategies for testing developmental hypotheses. Lerner [1998] explains the potential of this approach. By studying systematic changes in characteristics of the proximal or distal ecology, developmental scientists can begin to understand how variations in person-context relations influence actual or to-be-actualized developmental trajectories. In turn, the transactional linkages between individuals and settings can be opened to investigation. Presumably, theoretically based interventions modifying characteristics of the environments in which children are raised can enhance our understanding of developmental plasticity. Ultimately, that understanding may translate into variations in home, school, and neighborhood characteristics designed specifically to enhance the development of cognitive, emotional, and interpersonal strengths.

An even more creative and potentially valuable approach is offered by Turkheimer and Gottesman [1996]. By developing computer simulation models (similar to those designed for forecasting weather patterns, economic trends and other phenomena that result from highly complex interactions among numerous variables which cannot readily be experimentally manipulated), these developmental scientists have created a biometric environment in which variations in genetic and environmental factors can be simulated and their effects on behavioral outcomes estimated. This technology, as alien as it is promising, appears to offer an important window into hypothesis generation and testing about human behavioral adaptation. Potentially, the aforementioned variations in proximal and distal characteristics of the environment that are hypothesized as contributing to the development and maintenance of human strengths can be manipulated in virtual reality prior to undertaking complex and highly expensive actual studies.

Thus, wellness truly represents a conceptual, methodological, and political new frontier for the mental health sciences. Its exploration promises to challenge a significant portion of the major assumptions underlying existing work in our disciplines, to move us closer to our social, behavioral, and physical science colleagues and, especially, to bring us to issues of *health* rather than pathology. Like any voyage into uncharted territory, its outcome is uncertain, but its potential payoff appears well worth the associated risks.

## References

Agar, M. H. (1986). *Speaking of ethnography.* Beverly Hills, CA: Sage.

Albee, G. W. (1982). Preventing psychopathology and promoting human potential. *American Psychologist, 37,* 1043–1050.

Albee, G. W. (1986). Advocates and adversaries of prevention. In M. Kessler & S. E. Goldston (Eds.) *A decade of progress in primary prevention* (pp. 309–332) Hanover, NH: University Press of New England.

American Psychiatric Association (1994). *Diagnostic and statistical manual of mental disorders* (4th ed.). Washington, DC: Author.

Arnett, J. J. (1999). Adolescent storm and stress, reconsidered. *American Psychologist, 54,* 317–326.

Audy, J. R. (1971). Measurement and diagnosis of health. In P. Shepart & D. McKinley (Eds.), *Environmental essays on the planet as a home* (pp. 140–162). Boston: Houghton-Mifflin.

Barker, R. G. & Wright, H. F. (1951). *One boy's day.* New York: Harper & Row.

Barker, R. G. & Wright, H. F. (1955). *Midwest and its children.* New York: Harper & Row.

Barker, R. G. (1968). *Ecological psychology: Concepts and methods for studying the environment of human behavior.* Stanford, CA: Stanford University Press.

Brenner, C. (1974). *An elementary textbook of psychoanalysis.* New York: Doubleday.

Brodsky, A. E. (1996). Resilient single mothers in risky neighborhoods: Negative psychological sense of community. *Journal of Community Psychology, 24,* 347–364.

Bronfenbrenner, U. (1979). *The ecology of human development.* Cambridge, MA: Harvard University Press.

Caplan, G. (1964). *Principles of preventive psychiatry.* New York: Basic Books.

Coie, J. D., Watt, N. F., West, S. G., Hawkins, J. D., Asarnow, J. R., Markman, H. J., Ramey, S. L., Shure, M. B., & Long, B. (1993). The science of prevention: A conceptual framework and some directions for a national research program. *American Psychologist, 48,* 1013–1022.

Cowen, E. L. (1973). Social and community interventions. In P. Mussen & M. Rosen (Eds.) *Annual Review of Psychology, 24,* 423–472.

Cowen, E. L. (1991) In pursuit of wellness. *American Psychologist, 46,* 404–408.

Cowen, E. L. (1994). The enhancement of psychological wellness: Challenges and opportunities. *American Journal of Community Psychology, 22,* 149–180.

Cowen, E. L. (1996). The ontogenesis of primary prevention: Lengthy strides and stubbed toes. *American Journal of Community Psychology, 24,* 235–250.

Crabtree B. F. & Miller, W. L. (1992). *Doing qualitative research: Research methods for primary care.* (Vol. 3). Newbury Park: Sage Publications.

Dawes, R. M. (1994). *House of cards: Psychology and psychotherapy built on myth.* New York: Free Press.

Dumont, M. (1968). *The absurd healer: Perspectives of a community psychiatrist.* New York: Science House.

Durlak, J. A. & Wells, A. M. (1997). Primary prevention programs for children and adolescents: A meta-analytic review. *American Journal of Community Psychology, 25,* 115–152.

Durlak, J. A. & Wells, A. M. (1998). Evaluation of indicated preventive intervention (secondary prevention) mental health programs for children and adolescents. *American Journal of Community Psychology, 26,* 775–802.

Ellis, A. (1973). *Humanistic psychotherapy: The rational-emotive approach.* New York: McGraw-Hill.

Erikson, E. H. (1963). *Childhood and society* (2nd ed.). New York: Norton.

Fetterman, D. M. (1989). *Ethnography step by step.* Newbury Park: Sage Publications.

Freud, S. (1956). *A general introduction to psychoanalysis.* New York: Perma Books.

Ginsburg, H. & Opper, S. (1969). *Piaget's theory of intellectual development: An introduction.* Englewood Cliffs, NJ: Prentice Hall.

Gottlieb, G. (1992). *Individual development and evolutions: The genesis of novel behavior.* New York: Oxford University Press.

Helmstadter, G. C. (1964). *Principles of psychological measurement.* New York: Appleton-Century-Crofts.

Kellam, S. G., Branch, J. D., Agrawal, K. C. & Ensminger, M.E. (1975). *Mental health and going to school.* Chicago: University of Chicago Press.

Kellam, S. G. & Rebok, G. W. (1992). Building developmental and etiological theory through epidemiologically based preventive trials. In J. McCord & R. E. Tremblay (Eds.), *Preventing antisocial behavior: Interventions from birth through adolescence* (pp. 162–195). New York Guilford Press.

Kelly, J. G. (1974). Toward a psychology of healthiness. Icabod Spencer Lecture, Union College, Schenectady, NY: May.

Kirk, J. & Miller, M. L. (1986). *Reliability and validity in qualitative research.* Beverly Hills, CA: Sage Publications.

Kringy-Westergaard, C. & Kelly, J. G. (1990). A contextualist epistemology for ecological research. In P. Tolan, C. Keys, F. Chertak, & L. Jason (Eds.), *Researching community psychology: Issues of theory and methods* (pp. 23–31). Washington, DC: American Psychological Association.

Lerner, R. (1998). Theories of human development: Contemporary perspectives. In R. M. Lerner (Ed.), *Handbook of Child Psychology: Theoretical models of human development* (pp. 1–24). New York: Wiley.

Levine, M. & Perkins, D. V. (1997). *Principles of community psychology.* New York: Oxford University Press.

Lorion, R. P. (1990). Developmental analyses of community phenomena. In P. Tolan, C. Keys, F., Chertak, & L. Jason (Eds.), *Researching community psychology: Issues of theory and methods* (pp. 32–41). Washington, DC: American Psychological Association.

Lorion, R. P., Price R. H., & Eaton, W. W. (1989). The prevention of child and adolescent disorders: From theory to research. In D. Shaffer, I. Phillips & N. B. Enzer (Eds.), *Prevention of mental disorders, alcohol and other drug use in children and adolescents* (DHHS Publication No. (ADM) 89–1646)(pp. 55–96). Washington, DC: U.S. Government Printing Office.

Lorion, R. P. & Saltzman, W. (1993). Children's exposure to community violence: Following a path from concern to research to action. *Psychiatry, 56,* 55–65.

Matsen, A. S. & Coatsworth, J. D. (1998). The development of competence in favorable and unfavorable environments. *American Psychologist, 53,* 205–220.

Mishler, E. G. (1986). *Research interviewing: Context and narrative.* Cambridge, MA: Harvard University Press.

Mrazek, P. J. & Haggerty, R. J. (Eds.) (1994). *Reducing risks for mental disorders: Frontiers for preventive intervention research.* Washington, DC: National Academy Press.

Piaget, J. (1952). *The origins of intelligence in children.* New York: International Universities Press.

Public Health Service (1979). *Healthy people: The surgeon general's report on health promotion and disease prevention* (DHEW (PHS) Publication No. 79-55071). Washington, DC: U.S. Government Printing Office.

Rappaport, J. (1977). *Community psychology: Values, research and action.* New York: Holt, Rinehart and Winston.

Sameroff, A. J. & Chandler, M. J. (1975). Reproductive risk and the continuum of caretaking casualty. In F. D. Horowitz, M. Hetherington, S. Scarr-Salapatek, & G. Siegel (Eds.), *Review of child development research.* (pp. 187–244). Chicago: University of Chicago Press.

Sameroff, A. J. & Fiese, B. H. (1989). Conceptual issues in prevention. In D. Shaffer, I. Phillips, & N. B. Enzer (Eds.), *Prevention of mental disorders, alcohol and other drug use in children and adolescents* (DHHS Publication No. (ADM) 89-1646) (pp. 23–53). Washington, DC: U. S. Government Printing Office.

Sarason, S. B. (1978). The nature of problem solving in social action. *American Psychologist, 33,* 370–380.

Sarason, S. B. (1984). If it can be studied or developed, should it be? *American Psychologist, 39,* 477–485.

Scheff, T. J. (1984). *Being mentally ill: A sociological perspective.* Chicago: Aldine.

Seligman, M. E. P. (1998a). Building human strength: Psychology's forgotten mission. *APA Monitor, 29* (#1), 2.

Seligman, M. E. P. (1998b). Building human strength: Psychology's forgotten mission. *APA Monitor, 29* (#4), 2.

Sroufe, L. A. (1997). Psychopathology as an outcome of development. *Development and Psychopathology, 9,* 251–268.

Trickett, E. J. (1996). A future for community psychology: The contexts of diversity and the diversity of contexts. *American Journal of Community Psychology, 24,* 209–234.

Trickett, E. J., Watts, R , & Birman, D. (1993). Human diversity and community psychology: Still hazy after all these years. *Journal of Community Psychology, 21,* 264–279.

Turkheimer, E. & Gottesman, I. I. (1996). Stimulating the dynamics of genes and environment in development. *Development and Psychopathology, 8,* 667–678.

Wakefield, J. C. (1997). When is development disordered? Developmental psychopathology and the harmful dysfunction analysis of mental disorder. *Development and Psychopathology, 9,* 269–290.

Weiss, R. S. (1994). *Learning from strangers: The art and method of qualitative interview studies.* New York: The Free Press.

Wolpe, J. & Lazarus, A. A. (1966) *Behavior therapy techniques: A guide to the treatment of neuroses.* New York: Pergamon Press.

Zax, M. & Cowen, E. L. (1972). *Abnormal psychology: Changing conceptions.* New York: Holt, Rinehart & Winston.

# 2

## Adolescent Wellness: In the Eye of the Beholder?

*Suniya S. Luthar and Jacob A. Burack*

Opinions regarding competence or maladjustment imply a convergence of actual behaviors and the lens through which they are viewed. The lens, in turn, is inevitably colored by the viewers' backgrounds, such that the same behavior may be seen as seriously deviant in one culture, but relatively normal or even adaptive in another [Weisz et al. 1997]. In parallel fashion, what is perceived as adaptive in one setting may often be viewed negatively in another ecocultural context.

This chapter is based on the premise that definitions of successful adaptation among adolescents vary considerably, depending on whose perspective is sought. In particular, our focus is on the discrepancy between conceptualizations of positive adolescent adjustment within mainstream Western society—also reflected in traditional developmental psychology theories—and views of competence in the subculture of contemporary inner cities.[1] Issues relating to this schism are discussed in six sections. In the first, we sketch broad conceptions of positive outcomes among adolescents from the perspectives of both classical child development theories and individuals in socioeconomically disadvantaged settings. In the second, we present results of recent empirical studies that have shown that not only do these two sets of views have little in common, but in point of fact, are often diametrically opposed. In the third and fourth sections respectively, we appraise the implications of these divergent perspectives for conceptual definitions of competence and consider whether dissonance of this kind represents an "inner-city" phenomenon as opposed to, more broadly, an "adolescent" one. The two concluding sections include discussions on future directions for empirical research involving youngsters in poverty, and for intervention programs to maximize positive outcomes among these at-risk youth.

## Conceptions of Competence: Views from the Mainstream and from the Inner City

Developmental psychologists consider social competence to be a particularly useful indicator of children's overall positive adaptation or wellness [Luthar & Zigler 1991; Zigler & Trickett 1978]. This construct is typically understood as connoting individuals' success at meeting major societal expectations relevant to their particular stage of development, and is generally assessed based on overt, behavioral indicators as opposed to covert, intrapsychic ones [Havighurst 1972; Masten & Coatsworth 1998; Waters & Sroufe 1983]. Thus, social competence among toddlers may be evaluated based on their success at basic daily living tasks (e.g., eating independently or toileting) and behaviors reflecting secure attachment with caregivers. Among older children, appropriate indicators would include the ability to get along with age-mates and adults, and to learn effectively and behave appropriately at school.

Such theoretical views on social competence have formed the bedrock of much contemporary research on wellness among children at risk [Cowen 1994]. Pioneering studies on child resilience—including Norman Garmezy's Project Competence [Garmezy et al. 1984] and Emory Cowen's Rochester Child Resilience Project [Cowen et al. 1996]—have involved assessments of overall positive adaptation that are based in children's success at specific stage-salient tasks. The focus in both these projects was on elementary school children, and major competence indicators included adequate academic performance and satisfactory relationships with peers and with authority figures. Over time, these measurement strategies proved to be effective ones in capturing "overall" wellness: children's success in individual domains was strongly correlated with their levels of success in other major areas, both cross-sectionally as well as longitudinally over a period of several years [Cowen et al. 1997; Masten et al. 1995].

In studying resilience among at-risk adolescents, competence might theoretically be operationalized via some of the same indicators used with younger children, such as effective functioning at school [Masten & Coatsworth 1998]; various complications, however, can arise in this case. The use of similar competence indices would be predicated on the assumption that major societal expectations facing fourteen- and fifteen-year-olds are comparable to those facing their nine- or ten-year old-counterparts. Restated in Eriksonian terms, the presumption would be of adolescence as an extension of childhood: a period of hiatus before the young person is compelled to confront and undertake adult responsibilities and life choices.

Whereas such notions of adolescence as a moratorium may be relevant for many teenagers in mainstream Western society, they are often inapplicable in the context of contemporary urban poverty. For example, many disadvantaged African American teens are thrust into adult roles and do not experience adolescence as a transitional phase due to various sociocultural factors [Burton et al. 1995]. These include narrow age differences between themselves and their parents, blurred intergenerational boundaries, tendencies to accelerate the move from childhood to adulthood in response to perceptions of shortened life expectancies, and familial expectations to contribute to family finances. The adolescent stage is further blurred for inner-city teens who face the paradox of being treated as "grown children" at school, but are expected to take on adult responsibilities at home [Burton et al. 1995, p. 122]. In sum, the traditional theoretical view of adolescence as a distinct life stage, connoting a period of transition between childhood and adulthood, can be largely irrelevant to many young people from contemporary inner cities.

Similar dissonance is apparent when considering definitions of "adolescent competence" among families and children in inner-city settings, as compared to views prevailing in mainstream society. In their ethnographic research, Burton and her colleagues [1995] identified three categories of developmental outcomes considered successful by inner-city families. One of these entails indices of survival in a harsh and violent community, where success is viewed in terms of short-term goals and current well-being rather than long-term success. Relevant indices include physical survival, ability to make it out of the community, and external manifestations of cultural/situational success such as personal possessions and dressing well. The second category is the achievement of adult status, via economic independence (by traditional or illegal means) or parenthood. The third category includes comfort with gender-appropriate identities and as members of their own cultural and/or ethnic group.

Ethnographic data such as these suggest, then, that widespread conceptualizations of adolescent competence in traditional child development theory—which mirrors views of mainstream society—and those in the subculture of the inner city are often unrelated, or even sometimes at odds with each other. In the section that follows, we review results of quantitative research studies that buttress this suggestion.

## Empirical Evidence of Discrepant Conceptualizations of Wellness

Discrepancies between mainstream and inner-city conceptions of adolescent competence are particularly evident in empirical research where conventional benchmarks of adaptive functioning have been considered, including maintenance of (a) good academic performance, and (b) conforming, rule-abiding behaviors as opposed to disruptive, aggressive patterns. We consider each of these indices in relation to how they are viewed by youth in urban poverty, particularly in terms of prevalent attitudes in the adolescent peer group.

### Academic Achievement

For many teenagers outside mainstream, middle-class society, academic success is not a critical constituent of overall positive adaptation. Reviewing the literature on various facets of ethnic minority youngsters' well-being, for example, Steele [1997] showed that African American students typically display levels of global self-esteem that are similar to or higher than those of Caucasians, even though their academic performance is generally inferior. Interpreting these dual streams of apparently contrary evidence, Steele argued that the self-regard of minority youth is disassociated from success in domains that are evaluated negatively by their peers, including academics. Rather, these youngsters tend to prioritize domains that carry less threat of negative stereotyping such as identification with the peer group [Steele 1997].

Like minority students in particular, disadvantaged youth in general often experience negative stereotyping regarding academics [National Research Council 1993; Stipek 1997], and once again, their personal aspirations are not tied in heavily with scholastic success. This is illustrated in an investigation of two personality configurations, dependency and self-criticism, among inner-city high school students [Luthar & Blatt 1995]. The construct of dependency entails high preoccupation with personal relationships and concern about abandonment by others, whereas self-criticism refers to preoccupation with personal accomplishments and concern about failures. Several prior studies involving college students have established that these two personality configurations are linked with varying reactivity to different types of life events, such that students high on dependency display negative affect in the wake of difficult interpersonal events, whereas those high on self-criticism react strongly to failures in the realm of academics [Hammen et al. 1985; Zuroff & Mongrain 1987].

Among inner-city high school students, these findings were replicated for dependency but not self-criticism [Luthar & Blatt 1995]. In the presence of negative ratings by peers, greater levels of distress were found among disadvantaged youth high on the dependency factor as compared to their peers who scored lower on this factor. In contrast, inner-city teenagers high on self-criticism did not display the heightened reactivity to low grades that was evident among their more affluent college counterparts. Notwithstanding their tendencies to high personal ambition, then, self-critical youth in inner-city settings seemed to be relatively impervious to failures in the realm of academics.

There is accumulating empirical evidence, however, that academic success can not only be unrelated to disadvantaged adolescents' personal aspirations, but also that it can have negative implications—specifically, in terms of perceptions by peers. Cauce and colleagues [1982] reported inverse associations between academic achievement among these youngsters and the levels of informal support they received from friends. More recently, Arroyo and Zigler [1995] found that high-achieving inner-city youth seem to struggle with the conflict between excelling academically and achieving the approval of peers—suggestions further supported by Luthar's [1995] prospective findings that globally rated peer acceptance was linked with significant decrements in grades across the academic year. In the latter study, ninth grade students who were rated as highly sociable by their peers showed subsequent decreases in their grades. In parallel fashion, students initially viewed as being responsible, behaviorally conforming leaders received poor peer ratings on sociability by the end of the school year. Finally, individual-based analyses by Luthar and McMahon [1996] revealed a cluster of inner-city ninth graders who were viewed as highly sensitive and were generally isolated by their peers. These youngsters had significantly *better* grades and were viewed by teachers as being more task-oriented in the classroom, than were their classmates with more positive status in the wider peer group.

The apparent antipathy toward academic success among inner-city youth may partially reflect exposure to subculture-specific forces. (Note: Parallel issues among more mainstream youth are considered later in this chapter). As anthropologist John Ogbu and others have argued, disadvantaged youngsters are often unconvinced that success at school will lead to success in later life, given ongoing experiences with racism and marginalization, and perceptions of "job ceilings" which deny them access to jobs with prestige [see Nettles & Pleck 1994; Ogbu 1991; Spencer et al. 1993]. Many of these youth become deeply disenchanted with all that academics represents, a disillusionment probably reflected in increasing peer pressure away from academic striving over the years of childhood and adolescence [Cauce 1986; Luthar 1997].

### Aggression

As with academic performance, inner-city teenagers' location on the continuum of prosocial/responsible versus aggressive/disruptive behaviors is also frequently irrelevant to conceptions of their overall competence or lack thereof. In many urban areas with high poverty rates, patterns of behavior that may earn labels of "conduct disorder" from psychologists may be entirely normative, for verbal and physical aggression can be important for survival in crime-ridden neighborhoods [Coie & Jacobs 1993; Jensen & Hoagwood 1997; Prinz & Miller 1991; Wakefield 1997]. Richters and Cicchetti [1993] provide vignettes from the life histories of adult criminals, drawing attention to the persuasive draw of antisocial pursuits in their childhood environments. Underscoring the critical distinction between the moral implications of individuals' behaviors versus the concept of underlying psychopathology, these authors conclude that antisocial behaviors may often occur among essentially normally functioning individuals, reflecting their adaptation to the prevailing mores and norms of a counterculture subculture.

Beyond being just normative, aggression may also be *adaptive* for inner city youth, not only because of its value for sheer physical survival in dangerous territories, but also because it can have a positive valence among peers. Jarrett's [1990] review of ethnographic research has shown, for example, that in many childhood games, nondelinquent aggressive behaviors involving status leveling (victims for pleasure) and mutual verbal attacks in contest format ("rippin") can fulfill an important functional necessity, directly contributing to peer group solidarity—a critical source of support for many inner-city youth. Thus, some mild forms of verbal and physical aggressive behaviors (those which stop well short of delinquency) might be regarded as an important component of peer group identity and support, rather than unilaterally as indicators of disorder or psychopathology [Luthar 1999; Prinz & Miller 1991].

Recent studies have shown that aggressive behaviors may not only contribute to camaraderie among close friends, but further, that they are often viewed in a positive light by the wider peer group.[2] Whereas it is well known that deviant teens tend to form friendships with others also deviant [see Dishion et al. 1995; Kazdin 1995], several researchers have demonstrated that even the wider peer group may often endorse antiestablishment behaviors. In their study of disadvantaged eighth graders, Coie and colleagues reported positive links between accepted status among peers and tendencies to associate with deviant peers [Coie et al. 1995]. Among inner-city ninth-graders, Luthar and McMahon [1996] found that positive peer ratings were related to aggressive, disruptive behaviors in the classroom. Variable- and individual-based analyses in this study converged in indicating that whereas positive peer status was often linked with prosocial behavior and good grades, it equally often coexisted with disruptive patterns of behavior at school [see also Hoge et al.1996; Seidman et al. 1994].

Once again, the apparent endorsement of aggression by the peer group may partly derive from subcultural forces embedded in the context of poverty and restricted life opportunities [Hammond & Yung 1993]. In inner-city communities besieged by crime, aggressive behaviors may sometimes be linked with relatively high prestige [Coie & Jacobs 1993; Richters & Cicchetti 1993]. Behaviors which most adults would term as "deviant" are often the very behaviors that help adolescents in these communities maintain feelings of high self-esteem and status, as well as feelings of being included in (and possibly protected by) a valued group of peers in the community [Luthar 1999; Lynam et al. 1993].

## Interdomain Variations: Competing Conceptions of Competence

For the developmental scientist, empirical evidence that success in one major area of inner-city teens' adjustment (e.g., peer acceptance) can be detrimental for success in other important areas (behavioral conformity and good grades) evokes questions about which dimensions should be accorded priority in conceptually defining adolescent competence. In some instances, decisions are clear-cut, as when the negative ramifications of a particular outcome far outweigh the more immediate positive fallout. Thus, although membership in a criminal inner-city gang might foster short-term feelings of peer group solidarity, to view this as an overall adaptive outcome would be ludicrous given the real dangers that delinquent youth face themselves, as well as their potential to seriously harm others [Luthar 1999].

What, however, of less extreme adjustment patterns such as occasional indulgence in nondelinquent aggressive behaviors, or benign indifference to academic success—each of which is often related to high status in the peer group? Should a teenager who has marginal grades, yet has developed emotionally fulfilling, identity-affirming relationships with his age-mates be considered incompetent? We would argue against such absolutism in labeling. In view of the importance of peer relations during adolescence and clear long-term risks linked with academic failure, unequivocal labels of "incompetence" would be inappropriate for students who are ostracized by peers but excel scholastically, *and* for youth who are academically subaverage but receive substantial support and affirmation from their peers. Both profiles have clear drawbacks as well as benefits.

Acknowledging the benefits of these polarized profiles leads, logically, to the appeal of adaptation profiles that resonate with *both* microcosmic and macrocosmic value systems. Thus, whereas the teen who succeeds according to one set of societal values but fails according to the other (as in instances mentioned earlier) may display competence to some degree, such patterns of adaptation may arguably be viewed as hierarchically subordinate to those reflecting successful negotiation of both sets of mores. These integrated forms of wellness are reminiscent of the "bicultural" patterns described by Phinney [1990] and Spencer [Spencer & Markstom-Adams 1990], wherein ethnic minority individuals who identify with both their own ethnic group and the majority group tend to be at an advantage over those who identify with either one to the relative exclusion of the other ("assimilated" or "separated"). Analogously, among adolescents living in urban poverty, perhaps the most competent are those who retain major rewards of both worlds constituting their social surrounds, as exemplified by youth who excel academically yet retain the esteem of their inner-city peers [Luthar & McMahon 1996].

Conceptualizations of such biculturalism as the ultimate form of adolescent competence might be questioned, however, on at least three grounds. First, it may be argued that the imposition of mainstream society's values on inner-city youth is ethnocentric and disrespectful of local values and beliefs; the people's own perspectives should be given greatest priority in researchers' definitions of wellness [e.g., Prinz & Miller 1991]. While fully endorsing the need for respectful consideration of indigenous views, we believe that it is critical to consider also the disservice that can be done to disadvantaged youngsters if standards set for them were substantively different from those stipulated for others. The microcosm of the inner-city subculture does exist, after all, within the macrocosm of wider society, and poor children are far from immune to the rules of promising behavior that are drawn up by the more powerful majority—middle-class members of mainstream society.

Cautions similar to these have been raised by many in the context of educational practices and policies. Stipek [1997], for example, has written of the perils of setting lower achievement standards for children in disadvantaged schools than for others, noting that low adult expectations are frequently self-fulfilling. Similar issues are reflected in debates on bilingual education. While fostering foreign-born children's pride in their native languages, promoting their acquisition of English is also critical because knowledge of American language and culture is vital for long-term success in this country [Allen & Grobman 1996]. Returning to definitions of successful adaptation, then, we contend that while fully acknowledging the many serious obstacles inner-city adolescents face in life, it would be a mistake to (tacitly or otherwise) view them as living by a "different set of rules" as we consider what warrants labels of competence among them. While ignoring the children's own perspectives is unquestionably disrespectful, dismissiveness of mainstream society's expectations can eventuate in further disadvantaging a group of youngsters already at considerable risk.

The second question one might raise about bicultural patterns as an ultimate form of wellness is, given the antagonism between the two sets of value systems that economically disadvantaged youth encounter, how realistic is it that they can, in fact, be integrated? Is it even possible for more than a small handful of children to achieve such adjustment patterns? Apparently, it is. In research by Luthar and McMahon [1996], almost one-quarter of the over 300 inner-city teens assessed had peer ratings averaging almost a full standard deviation above sample means on peer-rated sociability *as well as* prosocial leadership; they also had significantly better academic grades than the normative or average cluster of teens. Furthermore, the absolute size of the prosocial-popular cluster was no smaller than the other two non-normative clusters—aggressive children with high peer status and high academic achievers who were isolated by peers. While clashes between macrocosmic and microcosmic systems may cause some inner-city youth to be strongly aligned with one value system and repudiate the other, therefore, these findings suggest that many are able to reap significant rewards of both.

A third question regarding bicultural adaptation is whether this may entail greater emotional costs than does competence that reflects subscription to just one value system. Constant efforts to live up to two sets of discordant standards can conceivably be stress-invoking, causing distress in the young person. To be sure, all adolescents might negotiate such tussles to some degree (as will be argued in the following section). Yet the ensuing strains are likely to be particularly pronounced for those in urban poverty, as they can often be in a position of persevering assiduously toward mainstream goals that command little respect from peers as well as, often, significant adults in their immediate surrounds.

It is also possible, on the other hand, that the strains of juggling both macro- and micro-systemic value systems are significantly offset by positive feelings that derive from retaining the major rewards of each. Preliminary support for the latter speculation is evident in Luthar and McMahon's [1996] findings that the cluster of prosocial, popular teenagers reported no greater depression or anxiety than did children in the normative cluster. In future research, longitudinal studies will be critical in illuminating both the strains and benefits that accompany some inner-city youngsters' apparently successful negotiation of major value systems that are often sharply at odds with each other.

## Peers versus Mainstream Society: An Inner-city Schism or an Adolescent Phenomenon?

Whereas antiestablishment peer group sentiments may partly derive from forces specific to poverty, it is also possible that much of what has been documented reflects an "adolescent" phenomenon rather than an exclusively "inner-city" one [Luthar 1997]. Steinberg [1987], for example, has noted that American teenagers in general, regardless of their sociocultural background, do not particularly admire hard work at school [see also Lepper et al. 1997]. Similarly, Moffitt [1993] has argued that during the developmental moratorium of adolescence in contemporary Western society, antisocial behaviors can take on a positive value among adolescents in general because they symbolize maturity and independence.

Suggestions such as these have received support in recent empirical work. For example, Wentzel and Asher [1995] demonstrated that even among middle-class youth, academic excellence tends to be linked with isolation by the peer group. Similarly, preliminary findings from our most recent research show that even among affluent high school students in suburban areas, peer acceptance is linked with various antiestablishment behavior patterns, including not just disruptiveness at school, but also students' use of cigarettes, alcohol, and marijuana [e.g., Luthar & D'Avanzo 1999].

Similarities such as these should not, however, be viewed as suggesting comparable phenomena across socioeconomic strata, because there are critical differences in environmental "safety nets" available for young people. Affluent adolescents tend to have access to resource-rich schools, good psychotherapists, and parents and teachers all strongly invested in pulling them toward conforming to mainstream mores. For these youngsters, therefore, long-term life trajectories are not inevitably imperiled by occasional lapses into what Moffitt [1993] calls adolescent-limited delinquency, for there is much to pull them back toward adherence to mainstream norms.

In inner-city settings, on the other hand, children who get drawn into antisocial lifestyles can confront relatively few external forces that will effectively and persuasively move them back toward conventional conformity. Quite to the contrary, negative peer pressure can be progressively *reinforced* by the other potent risks of life in chronic poverty, including resource-poor schools, overworked and demoralized teachers, limited family support for academic excellence, social and geographic segregation from mainstream society, and the incessant draw of crime to make quick money [Garcia Coll et al. 1996; Luthar 1999; Richters & Cicchetti 1993; Stipek 1997]. Viewed from organizational, transactional perspectives [Cicchetti & Schneider-Rosen 1986; Sameroff & Chandler 1975; Sroufe & Rutter 1984] therefore, the overall long-term repercussions of peer approval for rebellion can be substantially less benign for urban poor youth than for mainstream teens. In the years ahead, there is much to be gained from longitudinal studies on such multifinality in pathways [Cicchetti & Rogosch 1996], with documentation of the degree to which the same indicators (e.g., high peer status contingent on rebellious behaviors) might eventuate in vastly differing adult outcomes among economically disadvantaged youth as compared to their affluent counterparts.

## Additional Research Directions

Evidence of contradictions between mainstream and subcultural views of adolescent wellness suggests at least three other directions for future research, in addition to those previously mentioned (i.e., potential costs of bicultural adaptation, and multifinality in long-term adjustment outcomes). First, it would be useful to examine whether notions of competence among inner-city youth might show systematic variations across particular points in the developmental trajectory. Trends similar to those described among adolescents have been found among students in the first grade as well [Coie et al. 1991]; yet, findings at intervening developmental phases have been comparatively weak [see Dodge et al. 1990; Gonzales 1996]. Apart from interpretations resting on adolescence-specific forces [e.g., Moffitt 1993], trends such as these may partly reflect pressures that arise at times of transition and change, such as on entry into elementary or high school. As Caspi and Moffitt [1991] have argued, greater variations in successful or unsuccessful adaptation become apparent during life course transitions, when more innovative coping strategies are required. Concordantly, a peer cohort's collective view of members' assertive, dominating behaviors may fluctuate at times of change and transition, resulting in differing notions of what is considered acceptable or admirable across the childhood and adolescent years.

A second question involves a more fine-grained appraisal of the types of nonconformity that disadvantaged adolescents appreciate: precisely which forms and degrees of antiestablishment behaviors are approved of and which are disdained? Although academic striving is not prized, outright failure or dropping out of school may not earn the active respect of peers. Aggressiveness per se may not adversely affect peer status, yet it may be poorly tolerated if it reflects the use of force to acquire desired goals, or if it coexists with social insensitivity and self-regulation failures [Coie et al. 1995]. Similarly, Moffitt's [1993] thesis raises the important question of whether inner-city adolescents (or all adolescents) are as tolerant of flagrant delinquency as they appear to be of some mild disruptive or aggressive behaviors within the school setting.

Third, in studying "predictors of wellness" among disadvantaged youth, there is a need for greater contextual sensitivity, while delineating constructs of high potential salience in future research designs. Developmental psychologists must be attentive to indigenous perspectives in their selection not only of major indicators of competence ("outcome variables"), but also of salient risk and protective factors ("predictors or moderators"), for many constructs that generally serve protective functions can be rendered neutral or even deleterious by catalysts specific to the ecocultural setting of poverty. Aside from high peer status (as described in preceding discussions), several other ostensible assets have been shown to be involved in such conditional effects [see Luthar 1999]. Freitas and Downey [1998], for example, demonstrate that under conditions of unremitting economic deprivation, high intelligence can be applied toward increasingly artful schemes to evade the law, eventually proving to be counterproductive rather than beneficial for the individual's long-term welfare.

Fourth, we need more attention to the complexities of interrelationships across different forms of "successful adaptation" among disadvantaged youth, both cross-sectionally and longitudinally. Evidence that some subcultural views of wellness are antagonistic to those of wider society by no means implies that these two sets of perceptions are inevitably polarized, for several forms of adolescent competence—such as helping families and children in the local community—may be equally valued in both contexts. Thus, there needs to be greater empirical exploration of the specific spheres in which macrocosmic and microcosmic value systems operate in mutually antagonistic, relatively independent, or mutually facilitative ways, across the childhood years and subsequently through adulthood.

A final research direction entails conducting more developmental studies that include a focus on individuals and not exclusively variables [see Bergman & Magnusson 1997] and that provide qualitative insights in addition to quantitative ones [Jensen & Hoagwood 1997]. Particularly when working with groups little studied so far, quantitative psychological researchers would do well to incorporate methodologies from other social science disciplines—such as ethnographies, narratives, and case studies—that are integrally focused on understanding the meanings that people ascribe to events and circumstances in their lives [Cohler et al. 1995]. The incorporation of insights from qualitative studies can greatly increase both the subcultural relevance and the conceptual comprehensiveness of large-scale, expensive quantitative research aimed at testing specific hypotheses or predicting competent outcomes among children who live in poverty [Luthar 1999].

## Implications for Interventions

Underlying Emory Cowen's decades of research on wellness has been a steadfast conviction in the value of grounding preventive interventions in an understanding of the processes implicated in the development of competence among at-risk children and families [Cowen 1991, 1994; Cowen et al. 1996]. As we conclude this chapter, we consider implications for interventions targeting inner-city youth that derive from existing findings on diverging cultural views of competence.

First, there is a need to attend to the substantial imbalance in contemporary prevention approaches, wherein the focus on poor children's school performance vastly overshadows the emphasis on their mental health [see Knitzer, in press].[3] Without question, it is critical to promote school-based competence, for the negative long-term ramifications of academic failure are both pervasive and profound. Equally compelling, however, is the need to foster poor children's social-emotional well-being—if nothing else, because academic (and ultimately job) performance can rarely be sustained over time if coexistent with feelings of isolation, alienation, and hopelessness. For the 13-year-old in poverty—who has contended with scarce material and emotional resources at home, possibly parental psychopathology, and probably an unsafe, violent neighborhood—it must be a prodigious struggle to sustain academic diligence, if this entails revoking critical support from peers in her school and community.

Perhaps the obvious intervention strategy of choice, given such dilemmas, would be to move discrete environmental forces toward working in tandem rather than in mutual opposition, for example, by harnessing subcultural forces to maximize inner-city adolescents' conformity to prominent mainstream mores. Several psychologists, including John Coie [Coie & Jacobs 1993], Avshalom Caspi [1993], and Terrie Moffitt [1993], have noted that if deviant, highly visible peer leaders are provided with nondelinquent bases for authority, they can help alter an antiestablishment ethos within the peer group. Similarly, access to socially acceptable ways of approximating adult status, e.g., via legal employment or mentoring, can be critical in promoting adolescents' feelings of competence and efficacy [see Price et al. 1993; Takanishi 1993, 1996]. Although paid employment can compete with students' scholastic efforts, it can also confer various advantages in the transition to adulthood [see Shanahan et al. 1996], as it fosters feelings of dignity and discipline, as well as identification with a structured community that can be surprisingly supportive of continuing school involvement [Newman 1996].

For younger teens in poverty settings, there is value in increasing not just the quantity and quality, but also the diversity of extracurricular activities that are available in their schools and neighborhoods [see Natriello et al. 1990; Takanishi 1996]. Beyond organized sports (which undoubtedly carry much appeal for many teens), various other activities can effectively service major developmental needs of adolescence, e.g., allowing youth to achieve feelings of potency and prestige while interacting with peers in socially sanctioned ways. A compelling example lies in efforts by the U.S. Chess Center[4] based in Washington D.C., an organization that brings instruction in chess to schools and to public housing communities. In addition to providing the necessary equipment, professional teachers are sent to these communities on a regular basis, sometimes as often as once a week. The response has reportedly been positive, with many teenagers deciding to become tournament players, and some even attending national chess championship tournaments.

There also is value in community-based exposure to adult professional paths and to role models in diverse careers such as science, law, business, or medicine. Again, messages that commonly impinge on inner-city youth overwhelmingly emphasize success in sports as a viable route to long-term success. Furthermore, this is often at the cost of jeopardizing educational achievements, for many talented athletes from disadvantaged backgrounds are encouraged to forego educational opportunities in order to play professional sports. While applauding the financial opportunities that become available to star athletes, it is critical to recognize the pitfalls in messages wherein school is presented as an impediment, or at least a detour in the path, to a more lucrative lifestyle. Such messages are clearly inconsistent with the ubiquitous mainstream emphasis on the value of education, and over time, can prove to be harmful for the vast majority of disadvantaged youth who crave the fame and fortune of professional sport but, for any number of reasons, will never attain them.

While there are currently few large-scale attempts so far to systematically expose disadvantaged teens to diverse, prestigious mainstream career paths, useful directions for the future may be gleaned from some existing efforts. A case in point is the High School Summer Research Apprentice Program at the Yale University School of Medicine, in which inner-city high school students are placed, during their summer vacations, in research laboratories of Yale faculty. These experiences allow many bright, academically promising youth to interface with people and activities in research settings, providing exposure that few would have otherwise had as they define their own future professional goals.

Other possibilities are to organize community-based small group conversations with young adults who are on mainstream career trajectories and who themselves grew up in disenfranchised life circumstances (thus, individuals with whom the youngsters can personally identify). This strategy, exemplified in many existing mentorship programs for children in poverty, parallels the effective and commonly used approach in drug prevention programs, wherein older teens share relevant experiences with younger students from the same community [e.g., Botvin 1998].

A third and somewhat more personalized option is to provide individual mentors for teens at times of transition or heightened stress, such as when they enter high school. Natriello and colleagues [1990] describe one such program, which involves pairing incoming students with those who have been in the school for a while. The older students can provide critical mentorship and personal support to the younger ones, as the latter negotiate a developmental period that is not just stressful, but also often critically formative in terms of future life trajectories. Among the most appealing facets of such efforts is their implicit recognition of an issue all-too-often neglected in current interventions and policies: that in terms of their social and emotional needs, teenagers are *not* adults but have substantial needs for guidance, support, and nurturance, just as do their younger counterparts.

Finally, concerted efforts to involve adults in the families and schools are essential, for their commitment is critical in ensuring the long-term continuity of any prevention program in disadvantaged communities [Carnegie Council on Adolescent Development 1994; Comer 1988; Cowen et al. 1996; Knitzer, in press; Luthar 1999]. Involvement of adults, in turn, can be greatly facilitated with concerted attention to *their* salient, neglected needs. For example, disenfranchised mothers can derive substantial feelings of efficacy and empowerment if they are drawn into participating collaboratively in planning and implementing programs for their children. Substantive gains can also derive from services that directly target their needs pertaining to parenting, day care for younger children, or their own mental health difficulties [see Comer 1988; Conduct Problems Prevention Research Group 1992; Luthar & Suchman, in press; Zigler & Gilman 1996].

In a similar vein, there is a need to extend more support to teachers in inner-city schools. Many of these professionals care deeply for their students but feel overwhelmed by their own lack of training and available skills to deal with their students' diverse and substantial needs [Stipek 1997]. Again, support to teachers does necessitate large, expensive demonstration projects; there can be much value even in modest (and more easily implemented) efforts within particular communities. For example, faculty in university graduate programs of education, human development, or psychology could make important contributions by conducting occasional workshops for teachers in surrounding urban schools and by supervising practicum placements of their senior students within these schools. Many teachers in poverty settings chronically lack access to professional developmental opportunities, and as Stipek [1997, p. 89] has succinctly cautioned, "Until teachers are given the support *they* need to succeed, many children will continue to fail."

Finally, for those considering the development of new interventions for children and families in urban poor communities, it would be judicious to recognize once again that valuable directions regarding viable strategies can be gleaned by consulting the intended recipients. Whenever the intent is to intervene with individuals whose life trajectories are only modestly captured by conventional theories of psychology, in-depth attention to nuances of their everyday lives (e.g., via focus groups or ethnographic studies) can be critical in bolstering the effectiveness of the strategies envisioned. For example, critical directions can be identified by speaking with youngsters who seem to adeptly negotiate subcultural and wider society's mores, from teens firmly allied to one set of standards who disavow the other—and from the parents, teachers, school administrators, and providers of both formal services such as health care, as well as informal social support services such as ongoing after-school groups or local religious organizations. Expertise gleaned from these children and adults can prove to be invaluable in identifying potential impediments as well as reinforcements to planned intervention strategies, thus improving both cost-effectiveness of interventions over time, as well as the likelihood of their ultimate efficacy.

## Summary and Conclusions

This review has been focused on the frequently wide divide between views of adolescent competence in mainstream child development (based largely on work with white, middle-class youth), as compared to the views of wellness that predominate among many children and families in contemporary settings of urban poverty. The divide is evident, both in terms of indices that are accorded high versus negligible priority as signs of competence (e.g., academic success or socially conventional versus rule-thwarting behaviors) as well as in assumptions about the ramifications of "successful adaptation" in particular domains, for subsequent success in other spheres. Recent research evidence has shown that competence indicators valued by mainstream society versus those prized in the immediate subculture of poverty can often work in opposition, as exemplified by inverse associations between inner-city teenagers' academic striving/success and their status within the peer group.

Given substantive differences in ecocultural perspectives of competence, researchers concerned with wellness among inner-city teens confront decisions about which views should be accorded priority in operationalizing "overall competence." The most prudent strategy may be to assign greatest priority to the overarching category of wellness that represents an integration of *both* societal value systems concerned, the microcosmic and the macrocosmic.

Existing evidence on disparate competence indicators indicates several themes that warrant attention in future research. These include (a) potentials benefits and risks of "bicultural" adaptation profiles; (b) the degree to which dissonance between peer groups' and mainstream society's values characterizes inner-city teenagers more so than adolescents in general; (c) possible developmental variations in behaviors that the peer group tolerates or actively endorses; (d) the specific types and degrees of nonconforming behaviors that earn the admiration of inner-city peers; (e) contributions to wellness of risk and protective processes that are salient in disadvantaged settings specifically; and (f) relationships among different indices of competence, appraised both cross-sectionally and over time, and via both variable-based and individual-based analyses.

Despite the occasionally pronounced differences in macrocosmic versus microcosmic value systems encountered, a sizable number of inner-city youth do seem able to retain the major rewards of both worlds. For interventionists, the challenge ahead is to develop innovative, effective ways of reaching the thousands of youngsters in urban poverty who remain deeply alienated from mainstream standards and rewards. One route to accomplishing this can be via the peer group, for when deviant peer leaders are given access to socially conventional bases for authority, they can help alter a largely antiestablishment ethos in the wider peer group. Availability of diverse, high-quality, after-school extracurricular activities in school buildings or neighborhood centers can serve vital protective functions, and there is value also in providing inner-city youth with firsthand exposure to adult role models from varying professions considered prestigious in mainstream society. Collaborative involvement of adults who care for these youth—their parents and teachers—are critical for the long-term sustenance of any community-based intervention with these youngsters. Finally, there is an urgent need to achieve greater balance in our future interventions and social policies by bringing greater attention to poor children's emotional and mental well-being, bringing to the current (and incontrovertibly valuable) focus on poor children's school achievement, greater attention to their emotional and mental well-being as well. The risks to the psychological health of children in poverty are prodigious, and the support systems available to most of these youngsters, for too long, have remained dismally inadequate.

## Notes

1.   Within this paper, the term "inner-city" is used to refer to contemporary conditions of urban poverty in the United States. Most existing developmental research on poor families has been based in urban settings, areas in which minority families are disproportionately represented [Huston et al. 1994; Luthar 1999]. Accordingly, samples of studies cited here typically involve low SES urban individuals with an over-representation of ethnic minorities.

2.   Dissonance between mainstream society's and subcultural perspectives has been found in relation to several other indicators. For example, adolescent parenthood—conventionally viewed as both a sign and harbinger of adjustment problems—can be viewed positively by many urban poor youth, as it connotes a symbol of adult status and the opportunities for new intimate relationships and generational continu-

ity [Burton et al. 1995; Luthar 1999; see also Garcia Coll & Vasquez Garcia 1996]. Similarly, a high level of substance use is not inevitably a reflection of personal psychopathology among disadvantaged teens. On the other hand, this too has been found to be linked with relatively positive relations with peers [Luthar 1999; Wills et al. 1992].

3.   The extent of this imbalance is starkly illustrated in the contents of current social programs for poor children, which overwhelmingly target school readiness/performance and reduction of destructive behavior patterns such as delinquency or substance use [for an overview, see Crane 1998]. There is rarely explicit attention to the children's psychological difficulties, i.e., to internalizing problems such as depression and hopelessness, anxiety and fearfulness, and disturbances in sleep or appetite, all of which often arise from exposure to chronic urban poverty and can cause affected individuals (though not necessarily those around them) profound levels of distress [e.g., see Luthar 1999; Marans & Adelman 1997].

4.   A description of this program can be found on the World Wide Web at the following address: http://www.chessctr.org/schools.htm.

5.   This chapter was prepared with heartfelt appreciation of Emory Cowen, pioneer in the field of primary prevention, and mentor *par excellence.* Emory's magnanimity of spirit, compassionate caring, and incisive wisdom have benefited not only thousands of at-risk families but also scores of young researchers—to whom he has unstintingly offered his scientific guidance and personal support, always with delectable good humor. As a scientist, a senior colleague, and a person, Emory is truly an inspiration and deeply cherished role model.

# References

Allen, L. & Grobman, S. (1996). Multiculturalism and social policy. In E. F. Zigler, S. L. Kagan, & N. W. Hall (Eds.), *Children, families, and government* (pp. 355–377). New York: Cambridge University Press.

Arroyo, C. G. & Zigler, E. (1995). Racial identity, academic achievement, and the psychological well-being of disadvantaged adolescents. *Journal of Personality and Social Psychology, 69, 903–914.*

Bergman, L. R. & Magnusson, D. (1997). A person-oriented approach in research on developmental psychopathology. *Development and Psychopathology, 9,* 291–319.

Botvin, G. J. (1998). Preventing adolescent drug abuse through Life Skills Training: Theory, methods, and effectiveness. In J. Crane (Ed.),

*Social programs that work* (pp. 225–257). New York: Russell Sage Foundation.

Burton, L. M., Allison, K. W., & Obeidallah, D. (1995). Social context and adolescence: Perspectives on development among inner-city African-American teens. In L. J. Crockett & A. C. Crouter (Eds.), *Pathways through adolescence: Individual development in relation to social contexts* (pp. 119–138).

Carnegie Council on Adolescent Development (1994). *A matter of time: Risk and opportunity in the out-of-school hours.* Task Force on Youth Development and Community Programs. Washington, DC: Author.

Caspi, A. (1993). Why maladaptive behaviors persist: Sources of continuity and change across the life course. In D. C. Funder, R. D. Parke, C. Tomlinson-Keasey, & K. Widman (Eds.), *Studying lives through time.* Washington, DC: American Psychological Association.

Caspi, A. & Moffitt, T. E. (1991). Individual differences are accentuated during periods of social change: The sample case of girls at puberty. *Journal of Personality & Social Psychology, 61,* 157–168.

Cauce, A. M. (1986). Social networks and social competence: Exploring the effects of early adolescent friendships. *American Journal of Community Psychology, 14,* 607–628.

Cauce, A. M., Felner, R. D., & Primavera, J. (1982). Social support in high-risk adolescents: Structural components and adaptive impact. *American Journal of Community Psychology, 10,* 417–428.

Cicchetti, D. & Rogosch, F. A. (1996) Equifinality and multifinality in developmental psychopathology. *Development and Psychopathology, 8,* 597–600.

Cicchetti, D. & Schneider-Rosen, K. (1986). An organizational approach to childhood depression. In M. Rutter, C. Izard, & P. Read (Eds.), *Depression in young people: Clinical and developmental perspectives* (pp. 71–134). New York: Guilford.

Cohler, B. J., Stott, F. M., & Musick, J. S. (1995). Adversity, vulnerability, and resilience. Cultural and developmental perspectives. In D. Cicchetti & D. J. Cohen (Eds.), *Developmental Psychopathology, Vol. 2: Risk, disorder and adaptation* (pp. 753–800). New York: Wiley.

Coie, J. D., Dodge, K. A., Terry, R., & Wright, V. (1991). The role of aggression in peer relations: An analysis of aggression episodes in boys' play groups. *Child Development, 62,* 812–826.

Coie, J. D. & Jacobs, M. R. (1993). The role of social context in the prevention of conduct disorder. *Development and Psychopathology, 5,* 263–275.

Coie, J. D., Terry, R., Lenox, K., Lockman, J., & Hyman, C. (1995). Childhood peer rejection and aggression as predictors of stable patterns of adolescent disorder. *Development and Psychopathology, 7,* 697–713.

Conduct Problems Prevention Research Group. (1992). A developmental and clinical model for the prevention of conduct disorders: The Fast Track Program. *Development and Psychopathology, 4,* 509–527.

Cowen, E. L. (1991). In pursuit of wellness. *American Psychologist, 46,* 404–408.

Cowen, E. L. (1994). The enhancement of psychological wellness: Challenges and opportunities. *American Journal of Community Psychology, 22,* 149–179.

Cowen, E. L., Hightower, A. D., Pedro-Carroll, J. L., Work, W. C., Wyman, P. A., & Haffrey, W. G. (1996). *School-based prevention for children at risk: The Primary Mental Health Project.* Washington, DC: American Psychological Association.

Cowen, E. L., Work, W. C., & Wyman, P. A. (1997). In. S. S. Luthar, J. A. Burack, D. Cicchetti, & J. R. Weisz, (Eds.), *Developmental psychopathology: Perspectives on adjustment, risk, and disorder* (pp. 527–547). New York: Cambridge.

Crane, J. (Ed.). (1998). *Social programs that work.* New York: Russell Sage Foundation.

Dishion, T. J., Andrews, D. W., & Crosby, L. (1995). Antisocial boys and their friends in early adolescence: Relationship characteristics, quality, and interactional process. *Child Development, 66,* 139–152.

Dodge, K. A., Coie, J. D., Pettit, G. S., & Price, J. M. (1990). Peer status and aggression in boys' groups: Developmental and contextual considerations. *Child Development, 61,* 1289–1309.

Freitas, A. L., & Downey, G. (1998). Resilience: A dynamic perspective. *International Journal of Behavioral Development, 22,* 263–285.

Garcia Coll, C., Lamberty, G., Jenkins, R., McAdoo, H. P., Crnic, K., Wasik, B. H., & Vasquez Garcia, H. (1996). An integrative model for the study of developmental competencies in minority children. *Child Development, 67,* 1891–1914.

Garcia Coll, C. T., & Vazquez Garcia, H. A. (1996). Definitions of competence during adolescence: Lessons from Puerto Rican adolescent mothers. In D. Cicchetti & S. L. Toth (Eds.), *Rochester Symposium on Developmental Psychopathology* (Vol. 7) (pp. 283–308). New York: University of Rochester Press.

Garmezy, N., Masten, A. N., & Tellegen, A. (1984). Studies of stress-resistant children: A building block for developmental psychology. *Child Development, 55,* 97–111.

Gonzales, N. A., Cauce, A. M., Friedman, R., & Mason, C. A. (1996). Family, peer and neighborhood influences on academic achievement among African-American adolescents: One year prospective effects. *American Journal of Community Psychology, 24,* 365–387.

Hammen, C., Marks, T., Mayol, A., & deMayo, R. (1985). Depressive self-schemas, life stress, and vulnerability to depression. *Journal of Abnormal Psychology, 94,* 308–319.

Hammond, W. R. & Yung, B. (1993). Psychology's role in the public health response to assaultive violence among young African-American men. *American Psychologist, 48,* 142–154.

Havighurst, R. J. (1972). *Developmental tasks and education* (3rd ed.). New York: David McKay.

Hoge, R. D., Andrews, D. A., & Leschied, A. W. (1996). An investigation of risk and protective factors in a sample of youthful offenders. *Journal of Child Psychology and Psychiatry, 37,* 419–424.

Huston, A. C., McLoyd, V. C., & Garcia Coll, C. (1994). Children and poverty: Issues in contemporary research. *Child Development, 65,* 275–282.

Jarrett, R. L. (1990). *A comparative examination of socialization patterns among low-income African-Americans, Chicanos, Puerto Ricans, and whites: A review of the ethnographic literature.* Washington, DC: Social Sciences Research Council.

Jensen, P. S. & Hoagwood, K. (1997). The book of names: DSM-IV in context. *Development and Psychopathology, 9,* 231–249.

Kazdin, A. E. (1995). *Conduct disorders in childhood and adolescence* (2nd ed.). Thousand Oaks, CA: Sage.

Knitzer, J. (In press). Early childhood mental health services through a policy and systems perspective. In S. J. Meisels & J. P. Shonkoff (Eds.), *Handbook of early childhood intervention: Second edition.* New York: Cambridge.

Lepper, M. R., Sethi, S., Dialdin, D., Drake, M. (1997). Intrinsic and extrinsic motivation: A developmental perspective. In S. S. Luthar, J. Burack, D. Cicchetti, & J. Weisz (Eds.), *Developmental psychopathology: Perspectives on adjustment, risk, and disorder* (pp. 23–50). New York: Cambridge.

Luthar, S. S. (1995). Social competence in the school setting: Prospective cross-domain associations among inner-city teens. *Child Development, 66*, 416–429.

Luthar, S. S. (1997). Sociodemographic disadvantage and psychosocial adjustment: Perspectives from developmental psychopathology. In S. S. Luthar, J. A. Burack, D. Cicchetti, & J. R. Weisz (Eds.), *Developmental psychopathology: Perspectives on adjustment, risk, and disorder* (pp. 459–485). New York: Cambridge.

Luthar, S. S. (1998, August). *Resilience among at-risk youth: Ephemeral, elusive, or robust?* McCandless award presentation, Annual Convention of the American Psychological Association, San Francisco, CA.

Luthar, S. S. (1999). *Children in poverty: Risk and protective forces in adjustment.* Thousand Oaks, CA: Sage Publications.

Luthar, S. S. & Blatt, S. J. (1995). Differential vulnerabilities of dependency and self-criticism among disadvantaged teenagers. *Journal of Research on Adolescence, 5*, 431–449.

Luthar, S. S. & D'Avanzo, K. (1999). Contextual factors in substance use: A study of suburban and inner-city adolescents. *Development and Psychopathology, 11*, 845–867.

Luthar, S. S. & McMahon, T. (1996). Peer reputation among adolescents: Use of the Revised Class Play with inner-city teens. *Journal of Research on Adolescence, 6*, 581–603.

Luthar, S. S. & Suchman, N. E. (1999). Developmentally informed parenting interventions: The Relational Psychotherapy Mother's Group. In D. Cicchetti & S. L. Toth (Eds.), *Rochester Symposium on Developmental Psychopathology, Volume X: Developmental approaches to prevention and intervention.* Rochester, NY: University of Rochester Press.

Luthar, S. S. & Zigler, E. (1991). Vulnerability and competence: A review of research on resilience in childhood. *American Journal of Orthopsychiatry, 61*, 6–22.

Lynam, D., Moffitt, T., & Stouthamer-Loeber, M. (1993). Explaining the relation between IQ and delinquency: Class, race, test motivation, school failure, or self-control? *Journal of Abnormal Psychology, 102*, 187–196.

Marans, S. & Adelman, A. (1997). Experiencing violence in a developmental context. In J. D. Osofsky (Ed.), *Children in a violent society* (pp. 202–221). New York: Guilford.

Masten A. S. & Coatsworth, J. D. (1998). The development of competence in favorable and unfavorable environments: Lessons from research on successful children. *American Psychologist, 53,* 205–220.

Masten, A. S., Coatsworth, J. D., & Neemann, J. (1995). The structure and coherence of competence from childhood through adolescence. *Child Development, 66,* 1635–59.

Moffitt, T. E. (1993). Adolescence-limited and life-course persistent antisocial behavior: A developmental taxonomy. *Psychological Review, 100,* 674–701.

National Research Council. (1993). *Losing generations: Adolescents in high-risk settings.* Washington, DC: National Academy Press.

Natriello, G., McDill, E. L., & Pallas, A. M. (1990). *Schooling disadvantaged children: Racing against catastrophe.* New York: Teachers College Press.

Nettles, S. M. & Pleck, J. (1994). The multiple ecologies of risk and resilience in African American adolescents. In R. J. Hagerty, N. Garmezy, M. Rutter, & L. R. Sherrod (Eds.), *Stress, coping, & development: Risk and resilience in children.* New York: Cambridge University Press.

Newman, K. S. (1996). Working poor: Low-wage employment in the lives of Harlem youth. In J. A. Graber, J. Brooks-Gunn, & A. C. Petersen (Eds.), *Transitions through adolescence: Interpersonal domains and context* (pp. 323–343). Mahwah, NJ: Erlbaum.

Ogbu, J. U. (1991). Minority coping responses and school experience. *Journal of Psychohistory, 18,* 433–456.

Phinney, J. S. (1990). Ethnic identity in adolescents and adults: Review of research. *Psychological Bulletin, 108,* 499–514.

Price, R. H., Gioci, M., Penner, W., & Trautlein, B. (1993). Webs of influence: School and community programs that enhance adolescent health and education. In R. Takanishi (Ed.), *Adolescence in the 1990's: Risk and opportunity* (pp. 29–63). New York: Teachers College Press.

Prinz, R. J. & Miller, G. E. (1991). Issues in understanding and treating childhood conduct problems in disadvantaged populations. *Journal of Clinical Child Psychology, 20,* 379–385.

Richters, J. E. & Cicchetti, D. (1993). Mark Twain meets DSM-III-R: Conduct disorders, development, and the concept of harmful dysfunction. *Development and Psychopathology, 5,* 5–29.

Sameroff, A. J. & Chandler, M. (1975). Reproductive risk and the continuum of caretaker casualty. In F. D. Horowitz, M. Hetherington, S. Scarr-Salapatek, & G. Siegel (Eds.), *Review of child development research* (Vol. 4) pp. 187–244). Chicago: University of Chicago Press.

Seidman, E., Allen, L., Aber, J. L., Mitchell, C., & Feinman, J. (1994). The impact of school transitions in early adolescence on the self-system and perceived social context of poor urban youth. *Child Development, 65*, 507–522.

Shanahan, M. J., Elder, G. H., Burchinal, M., & Conger, R. D. (1996). Adolescent paid labor and relationships with parents: Early work-family linkages. *Child Development, 67*, 2183–2200.

Spencer, M. B., Cole, S. P., DuPree, D., Glymph, A., & Pierre, P. (1993). Self-efficacy among urban African American early adolescents: Exploring issues of risk, vulnerability, and resilience. *Development and Psychopathology, 5*, 719–739.

Spencer M. B. & Markstom-Adams, C. (1990). Identity processes among racial and ethnic minority children in America. *Child Development, 61*, 290–310.

Sroufe, L. A. & Rutter, M. (1984). The domain of developmental psychopathology. *Child Development, 55*, 17–29.

Steele, C. M. (1997). A threat in the air: How stereotypes shape intellectual identity and performance. *American Psychologist, 52*, 613–629.

Steinberg, L. (1987, April 25). Why Japan's students outdo ours. *New York Times*, p. 15.

Stipek, D. (1997). Success in school: For a head start in life. In S. S. Luthar, J. Burack, D. Cicchetti, & J. Weisz (Eds.), *Developmental psychopathology: Perspectives on adjustment, risk, and disorder* (pp. 75–92). New York: Cambridge.

Takanishi, R. (1993). *Adolescence in the 1990s: Risk and opportunity.* New York: Teachers College Press.

Takanishi, R. (1996). Changing images of adolescents: Rethinking our policies. In E. F. Zigler, S. L. Kagan, & N. W. Hall (Eds.), *Children, families, and government.* New York: Cambridge University Press.

Wakefield, J. C. (1997). When is development disordered? Developmental psychopathology and the harmful dysfunction analysis of mental disorder. *Development and Psychopathology, 9*, 269–290.

Waters, E. & Sroufe, L A. (1983). Social competence as a developmental construct. *Developmental Review, 3*, 79–97.

Weisz, J., McCarty, C. A., Eastman, K. L., Chaiyasit, W., & Suwanlert, S. (1997). Developmental psychopathology and culture: Ten lessons from Thailand. In S. S. Luthar, J. Burack, D. Cicchetti, & J. Weisz (Eds.), *Developmental psychopathology: Perspectives on adjustment, risk, and disorder* (pp. 568–592). New York: Cambridge.

Wentzel, K. R. & Asher, S. R. (1995). The academic lives of neglected, rejected, popular, and controversial children. *Child Development, 66*, 754–763.

Wills, T., Vaccaro, D., & McNamara, G. (1992). The role of life events, family support, and competence in adolescent substance use: A test of vulnerability and protective factors. *American Journal of Community Psychology, 20*, 349–374.

Zigler, E. F. & Gilman, E. (1996). Not just any care: Shaping a coherent child care policy. In E. F. Zigler, S. L. Kagan, & N. W. Hall (Eds.), *Children, families, and government: Preparing for the 21st century* (pp. 94–116). New York: Cambridge.

Zigler, E. & Trickett, P. K. (1978). IQ, social competence, and evaluation of early childhood intervention programs. *American Psychologist, 33*, 789–798.

Zuroff, D. C. & Mongrain, M. (1987). Dependency and self-criticism: Vulnerability factors for depressive affective states. *Journal of Abnormal Psychology, 96*, 14–22.

# Acknowledgments

This work was supported by Research Scientist Development Award K21-DA00202, P50-DA09241, RO1-DA10726, RO1-DA11498, and by funding from the William T. Grant Foundation (Luthar), and a research award from the Social Sciences and Humanities Research Council in Canada (Burack). The authors gratefully acknowledge suggestions on a prior draft from the editors of this volume.

# 3

# Empowerment, Wellness, and the Politics of Development

*Angela Wiley and Julian Rappaport*

> We have not yet given adequate attention to envisioning truly emancipatory knowledge-seeking. We have not yet found the space to step back and image up the whole picture of what science might be in the future. In our culture, reflecting on an appropriate model of rationality ... could produce a politics of knowledge-seeking that would show us the conditions necessary to transfer control from the "haves" to the "have nots. [Harding 1986, p. 19–20]

The notion of wellness, as explicated in both the theoretical and empirical scholarship of Emory L. Cowen [e.g. 1991, 1994, 1996, in press] is an alternative to the tendency of helping professionals to view people as their problems, their diagnoses, and their deficits. Its conceptual roots are in Cowen's earlier, now classic writing on a community psychology of prevention as opposed to repair [Cowen et al. 1967; Cowen 1973, 1977, 1980, 1982, 1985; Cowen et al. 1975]. Wellness as a construct has emerged from the prevention of illness movement and evolved to a promotion of health alternative, to a large extent in the context of the ambitions of a community psychology movement that has included in its agenda a concern with social justice and progressive politics [see, for example, Albee 1996; Albee et al. 1988; Heller et al. 1984; Joffe & Albee 1981; Kelly 1990, this volume; Levine & Perkins 1997; Rappaport 1977, 1981, 1992; Rappaport & Seidman, in press; Rappaport & Stewart 1997; Seidman & Rappaport 1986; Tolan et al. 1990; Trickett 1996, among many others].

Promotion of health in this context is an expansive, multidisciplinary task; as such, it opens a host of possible alliances among scholars and activists from various disciplines and their citizen partners, including the supposed beneficiaries of human services. A focus on wellness among children calls especially upon the work of developmental psychologists for both theory and data. In this alliance, there is much to be gained and also much at risk [Felner et al., in press]. With the insights of developmental psychology come certain assumptions and blindnesses common to mainstream psychology, many of which have been critiqued by community psychologists and others [Burman 1997; Fox & Prilleltensky 1997] interested in social change. Historically, community psychologists have been most critical of clinical psychology, partly because the field of community psychology emerged first among those who sought to break from clinical psychology's deep-seated assumptions and practices that were seen to limit both the reach and effectiveness of human services for those outside the mainstream [Cowen et al. 1967]. In this volume, Cowen continues to raise serious questions about clinical psychology's movement into "prevention science."

Community psychology's aim is to foster a more just society, where power is interrogated and there is full participation by people of color, class, and gender, who have neither been well represented nor understood by those who control our social institutions. For wellness to serve such purposes, the incorporation of developmental psychology's insights must be accompanied by the same progressive critical analysis that meets the clinician's analysis and practice.

Wellness research and scholarship emerging from Emory Cowen's four decades of programmatic work is largely, if not exclusively, a story about childhood. It is concerned with the well-being of children, albeit in the context of schools, families, and communities [see, for example, Cowen et al. 1996]. Whatever else the wellness metaphor evokes (indeed, it is a metaphor), it also conjures up the physical body and reminds us that we are in a profession (psychology) that considers itself to be a part of the health care delivery system, even if we work in places like schools and neighborhoods. The imagery of the health care professional exerts considerable, if unspoken, influence on what we see as social issues, how we look at those issues, the questions we ask, and the ways we carry out our work.

The idea of wellness fits a profession concerned with health (and illness), the training of experts, and a discipline interested in exploring the nature of human development. Health care, education, and human development are primary underpinnings for a psychology of wellness. Because children and families are a central focus of developmental psychology, it is reasonable that this research tradition should emerge as central to an elaboration of the wellness metaphor among psychologists. But children and families are also a center of political activity and interest. Much public discourse and policy intervention focuses on poor and minority children and families, especially those with the least exercised political power.

Developmental psychology brings more than "the facts" to wellness; it also brings its own distinct political point of view, usually couched in words that seem to make the course of children's development look "natural" and inevitable but for the inadequacies of their parents, their neighborhood culture, or their genetics [Fox & Prilleltensky 1997]. Psychology, perhaps especially developmental psychology, tends to focus our attention on individual children's "progress" (or lack of expected "normal" progress) in ways that can (but need not) conceal deeply held values such that we make it easier for policymakers to see "bad mothers, absent fathers, and broken homes" rather than "poverty, unemployment, and frustration" [Burman 1997, p. 142]. Children with problems in living are often explained by references to inadequate parents and impulsive or stupid children [see, for example, Aber & Rappaport 1994; Lykken 1994; Sklar 1995].

## Stories of Wellness and Empowerment

Within the wellness story, the child is the central hero in a romantic odyssey—acquiring attachments and overcoming circumstances to gain competencies and coping skills, usually with the aid of enlightened and skilled family members, experts who consult with direct care givers, and key significant others in positions of authority. Wellness tells an optimistic story to professional caregivers. It engenders hope in the face of adversity and faith in our own work as experts, consultants, advocates, and researchers. It says we can prevent problems in living before the fact of their occurrence by working with our children and their caretakers before, rather than only after, they are in trouble. This story has inspired a good deal of direct intervention with children, youth, and their caregivers [e.g., Cowen, et al. 1996], but it has not said much about empowerment, nor has the empowerment literature said much about wellness.

Empowerment is a construct that has been claimed by people who hold many divergent political aims. In the psychology and applied human services field, the term has been best defined by the Cornell University Empowerment Group [1989], whose definition we will return to in our conclusions section:

> "Empowerment is an intentional, ongoing process, centered in the local community, involving mutual respect, critical reflection, caring and group participation, through which people lacking an equal share of valued resources gain greater access to and control over those resources" [p. 2].

While Cowen [1994] theorizes on five different pathways to wellness enhancement, including a concern with settings and with empowerment, these have not been primary concerns central to the wellness story. The idea of empowerment as defined above evokes a different metaphor than wellness—one that is not necessarily child-centered, evocative of the physical body and biomedical expertise, nor quite so optimistic. It is a metaphor that draws us, quite directly, into the politics of helping and the politics of adults authorized to use their power to socialize others [Perkins & Zimmerman 1995]. Empowerment is a metaphor of the body politic, rather than the personal body. In this chapter we ask if it is useful to mix metaphors like wellness, (designed to provide a vehicle for thinking about the person as a bio-social organism) with metaphors like empowerment. Empowerment is invoked to think about persons as behaving in contexts defined by social, cultural, organizational, political, and economic power, as well as "a stronger awareness of the connection between proximal conditions and distal events in the larger society, and actions directed at these less local conditions" [Saegert & Winkel 1996, p. 521].

Empowerment turns our attention to the power and politics of life circumstances and to the organizational characteristics that describe settings [Maton & Salem 1995]. Developmental psychology, like most of psychology, tends to either ignore the sociopolitical realities that contextualize human development, or assume that competent individuals can overcome these realities. Empowerment tends to assume that the nature of power is such that those who hold it have the advantage of interpreting the meaning of behavior in ways that define development and competence, and that this in turn has a reciprocal relationship with respect to further development of competent individuals.

Whereas wellness tells a romantic story, the empowerment story is often ironic rather than romantic. Its characters, including the narrators of the story (writers, scholars, and researchers), are full of contradictions and inconsistencies. It is a metaphor that calls one to divergent, rather than convergent thinking. Those who adopt the empowerment social agenda are wary of "programs" designed by experts who claim to fix things, and are more concerned about who has a voice in the conversation and a place at the table [Fowers & Richardson 1996; Rappaport 1990, 1994, 1998; Stewart & Rappaport 1997; Thomas & Rappaport 1996]. The metaphor of empowerment has been described as paradoxical [Rappaport 1981]. Sometimes there are no heroes in this story. Its central characters are more flawed and less innocent than children, although children and families are often the point of their concerns. The experts in this story often fix one difficulty only to cause a different problem elsewhere. As Sarason [1986] has put it, there are no final solutions that solve a social problem now and forevermore. In the empowerment story, citizen rights and stakeholder conflict are more central, even encouraged, than in the wellness story. The empowerment story is about a political process. It asks, "Who gets to make decisions and how?" The empowerment story is also about culture and asks, "Whose way of doing (and seeing) things counts as important?" Empowerment often highlights community, as opposed to only individual development [Rappaport 1995; Riger 1993].

Thus, while children and families are a central focus of developmental psychology, children and families are also the centers of great political activity and interest. Interpretations of childhood and family interactions are frequently the subject of contentious public discourse with high stakes. Much recent public discourse and policy interventions have focused on poor and minority children and families—those with the least exercised political power. What, we ask here, might the metaphor of empowerment ask of the wellness metaphor and of developmental psychology—if developmental psychology is to be its underpinning?

## Logic of Science and Politics in Developmental Psychology

There is a relationship between science and politics that conforms to its own internal logic: (a) Interpretation contributes to our understanding of human development; (b) What is interpreted is done so within the realm of power and politics: and (c) Thus, power and politics are inherent in our understanding of human development. Following this thought to its logical end indicates to us that developmental psychology is an inherently political undertaking. But then, "science has always been a social product" [Harding 1986, p. 137], and thus it is inevitable that culture and history contribute to our interpretation of human development [Dilworth-Anderson & Burton 1996; Fisher et al. 1998; Sampson 1993].

Empowerment theory suggests that, if developmental psychology is to provide a legitimate empirical basis for understanding human development in general and wellness in particular, in a diverse society we will need to make its politics transparent and open to public scrutiny. If developmental psychology is to be the underpinning of a wellness perspective such that it deserves to be applied to political decisions of great weight (such as the allocation of resources in the education and human services arena) and put into practice (in ways that affect the lives of real children), we are morally obligated to explore the range of normative but distinct paths of development that exist in different communities [see, for example, Elder et al. 1993; Miller et al. 1997].

As the population of the United States becomes more and more diverse, it is critical to understand what that diversity means for human psychology and functioning [Albert 1988; Dilworth-Anderson & Burton 1996; Trickett et al. 1994]. Greenfield [1994] has argued that we must move "toward the construction of a truly universal theory of development through the empirical and theoretical understanding of human diversity" [p. 1]. Without exploring here if it is in fact either desirable or possible to construct a "truly universal theory of development," it is obvious that diversity exists in a world of politics and not all groups have equal access to resources and opportunities. This political reality makes it necessary to interpret the facts of human development in light of the particulars of social, economic, and cultural power, and in light of the tendencies of organizations, institutions, and communities to apply power in their own perceived self interest.

McLoyd [1990, 1994] has argued that it is inexcusable for developmentalists to fail to consider how to prevent the disruption of natural developmental processes. Further, she has implied, and we agree, that it is within the mandate of developmental psychology to do work that actually facilitates the development of poor children and children from minority groups. This requires making the transition from research to practice and policy. But such transition requires considerably more than the direct application of empirical research from one context to another, a serious problem for laboratory-based science, or even for a science that assumes generalizability across field contexts.

Psychology, as a discipline, has operated on the assumption that the social, cognitive, and behavior patterns of Caucasian Americans are the norm [LaFromboise et al. 1993]. In line with this, one way that mainstream developmental psychology has protected itself from the politics of the surrounding world is by focusing almost exclusively on the development of Caucasian, middle-class children [Fisher & Brennan 1992; Graham 1992; Hagen et al. 1990; Loo et al. 1988; Luthar & Burack, this volume]. In Graham's [1992] analyses, studies including minority samples have frequently lacked methodological rigor (for example, many have confounded race and socioeconomic class and/or have failed to measure SES adequately). More frequently, research published in mainstream developmental psychology journals has simply glossed over sample ethnicity or has sampled from only the ranks of lower socioeconomic class minorities [Fisher & Brennan 1992; Hagen et al. 1990]. This latter strategy is entwined with both a focus on the deficits rather than the strengths of minority communities, as well as an emphasis on the homogeneity of minority communities rather than acknowledgment of their diversity [Kelley et al. 1992]. Additionally, there is an implication in the pattern of developmental research and its interpretation that suggests that minority development is a delayed form of Caucasian middle-class development. In other words, given time and proper grooming, minority child development will come to resemble the normative development of middle-class Caucasian children. The methodological focus on Caucasian middle-class children paired with the universal generalization is both ethically objectionable and scientifically faulty [Lerner 1993]

Some people have begun to make connections between developmental science and social problems. The relatively young science of developmental psychopathology is one example [see Cicchetti 1984, 1989, 1993; Cicchetti & Toth 1992; Hoagwood & Jensen 1997; Rutter & Garmezy 1983; Sroufe & Rutter 1984]. The foundation of this approach includes a concern to link the frequently distant realms of developmental research and real world practice and application [Cicchetti & Toth 1998]. The basic focuses of developmental psychopathology, laid out clearly in Toth & Cicchetti [1999], include: consideration of normal and abnormal development as these inform one another; emphasis on interdisciplinary approaches; focus on prevention as well as intervention; and attending to the diversity in both processes and outcomes of development, as well as the contextual and cultural influences on these.

Another example is apparent in the emerging realm of "applied developmental psychology" [Morrison et al. 1984; Sigel & Cocking 1980; Zigler & Finn 1984]. Some researchers in this relatively young field focus on knowledge application and others on knowledge generation with an eye toward application [Fisher & Tryon 1988; Morrison et al. 1984; Scholnick et al. 1988]. Fisher and Murray [1996] have argued that, to adequately meet the needs of society, developmental science must engage the surrounding community and other disciplines. They discuss the importance of doing research in the service of enhancing human development, particularly among those diverse populations whose development has been neglected in the past

[Fisher 1998]. This focus, while familiar to community psychology, has not been deeply embedded in the traditions of developmental psychologists' training or disciplinary rhetoric. Work in these burgeoning areas holds promise for expanding the scope of mainstream developmental psychology and increasing its impact in the real world of children and families.

Some mainstream developmental researchers have done research within disempowered populations (such as ethnic minorities and economically-depressed communities), but most of this research has been undertaken and left in a vacuum, thus allowing it to be used in the political realm of real life without researcher input or framing. A great deal of research concerning disempowered groups has focused on their presumed deficits and their involvement in societally-disapproved behaviors such as substance abuse, teen pregnancy, continued poverty, poor child rearing, academic underachievement, and criminal or delinquency rates. Relatively less research has focused on strengths, ability to survive and thrive, and the ways in which communities can and do provide unique and healthy contexts for development [see Wyman et al., this volume]. There is an important exception to this common focus on what disempowered groups lack. A growing community of scholars are interested in resilience, defined as positive adaptation despite significant adversity [see Luthar et al., in press, for a comprehensive review; also, Cicchetti & Garmezy 1993; Garmezy 1990; Luthar & Zigler 1991; Masten et al. 1990; Rutter 1990; Werner & Smith 1982, 1992]. There has also been increasing interest in the protective processes that may underlie resilience [Cowen et al. 1997; Luthar 1999]. Others have begun examining resiliency as the intersection between the person and her context, such as neighborhood context [Aber & Nieto, this volume]. Such researchers are interested in the degree to which contextual factors account for positive outcomes in spite of adversity.

This work on the factors and processes implicated in positive outcomes for disempowered children and families represents a significant step in the right direction. Even so, very little research has centered on locating resources, or featured collaboration with local people in collegial efforts at social and institutional change pertinent to development [Sklar 1995]. This kind of research has an empowering potential. Wellness points us in that direction. Empowerment asks, "How do we get there?"

There are at least four conceptual issues that should be made explicit when trying to reframe our ways of knowing about the development of diverse families [Dilworth-Anderson & Burton 1996] and the development of children within them. (1) What basic conceptual frameworks inform our thinking and form a foundation for our research? Our conceptual frameworks are our assumptions and ideas about how the social world works, about what is "normal." Do we think we are "color blind," or do we think about that question at all? We must challenge these basic frameworks if we are to research with an open mind.( 2) What values do we bring to the research process? Values have an enormous impact on the questions that researchers propose and the ways they go about answering these [for example, Gates 1992; Scarr 1985]. Acknowledging our values and our place in the social order (race, gender, class, culture), and exploring the meaning of this placement vis-à-vis our research, is a first step in rendering our values manageable. (3) What are our theoretical assumptions and how have these come to be? Theoretical assumptions, which underpin research, are often implicit and thus go unexamined. They are informed by training, and the culture and history of disciplines and the society at large, with all its political and historical concerns. (4) Are we assuring a methodological fit between our research methods and our sample populations? Measures and procedures created with and for one group (primarily middle-class Caucasians) will not necessarily be valid with other groups. Trying to force a fit where one does not exist is a sure way to support the status quo and contribute further to disempowering already overwhelmed communities.

## Some Starting Points for Empowering Research

There are many topics within the existing disciplinary confines of developmental psychology that would be appropriate for reexamination from an empowerment perspective. There are two related areas that represent particularly obvious opportunities for developmental researchers to engage in empowering inquiry. In both content areas, there is already an impressive amount of data and theory, far too much for a thorough review in this chapter. We highlight some of the work on both topics, focusing on the paucity of systematic data in minority groups and on the missed opportunities thus far in both areas for empowerment of children and families.

## Attachment Theory and Research

Attachment is an important construct in modern developmental psychology [Ainsworth et al. 1978; Bowlby 1969, 1973, 1980]. Attachment theory holds that humans have evolved with a biologically-based tendency to form long-lasting bonds with a mother figure during infancy [Ainsworth & Marvin 1995]. Attachment behaviors appear as organized patterns, particularly in times of heightened stress, presumably to maximize safety and comfort [Carlson et al. 1989]. Attachment bonds are critical for many aspects of normal, healthy development, both within childhood and far beyond [Bretherton 1985; Elicker et al. 1992; Zeanah et al. 1993 provides a review]. The quality and strength of attachment relationships are typically assessed in a laboratory method, the Strange Situation [Ainsworth & Wittig 1969] and are categorized as secure, avoidant, or resistant [Carlson et al. 1989 discuss the categories in detail]. Recently a fourth category, disorganized/disoriented, has been added that is characteristic of children who have been maltreated [Carlson et al. 1989; Main & Solomon 1990; Main & Hesse 1990]. See Cicchetti, Toth, and Rogosch [this volume] for application of attachment theory to considerations of maltreatment.

Waters, Vaughn, Posada, and Kondo-Ikemura [1995] have summarized recent consensus on the construct by noting that, among other accepted characteristics, attachment is thought to involve a typology that is universally applicable and to depend on adequate maternal sensitivity to the infant [Ainsworth & Bell 1970; Ainsworth & Marvin 1995]. Typically, accepted findings conclude that lower-class children are less securely attached (minority children are often lumped into this category) than middle-class children [Van Ijzendoorn

& Kroonenberg 1988]. From an empowerment perspective, the unexamined assumption that minority children (even those from economically poor life circumstances) are necessarily "at risk" for less than secure attachments to significant others is as damaging a stereotype as the earlier (no longer socially acceptable) assumptions that economically poor or minority children are less moral or less intelligent than their more affluent, Caucasian counterparts. These are simply different expressions of the same (usually unexamined) assumptions.

Although the seminal work on attachment was done in Uganda [Ainsworth 1967], most subsequent work specifying attachment patterns has been done with middle-class, Caucasian American families or with small numbers of minority families added to the mix, making valid interpretations for minority families impossible [for a recent exception, see Barnett 1998]. We know precious little about the distribution of attachment behaviors within various minority populations. This has not prevented conclusions from being drawn about minority populations based on the scanty research. For example, some have argued that there are likely to be more insecurely attached minority infants because minorities are overrepresented among the ranks of the poor and are thus disproportionately exposed to the stressing conditions of poverty [Broussard 1995].

Fisher et al. [1998] present a detailed critique of conventional attachment theory, beginning with its evolutionary assumptions about probable early hominoid life and behavior. They argue that recent understandings of the organization and patterns of hunter-gatherer societies lead to the conclusion that human infants are more likely to have evolved a tendency to form flexible attachments to multiple figures rather than the dyadic bonds assumed to be normal by conventional attachment theory. Interestingly enough, there is notable shared responsibility for child rearing in African American, American Indian, and Latin American families [Carson et al. 1990; Chatters 1994; Crawley 1988; Dilworth-Anderson 1992; London & Devore 1988; Martinez 1988; Martinez 1993; McAdoo 1993; Redhorse 1980; Vega 1990], leaving open the possibility that children in these subcultures form multiple attachments. Further, African American children have been observed to demonstrate multiple bonds to a range of caregivers [Shimkin et al. 1978].

Some researchers have begun to note the awkward fit of attachment models to the family structures and patterns of minority families. Expectations based on attachment theory do not seem to hold up in systematic observations of poor, mostly African American families involved in the child welfare system [Haight, personal communication, February 16, 1998]. Contradictory patterns appear when attachment categories are used with Latin American families [Fracasso et al. 1994] and African American families [Bakeman & Brown 1980; Jackson 1986, 1993; Kennedy & Bakeman 1984]. This work, although rarely mentioned in standard lectures on attachment, points to the improbability that one typology of parent-child attachment can hold across all cultural groups or in all circumstances. While attachment probably is an inherent part of human child development, serving a common function, there is growing support that the particular forms of the phenomenon are likely to be cultural-specific. Because detailed understanding of how young children and their parents relate to one another is clearly important, more attention should be focused on attachment relationships for families outside the middle-class, Caucasian American mainstream. There is a marked need in developmental psychology for what Fisher et al. [1998] refer to as "culturally anchored conceptions of attachment." Such conceptions will have to be created and tested from a bottom-up perspective, taking into account the family structures and caregiving traditions within distinct communities.

Developmental psychology has spent a great deal of time and energy exploring various aspects of the early socioemotional bonds between parents and children without a strong or systematic effort to put these findings into practice. Next we move to consider the empowerment potential in a related but more clearly practice-oriented realm of inquiry—developmental investigations around the phenomenon of child abuse and the resulting practice of foster care.

## Child Abuse and Foster Care Research

In 1995, in this country alone, 2.96 million children were reported as abused or neglected, and 996 died at the hands of caregivers [Petit & Curtis 1997]. These frightening figures speak to a practical need for detailed understanding of the causes, correlates, and consequences of child abuse and neglect, particularly because there is convincing general evidence that maltreated children do suffer long beyond the actual incidence of the abuse or neglect [Cicchetti et al., this volume; Coster & Cicchetti 1993; Salzinger et al. 1993]. As yet, a systematic and replicated theory of child maltreatment that can inform practice and policy has not emerged [Cicchetti & Toth 1993], nor has "a coordinated approach and general conceptual framework that can add new depth to our understanding of child maltreatment" [National Research Council 1993, p. 43; but see Cicchetti et al., this volume].

A significant body of research has focused on several levels of correlates, including characteristics of abusive parents, of abused children, and of abusive families. Abusive parents, for example, often have a history of maltreatment in their family of origin, harbor unrealistic desires for children to meet their emotional needs, exhibit poor control of aggressive impulses, express distaste for parenthood, and are emotionally distressed or depressed [Kempe et al. 1962; McLoyd 1990; Panaccione & Wahler 1986; Patterson 1982; Spinetta & Rigler 1972; Trickett et al. 1991]. Premature children or those with difficult temperaments or health or developmental problems are more likely to be the victims of abuse, although these factors often interact with parental characteristics [Pianta et al. 1989]. Families that live in isolation, without a safety net of social support, are more likely to abuse their children [Thompson 1995]. Families experiencing economic stress are more likely to have children who are abused [Daniel et al. 1983; Garbarino 1976; Parke & Collmer 1975] or neglected [Giovannoni & Billingsley 1970].

Although the National Clearing House on Child Abuse and Neglect [1995] has published general guideline definitions for the major types of abuse and neglect, a systematically employed definition of child maltreatment has not arisen, likely due to the general lack of coordinated research attention to the problem. Over time and across geography, different practical definitions have been used in the interest of simply addressing the pressing social and legal problem of child abuse and neglect [National Research Council 1993]. While this lack of consensus in terminology has hindered progress in creating a theory of maltreatment, in some senses it has probably been a blessing. Unlike the case of the commonly accepted and often universally-applied attachment model, there is still acknowledgment among many child welfare practitioners that the problem of maltreatment stems from a complex set of factors that may not be the same in every cultural group. The National Research Council [1993] has called for carefully conceived and controlled research that addresses cultural differences in maltreatment and the large, related constellation of topics such as culturally-situated parenting practices and beliefs and culturally-specific family structures. One promising effort to create and validate a definition of child maltreatment is being undertaken by proponents of the developmental psychopathology approach [Barnett et al. 1993; Cicchetti & Barnett 1991; Cicchetti et al., this volume]. These researchers recommend a multidimensional approach that includes a consideration of the abused child's developmental stage, as well as the family's cultural context.

Folk wisdom apart from research leads to the expectation that poor people and people of color are more likely to maltreat their children. Adding support to this, African American children are clearly represented in the ranks of those reported as abused and neglected disproportionate to their numbers in the general population. This has been a historical pattern since figures have been reported [Hampton 1991]. There is some evidence, though, that these official figures do not tell the whole story, and that African American families (as well as poor families) may be more likely to be the *subjects* of reports and may be more likely to have those reports substantiated by the legal and child welfare systems [for example, see Gelles 1975; Gill 1970; Turbett & O'Toole 1980]. Misunderstandings of cultural differences in child rearing, discipline, and parent-child roles can lead to unnecessary removal of children from their home [Stehno 1982]. This problem that is heightened when there is social distance (i.e., differences in class, race, or ethnicity) between the professional and the alleged abuser [Hampton 1986] or when professional decision making and service provision is not carefully couched in paradigm conducive to family and community empowerment [Leashore et al. 1991]. Joel Handler [1990], a law professor, has suggested that a problem for much of the human services system lies in its structure as a "legal-bureaucratic" rather than a "participatory" relationship between citizen and state. Handler suggests that a system designed with participatory decision making in mind is both desirable and feasible. All of these dynamics need further research and attention.

Although developmental psychology has not ignored the phenomenon of child maltreatment, we know very little conclusively about the causes, correlates, and consequences of child maltreatment in minority populations. Within-group analyses of ethnic group populations controlled for socioeconomic class have been rare. In one counter example, Daniel et al. [1983] examined a subsample of poor African American families and found that abusive mothers were more likely than nonabusive mothers to be very poor, to suffer from more social isolation, to have higher general levels of stress, and to have recently experienced highly stressful events in their personal lives (such as death of a close family member). In contrast to common perceptions and reporting statistics, when poverty is held constant, there is no difference between African Americans and Caucasians on interfamily violence [Bell & Chance-Hill 1988]. Supporting this, the National Center on Child Abuse and Neglect [1988] reported that there is no correlation of race or ethnicity with child maltreatment. In fact, flying in the face of conventional wisdom, there is research suggesting that African American parents are *less* likely to abuse their children than Caucasian parents [Zuravin & Greif 1989].

One line of research has posed an additional challenge to the conventional wisdom that minorities are more abusive. In a study that had African American, Latin American and Caucasian American families rate vignettes describing abusive and potentially abusive circumstances, minority families rated abusive and potentially abusive stories as more serious than did the Caucasian American parents [Giovannoni & Becerra 1979]. These findings were replicated and expanded by Ringwalt & Caye [1989], who also found that lower SES adults were more likely than those of higher SES circumstances to view abusive situations as serious. Fisher et al. [1998] interpret these and some other studies in this area as indicating that minority status acts as a buffer against child maltreatment amid the poverty and ensuing chaos that rocks so many families. Clearly, normative parenting as well as child maltreatment in minority groups require more in-depth, within group, and ethnographically sensitive research.

Within child welfare practice and policy, foster care has been called one success story in the ongoing saga of the developmental research-practice relationship [Shore 1998]. Shore notes that attachment theory, and the research that resulted from it, sprung from a crisis in how children were treated in hospital-stay situations (they were traditionally ripped away from parents and isolated, with no respect for their obvious distress). Attachment theory and research from the field of developmental psychology was combined with the experiences of myriad practitioners to alter the way that foster care is done. "The recognition of the child's need for continuity and stability has resulted in federal legislation ... to encourage permanency planning and early adoption of foster children, thus preventing the development of severe psychological problems," [p. 476]. In spite of this successful integration, research on the utility and ultimate success of foster care and other protective services as interventions is scant and generally unreliable [Melton 1984]. Recently, there has been growing attention to the subset of kinship foster care, an area of particular relevance for the empowerment of minority communities.

"Kinship care" refers to those situations where children who have been removed from the homes of their parents, usually as a consequence of maltreatment, and are placed with relatives, although legal custody remains with the state. Partially due to the enormous influx of cases into the child welfare system in the late 1980s, kinship care is a rapidly growing form of out-of-home care across the country [Berrick 1997], with an average of over 31% of all children in care placed in relative homes [Kusserow 1992]. African American children make up the bulk of those involved in this type of care [Berrick et al. 1994]. Many African American families utilize extensive kinship care in everyday life, with grandmothers and aunts playing a significant role in child rearing [Chatters et al. 1994; Crawley 1988; Dilworth-Anderson 1992; McAdoo 1980, 1993; Stack 1974; Sudarkasa 1988]. This tradition has led a number of African American scholars and practitioners to advocate for kinship care as a central component of family preservation services to African American families [Black Administrators in Child Welfare 1994; Danzy & Jackson 1997]. There is a growing sense that kinship care represents an indigenous resource for the African American community, a natural system of care that must somehow be fitted into the unnatural situation that arises from contact with the child welfare system [Danzy & Jackson 1997].

In spite of its intuitive appeal as a culturally-sensitive placement option and its acceptance by many within the African American community as a critical part of family preservation, child welfare systems across the country have been very slow to make kinship care a stable part of their family preservation and support services rather than treating it as a makeshift solution to a crisis. Surprisingly, there has been very little research on kinship care relative to its growing importance generally and for African American children in particular [Berrick 1997; Davidson 1997; Gebel 1996], and even less for children in other minority communities. Very few studies have compared kinship care children with nonrelative foster care [for exceptions see, Benedict et al. 1996; Berrick 1997; Berrick et al. 1994; Iglehart 1994]. As an example, Iglehart's [1994] study in California included African American and Latino children, but did not interview them or their kin caregivers directly or focus on their experiences.

Some interesting findings have emerged from the existing litera-ture, findings that will require additional research for their interpre-tation. For example, it is documented that, on average, children remain in kinship foster homes longer prior to reunification with their parents than do children in nonrelative foster care [for example, see Benedict & Caucasian 1991; Courtney & Needell 1997; Wulczyn & Goerge 1992]. While the positive side of this is that kinship place-ments are often more stable than nonkinship placements, researchers are only beginning to delve into potential reasons for and conse-quences of such findings. Until further research is completed, it is clearly premature to assume that kinship care is the optimal option for all children in spite of its popular appeal.

In general, a review of child welfare literature will demonstrate that scholars in this field have a limited knowledge of work in developmental psychology. Developmental researchers could add a great deal to the debate on questions about child maltreatment and out-of-home placement and in a way that empowers the rising numbers of children and families for whom these terrible experiences are a reality. Surely developmental psychologists do not view themselves as members of a discipline that focuses exclusively on the development of the majority (putting aside for a moment the likely fallacy that development has a single normative path, even in the statistical and political majority). Issues of attachment and socioemotional development, identity formation, self-esteem, wellness, and the many contextual influences on development are a few of the developmental issues that have direct relevance for child welfare problems. Developmental and wellness researchers are in a unique position to apply their knowledge of children's development across a wide range of domains to some very real and pressing problems in the lives of many children and families. We do not imply that wellness researchers should have all the responsibility for research that deals with children, families, social service provision, etc. We also do not imply that developmental researchers ought to be practitioners in the traditional sense. Rather, we are encouraging a much greater degree of interdisciplinary collaboration than has existed in the past and, more importantly, we are calling for a reconceptualization of the researcher as an advocate and agent of empowerment.

## The Relationship of Developmental Science to Advocacy

The work of developmental psychologists is of interest to the wider world: to parents, to practitioners, to policymakers, and to the media. While the full complexity of research (alpha levels, statistical signifi-cance, reliability, etc.) may be of less interest and may be less accessible to the nonscientist, many developmental findings, includ-ing those concerned with the concept of wellness, will make their way, in some form, to portions of the general public. Given this inevitabil-ity, we argue that developmental science should involve advocacy, a critical responsibility accepted by the empowerment oriented re-searcher. Shore [1998] defines advocacy as "[providing] a voice for the underserved and powerless children, the disenfranchised, those with severe handicaps, the poor, and others who need someone to speak for them and their needs" [p. 474]. We find this definition to be paternalistic, if well-meaning. Advocacy involves creating contexts

that empower groups and individuals within them to *speak for themselves* as much as possible. This might mean facilitating or bridging
access of disempowered groups to resources [Good et al. 1997; Kloos
et al. 1997] or translating for voices that are so rarely heard that their
vocabulary is little known [see Fine 1994 for a discussion of how
difficult this can be). Such work can only emerge from a close working
relationship between researchers and the people being researched, a
central point of the empowerment perspective to which we return in
our conclusions, below.

We agree with Shore that advocacy involves the integration of
theory, research, and practice (or action). Theory, carefully examined
and modified as necessary [Dilworth-Anderson & Burton 1996],
serves to organize the knowledge base and provides a springboard for
planning questions and interpreting findings. Research, carried out
with appropriately fitting methods, should contribute to the knowledge base. Research should approach the existing knowledge base
with as clear and unobstructed a vision as possible, creatively framing
questions about it, and altering it where necessary without hesitation.
Finally, practice provides the context for application or action, the
realm where the issues for research are apparent and where the
domains and dynamics of change can be seen. We are arguing that the
realm of practice is an action domain that is appropriate for all
developmental researchers interested in wellness and empowerment,
be they clinical, community, applied, or basic.

## Conclusions

A developmental psychology that makes a serious commitment to put
its findings and theories into action and advocate as necessary for
those whom it studies will seek to empower children and their
families, especially those who have been routinely deprived of a say in
their own communities and schools. We may well have to start by
emphasizing the needs of disempowered children and families as a
proper arena for scientific inquiry. Prior to engaging in the research
process, we will have to explore our own values as individual researchers and as a discipline. Without this step, our studies of multicultural

families run the risk of simply replicating the status quo [Dilworth-Anderson et al. 1993]. Once we have adjusted the domain, we will need to approach our questions and methods with an open mind, perhaps adapting them as necessary to fit the cultural backgrounds and environmental circumstances of disempowered populations. This will involve a reconceptualization of "good research" that acknowledges the necessity of interweaving scientific process with cultural characteristics [see Rogler 1989, for a similar argument]. Concretely, developmental psychology should act as an agent of empowerment by making research responsive to the real life needs of the underserved (minority children, poor children, and their families). This empowering responsiveness would need to be manifested in all areas: research content, methods, interpretation and application.

## Content

There can be little doubt that the selection of research questions is likely to be related to the broader social context in which any science exists [Harding 1986]. In general, the field of development must ask questions about the differences between individuals, about variations that appear within the individual across the lifespan and in response to contextual changes, and about the differences and similarities that exist between cultural and subcultural groups. Particular areas requiring attention include ethnic identity, especially that of mixed background individuals [Phinney 1990]; understandings of prejudice that take into account the experiences and characteristics of those experiencing it [Gaines & Reed 1995; LaFramboise et al. 1993]; alternative developmental pathways [see Miller et al. 1997; Wiley et al. 1998]; alternative family structures [Billingsley 1992; Daley et al. 1995; Stack 1974]; and the impact of various policy issues, such as day care, on all families, but particularly ethnic minority families [Jackson 1993]. This change in content focus would also include an examination of the many strengths despite oppression that exists in the disempowered communities [Hill 1971]. It is disheartening to note that while changes have occurred, in large part the developmental research community has not heeded Robert Hill's observation in 1971 from his book, *The Strengths of Black Families*: "Most discussions of black families tend to focus on indicators of instability and weakness. With few exceptions, most social scientists continue to portray black families as disorganized, pathological and disintegrating" [p. 37]. [See also Baratz & Baratz 1970; Ginsburg 1972.]

*Methodological Adjustment*

Research must be constructed and carried out in such a way as to examine disempowered populations carefully in their own historical, cultural, and economic contexts (without invidious comparisons and homogenous universal expectations). We may have to think outside of our mainstream methodological approaches since traditional science's norms and methods may not be suitable in and of themselves for eliminating inherent biases, since these are central parts of the problem [Harding 1986]. Current methodological conventions often have led researchers to misconstrue normative patterns in minority populations simply because these do not match patterns based in the Caucasian middle class [Padilla 1995]. "In the study of ethnic identity development ... constructs selected for measurement may represent self attributes that are desirable in the dominant society, but not in the particular ethnic minority cultures" [Fisher et al. 1998]. This holds true, no doubt, beyond the study of identity development.

The work of Stevenson [1993, 1994, 1995] on the socialization of racial identity is an excellent example of work that approaches an ethnic community on its own ground, carefully creating methodological categories that fit their experiences. In another example, there has been much discussion of the individual-collective distinction in identity development [Greenfield 1994; Markus & Kitayama 1991; Triandis 1989]. The kernel of the idea is that all cultures must deal with the issue of how people within the culture relate to one another. Some cultures settle this by valuing characteristics of the individual such as autonomy, initiative, and independence, while others focus on affiliation, interdependence, and group functioning [Triandis 1989]. Some have linked the autonomy emphasis to Western cultures and the connected affiliation to non-Western cultures [Greenfield 1994]. Of course, all cultures have both individuals and collectives, so both of these ideas are generally present [Kim & Choi 1994; Turiel 1994], allowing for variation within cultural groups and societies composed of multiple subcultures [Fisher et al. 1998]. It is critical to understand that African American and Latin American and other families differ from Caucasian families on these dimensions, and that each of these groups contains patterned variation within it. Wiley et al. [1998] have argued that there is class-based variation in constructs of autonomy within Caucasian culture. Consideration of inter- and intra-group variation can permit a better understanding of attachment patterns and family interactions, as well as how these interface with schooling and, later, relationships and employment.

There are some existing methodological models that focus on contexts, particularly the life span, ecological, developmental contextual, and applied developmental approaches [Baltes 1987; Bronfenbrenner 1977; Cicchetti & Lynch 1993; Lerner 1991; Seidman 1987; Sigel & Cocking 1980]. These approaches do not inform the majority of developmental researchers. There is an overpowering need for research on the developmental pathways of disempowered children and families at what Bronfenbrenner [1977] has called the macro- and exo-contextual levels.

## Interpretations of the Findings

Science is not objective or "decontextualized," although some from within the scientific community and many lay people still hold dear this misconception. Researchers *always* do their work from a position informed by their own political and social background. Interpretations of findings will thus never occur in a political vacuum. Rather than disputing this or reaching for an impossible ideal objectivity, it is preferable to make clear our political positions and agendas as developmental scientists.

It is exciting to consider that "some politics—[for example] the politics of movements for emancipatory social change—can increase the objectivity of science" [Harding 1986, p. 162] by challenging implicit assumptions. By this we mean that past research has often shored up the claims to power of society's dominant groups under the shroud of "objectivity," without raising questions about why issues are framed in ways that benefit some at the expense of others. In challenging this fiction, and openly conducting our research and interpreting our findings from an empowerment and wellness perspective, we should improve our research by interrogating it. When we are able to openly acknowledge our politics, we are freed to go about the business of seeking knowledge and determining how it relates to empowering vulnerable children and families.

In the interest of clarity, we do not mean that developmental researchers need to issue statements on their political party affiliation or stance on specific pieces of legislation. Rather, we are positing that developmental researchers concerned with wellness and empowerment will start by asking questions and designing studies with those priorities in mind. Even further, they will interpret findings and draw conclusions that are informed by this clearly political agenda.

## Application of Research Findings

This is the critical action step where researchers, who best understand the implications and limitations of the work, engage in interpretation and translation of the work for application and advocacy. This is the arena in which mainstream developmental science has the least experience.

The practice of community psychology is steeped in the traditions of "action research." In this world view, research and practice are not discrete, and social action is an important part of the tradition. The empowerment social agenda calls for a far more collaborative relationship in setting the goals of research (which philosophers of science tell us predetermines the answers), and sometimes requires a very different methodology than the typical psychological study [Rappaport 1990]. Consider the definition of empowerment cited above, which we repeat here for convenience:

> Empowerment is an intentional, ongoing process, centered in the local community, involving mutual respect, critical reflection, caring and group participation, through which people lacking an equal share of valued resources gain greater access to and control over those resources. [Cornell University Empowerment Group 1989, p.2]

Empowerment requires that our work involve both "mutual respect" and "group participation." This is intended to mean that the voices of the people being studied will actually be reflected in the work being done. Translated into research terms, it means that the very conceptualization of "wellness," for example, must involve the people to whom it is being applied, an assurance that it will be defined in different ways by different people in different contexts (recall also the discussion of "attachment," above). In the psychological meaning of wellness, there is surely enough ambiguity (as there is in the term "mental health") to assure us that we will discover multiple meanings, if we are attentive to contexts. Isn't this the point of a culturally anchored methodology? [See for example, Fisher et al. 1998; Seidman et al. 1993.]

To take this seriously, rather than as a palliative to political correctness, most researchers will need to spend considerable time (perhaps in the mode of ethnographic and qualitative researchers) living and working in context before they will understand the meaning of wellness in unfamiliar places. Even in school settings, where researchers have spent considerable time, advocating for collaboration and group participation as an "ongoing process, centered in the local community" requires a kind of intentionality and commitment to working with (rather than on or for) children and their families that is uncommon in psychological research. More typically we want to "help" children to fit in, rather than argue for changes they and their families want, changes that might make schooling more responsive to the real lives of the people schools are presumed to serve. Sometimes this approach will require us to deal with issues that are disturbing to the powerful people who operate schools. This may require us to share in the risks taken by the people we work with and study. For example, accusations of institutionalized racism in the very practices of schooling [see for example, Delpit 1995] can make for conflict rather than cooperation. When we mix the metaphors of empowerment and wellness, the result may be disruptive of the status quo, rather than conciliatory, and focused on settings rather than on individual adjustment.

"Change" understood this way is not limited to individual change, but calls attention to institutionalized practices as well. Aligning ourselves with group-based arguments for change in the status quo of the settings in which we work makes us less likely to reflexively align ourselves with the views of the most powerful as to what constitutes doing well, or with their views on how to create settings that facilitate doing well. This requires that we engage, together with the people with whom we are working, in a social, political, and economic analysis that contextualizes the psychological experience of education. This is what is meant by "critical reflection" in the definition of empowerment presented above.

The last phrase in the empowerment definition refers to an ongoing process "through which people lacking an equal share of valued resources gain greater access to and control over those resources," an outright acknowledgment that we intend to advocate for a redistribution of resources of all kinds—material, social, and psychological. This puts us squarely in touch with the values of social justice. If wellness reminds us that we are practicing in the traditions of a health care profession, empowerment forces us to attend to the politics of our practices. Together these metaphors can lead us to use, and be used by, developmental psychology in a conscious effort to inform our knowledge base and to further the well-being of children and families currently outside the mainstream of North America's bountiful society.

## Notes

Throughout this chapter, we use "minority" to refer to groups that have been systematically stripped of their rights to full participation in the Caucasian society of North America. This includes racial/ethnic groups and socioeconomically depressed groups. We do not imply that there is no distinction within and among these groups and refer the reader to Fisher et al. [1998] for an excellent review of the topic.

## References

Aber, M. S. & Rappaport, J. (1994). The violence of prediction: The uneasy relationship between social science and social policy. *Applied and Preventive Psychology, 3*, 43–54.

Adoption Assistance and Child Welfare Act of 1980, P.L. 96-272, 94 U.S. Statutes at Large § 500 (1980).Ainsworth, M. D. (1967). *Infancy in Uganda: Infant care and the growth of love*. Baltimore: Johns Hopkins Press.

Ainsworth, M. D. S. & Bell, S. M. (1970). Attachment, exploration, and separation: Illustrated by the behavior of one-year-olds in a Strange Situation. *Child Development, 41,* 49–67.

Ainsworth, M. D. S., Blehar, M. C., Waters, E., & Wall, S. (1978). *Patterns of attachment.* Hillsdale, NJ: Erlbaum.

Ainsworth, M. D. S. & Marvin, R. S. (1995). On the shaping of attachment theory and research: An interview with Mary D. S. Ainsworth (Fall 1994). *Monographs of the Society for Research in Child Development, 60*(2–3), 3–21.

Ainsworth, M. D. S. & Wittig, B. (1969). Attachment and the exploratory behavior of one-year-olds in a strange situation. In B. M. Foss (Ed.), *Determinants of Infant Behavior: Vol. 4.* (pp. 113–136). London: Methuen.

Albee, G. W. (1996). Revolutions and counterrevolutions in prevention. *American Psychologist, 51,* 1130–1133.

Albee, G. W., Joffe, J. M., & Dusenbury, L. A. (Eds.). (1988). *Prevention, powerlessness, and politics: Readings on social change.* Beverly Hills, CA: Sage.

Albert, R. (1988). The place of culture in modern psychology. In P. Bronstein, & K. Quina (Eds.), *Teaching a psychology of people: Resources for gender and sociocultural awareness* (pp. 12–18). Washington, DC: American Psychological Association.

Bakeman, R. & Brown, J. V. (1980). Early interaction: Consequences for social and mental development at three years. *Child Development, 51,* 437–447.

Baltes, P. B. (1987). Theoretical propositions of life-span developmental psychology: On the dynamics between growth and decline. *Developmental Psychology, 23,* 611–626.

Baratz, S. & Baratz, J. C. (1970). Early childhood intervention: The social science base of institutional racism. *Harvard Educational Review, 40,* 29–50.

Barnett, D., Kidwell, S. L., & Leung, K. H. (1998). Parenting and preschooler attachment among low-income urban African American families. *Child Development, 69,* 1657–1671.

Barnett, D., Manly, J. T., & Cicchetti, D. (1993). Defining child maltreatment: The interface between policy and research. In D. Cicchetti & S. L. Toth (Eds.), *Child abuse, child development, and social policy* (pp. 7–73). Norwood, NJ: Ablex.

Bell, C. C. & Chance-Hill, G. (1988). Treatment of violent families: Annual meeting of the American family therapy association. *Journal of the National Medical Association, 83,* 203–208.

Benedict, M. I. & White, R. B. (1991). Factors associated with foster care length of stay. *Child Welfare, 70,* 45–57.

Benedict, M. I., Zuravin, S., & Stallings, R. Y. (1996). Adult functioning of children who lived in kin versus nonrelative family foster home. *Child Welfare, 75,* 529–549.

Berrick, J. D. (1997). Assessing quality of care in kinship and foster family care. *Family Relations, 46,* 273–280.

Berrick, J. D., Barth, R. P., & Needell, B. (1994). A comparison of kinship foster homes and family foster homes: Implications for kinship as family preservation. *Children and Youth Services, 16,* 7–13.

Billingsley, A. (1992). *Climbing Jacob's ladder: The enduring legacy of African-American families.* New York: Simon & Schuster.

Black Administrators in Child Welfare, Inc. (1994). *Policy statement on kinship care.* Washington, DC: Child Welfare League of America.

Bowlby, J. (1969). *Attachment and loss: Vol. 1. Attachment.* New York: Basic Books.

Bowlby, J. (1973). *Attachment and loss: Vol. 2. Separation, anxiety and anger.* New York: Basic Books.

Bowlby, J. (1980). *Attachment and loss: Vol. 3. Loss, sadness and depression.* New York: Basic Books.

Bretherton, I. (1985). Attachment theory: Retrospect and prospect. *Monographs of the Society for Research in Child Development, 50*(1–2), 3–35.

Bronfenbrenner, U. (1977). Toward an experimental ecology of human development. *American Psychologist, 32,* 513–531.

Broussard, E. R. (1995). Infant attachment in a sample of adolescent mothers. *Child Psychiatry and Human Development, 25,* 211–219.

Burman, E. (1997). Developmental psychology and its discontents. In D. Fox, & I. Prilleltensky (Eds.), *Critical psychology: An introduction* (pp. 134–149). Thousand Oaks, CA: Sage.

Carlson, V., Cicchetti, D., Barnett, D., & Braunwald, K. (1989). Disorganized/disoriented attachment relationships in maltreated infants. *Developmental Psychology, 25,* 525–531.

Carson, D. K., Dail, P. W., Greely, S., & Kenote, T. (1990). Stresses and strengths of Native American reservation families in poverty. *Family Perspective, 24,* 383–400.

Chatters, L. M., Taylor, R. J., & Jayakody, R. (1994). Fictive kinship relations in Black extended families. *Journal of Comparative Family Studies, 25*, 297–312.

Cicchetti, D. (1984). The emergence of developmental psychopathology. *Child Development, 55*, 1–7.

Cicchetti, D. (1989). Developmental psychopathology: Past, present, and future. In D. Cicchetti (Ed.), *Rochester Symposium on Developmental Psychopathology: Vol. 1. The emergence of a discipline* (pp. 1–12). Hillsdale, NJ: Erlbaum.

Cicchetti, D. (1993). Developmental psychopathology: Reactions, reflections, projections. *Developmental Review, 13*, 471–502.

Cicchetti, D. & Barnett, D. (1991). Toward the development of a scientific nosology of child maltreatment. In W. Grove & D. Cicchetti (Eds.), *Thinking clearly about psychology: Essays in honor of Paul E. Meehl: Vol. 2. Personality and psychopathology* (pp. 346–377). Minneapolis: University of Minnesota Press.

Cicchetti, D. & Garmezy, N. (Eds.). (1993). Milestones in the development of resilience [Special issue]. *Development and Psychopathology, 5*, 497–774.

Cicchetti, D. & Lynch, M. (1993). Toward an ecological/transactional model of community violence and child maltreatment: Consequences for children's development. *Psychiatry, 56*, 96–118.

Cicchetti, D. & Toth, S. L. (1992). The role of developmental theory in prevention and intervention. *Development and Psychopathology, 4*, 489–728.

Cicchetti, D. & Toth, S. L. (1993). Child maltreatment research and social policy: The neglected nexus. In D. Cicchetti & S. L. Toth (Eds.), *Child abuse, child development, and social policy* (pp. 1–6). Norwood, NJ: Ablex.

Cicchetti, D. & Toth, S. L. (1998). Perspectives on research and practice in developmental psychopathology. In W. Damon (Series Ed.) & I. Sigel & K. A. Renninger (Vol. Eds.), *Handbook of child psychology: Vol. 4. Child psychology in practice* (5th ed.) (pp. 479–593). New York: Wiley.

Cornell University Empowerment Group. (1989, October). *Networking Bulletin, 1*(2).

Coster, W. & Cicchetti, D. (1993). Research on the communicative development of maltreated children: Clinical implications. *Topics in Language Disorders, 13*, 25–38.

Courtney, M. E. & Needell, B. (1997). Outcomes of kinship care: Lessons from California. In J. D. Berrick, R. P. Barth, & N. Gilbert (Eds.), *Child welfare research review, Vol. II* (pp. 130–149). New York: Columbia University Press.

Cowen, E. L. (1973). Social and community interventions. In P. Mussen & M. Rosenzweig (Eds.), *Annual Review of Psychology, 24,* 423–472.

Cowen, E. L. (1977). Baby-steps toward primary prevention. *American Journal of Community Psychology, 5,* 1–22.

Cowen, E. L. (1980). The wooing of primary prevention. *American Journal of Community Psychology, 8,* 258–284.

Cowen, E. L. (1982). Research in primary prevention in mental health. [Special Issue]. *American Journal of Community Psychology, 10*(3).

Cowen, E. L. (1985). Person-centered approaches to primary prevention in mental health: Situation-focused and competence-enhancement. *American Journal of Community Psychology, 13,* 31–48.

Cowen, E. L. (1991). In pursuit of wellness. *American Psychologist, 46,* 404–408.

Cowen, E. L. (1994). The enhancement of psychological wellness: Challenges and opportunities. *American Journal of Community Psychology, 22,* 149–179.

Cowen, E. L. (1996). The ontogenesis of primary prevention: Lengthy strides and stubbed toes. *American Journal of Community Psychology, 24,* 235–249.

Cowen, E. L. (2000). Community psychology and routes to psychological wellness. In J. Rappaport & Edward Seidman (Eds.), *Handbook of community psychology* (pp. 79–99). New York: Klewer/Plenum.

Cowen, E. L., Gardner, E. A., & Zax, M. (Eds.). (1967). *Emergent approaches to mental health problems.* New York: Appleton-Century-Crofts.

Cowen, E. L., Hightower, A. D., Pedro-Caroll, J. L., Work, W. C., Wyman, P. A., & Haffey, W. G. (1996). *School-based prevention for children at risk: The primary mental health project.* Washington, DC: American Psychological Association.

Cowen, E. L., Trost, M. A., Lorion, R. P., Dorr, D., Izzo, L. D., & Isaacson, R. V. (1975). *New ways in school mental health: Early detection and prevention of school maladaption.* New York: Human Sciences.

Cowen, E. L., Wyman, P. A., Work, W. C., Kim, J. Y., Fagen, D. B., & Magnus, K. B. (1997). Follow-up study of young stress-affected and stress-resilient urban children. *Development and Psychopathology, 9,* 564–577.

Crawley, B. (1988). Black families in a new-conservative era. *Child Development, 65,* 415–419.

Daley, A., Jennings, J., Beckett, J. O., & Leashore, S. (1995). Shared family care: Child protection and family preservation. *Social Work, 40,* 145–288.

Daniel, J. H., Hampton, R. L., & Newberger, E. H. (1983). Child abuse and accidents in Black families: A controlled comparative study. *American Journal of Orthopsychiatry, 53,* 645–653.

Danzy, J. & Jackson, S. M. (1997). Family preservation and support services: A missed opportunity for kinship care. *Child Welfare, 76,* 31–44.

Davidson, D. (1997, Sept./Oct.). Service needs of relative care givers: A qualitative analysis. *Families in Society,* 502–510.

Delpit, L. (1995). *Other people's children: Cultural conflict in the classroom.* New York: New Press.

Dilworth-Anderson, P. (1992). Extended kin networks in Black families. *Generations, 16,* 29–32.

Dilworth-Anderson, P. & Burton, L. M. (1996). Rethinking family development: Critical conceptual issues in the study of diverse groups. *Journal of Social and Personal Relationships, 13,* 325–334.

Dilsworth-Anderson, P., Burton, L. M., & Turner, W.L. (1993). The importance of values in the study of culturally diverse families. *Family Relations, 42,* 238–242.

Elder, G. H., Modell, J., & Park, R. D. (1993). *Children in time and place: Developmental and historical insights.* New York: Cambridge University Press.

Elicker, J., Egeland, M., & Sroufe, L. A. (1992). Predicting peer competence and peer relationships in childhood from early parent-child relationships. In R. D. Parke & G. W. Ladd (Eds.), *Family-peer relationships: Modes of linkage* (pp. 77–106). Hillsdale, NJ: Erlbaum.

Felner, R. D., Felner, T. J., & Silverman, M. (2000). Conceptual and methodological issues in the evolution of the science and practice of prevention. In J. Rappaport & E. Seidman (Eds.), *Handbook of community psychology,* (pp. 9–42). New York: Plenum.

Fine, M. (1994). Working the hyphens: Reinventing self and others in qualitative research. In D. K. Denzin & L. S. Guba (Eds.), *Handbook of qualitative research* (pp. 70–82). Thousand Oaks, CA: Sage.

Fisher, C. B. & Brennan, M. (1992). Applications and ethics in developmental psychology. In R. M. Lerner & M. Perlmutter (Eds.), *Life span development and behavior* (Vol. 11) (pp. 189–219). Hillsdale, NJ: Erlbaum.

Fisher, C. B., Jackson, J. F., & Villarruel, F. A. (1998). The study of African American and Latin American children and youth. In W. Damon, I. E. Sigel, & K. A. Renninger (Eds.), *Handbook of child psychology: Vol. 4. Child psychology in practice* (5th ed.) (pp. 1145–1207). New York: Wiley.

Fisher, C. B. & Murray, J. P. (1996). Applied developmental science comes of age. In C. B. Fisher, J. P. Murray, & I. E. Sigel (Eds.), *Applied developmental science: Graduate training for diverse disciplines and educational settings* (pp. 1–22). Norwood, NJ: Ablex.

Fisher, C. B. & Tryon, W.W. (1988). Ethical issues in the research and practice of applied developmental psychology. *Journal of Applied Developmental Psychology, 9*, 27–39.

Fowers, B. J. & Richardson, F.C. (1996). Why is multiculturalism good? *American Psychologist, 51*, 609–621.

Fox, D. & Prilleltensky, I. (Eds.). (1997). *Critical psychology: An introductory handbook*. Thousand Oaks, CA: Sage.

Fracasso, M. P., Busch-Rossnagel, N. A., & Fisher, C. (1994). The relationship of maternal behavior and acculturation to the quality of attachment in Hispanic infants living in New York City. *Hispanic Journal of Behavioral Sciences, 16*, 143–154.

Gaines, S., Jr. & Reed, E. (1995). Prejudice from Allport to DuBois. *American Psychologist, 50*, 96–103.

Garbarino, J. (1976). A preliminary study of some ecological correlates of child abuse: The impact of socioeconomic stress on mothers. *Child Development, 47*, 178–185.

Garmezy, N. (1990). A closing note: Reflections on the future. In J. Rolf, A. Masten, D. Cicchetti, K. Nuechterlein, & S. Weintraub (Eds.), *Risk and protective factors in the development of psychopathology* (pp. 527–534). New York: Cambridge University Press.

Gates, H. L. (1992). *Loose canons: Notes on the culture wars*. New York: Oxford University Press.

Gebel, T. J. (1996). Kinship care and non-relative family foster care: A comparison of caregiver attributes and attitudes. *Child Welfare, 75*, 5–18.

Gelles, R. J. (1975). The social construction of child abuse. *American Journal of Orthopsychiatry, 43*, 363–371.

Gill, D. (1970). *Violence against children: Physical abuse against children in the United States*. Cambridge, MA: Harvard University Press.

Ginsburg, H. (1972). *The myth of the deprived child: Poor children's intellect and education.* Englewood Cliffs, NJ: Prentice Hall.

Giovannoni, J. M. & Becerra, R. M. (1979). *Defining child abuse.* New York: The Free Press.

Giovannoni, J. M. & Billingsley, A. (1970). Child neglect among the poor: A study of parental adequacy in families of three ethnic groups. *Child Welfare, 49,* 196–204.

Good, T., Wiley, A., Thomas, R. E., Stewart, E., McCoy, J., Kloos, B., Hunt, G., Moore, T., & Rappaport, J. (1997). Bridging the gap between schools and community: Organizing for family involvement in a low-income neighborhood. *Journal of Educational and Psychological Consultation, 8,* 277–296.

Graham, S. (1992). "Most of the subjects were white middle class": Trends in published research on African Americans in selected APA journals, 1970–1989. *American Psychologist, 47,* 629–639.

Greenfield, P. M. (1994). Independence and interdependence as developmental scripts: Implications for theory, research, and practice. In P. M. Greenfield & R. R. Cocking (Eds.), *Cross-cultural roots of minority child development.* Hillsdale, NJ: Lawrence Erlbaum Associates.

Hagen, J. W., Paul, B., Gibb, S., & Wolters, C. (1990, March). *Trends in research as reflected by publications in Child Development: 1930–1989.* Paper presented at the biennial meeting of the Society for Research on Adolescence, Atlanta, GA.

Hampton, R. L. (1986). Race, ethnicity, and child maltreatment: An analysis of cases recognized and reported by hospitals. In R. Staples (Ed.), *The Black family: Essays and studies* (3rd ed.) (pp. 172–185). Belmont, CA: Wadsworth.

Hampton, R. L. (1991). Child abuse in the African American community. In J. E. Everett, S. S. Chipungu, & B. R. Leashore (Eds.), *Child welfare: An Africentric perspective* (pp. 220–246). New Brunswick, NJ: Rutgers University Press.

Handler, J. F. (1990). *Law and search for community.* Philadelphia: University of Pennsylvania Press.

Harding, S. (1986). *The science question in feminism.* Ithaca, NY: Cornell University Press.

Heller, K., Price, R. H., Reinharz, S., Riger, S., & Wandersman, A. (1984). *Psychology and community change.* Pacific Grove, CA: Brooks/Cole.

Hill, R. (1971). *The strengths of Black families.* New York: Emerson Hall.

Hoagwood, K. & Jensen, P.S. (1997). Developmental psychopathology and the notion of culture: Introduction to the special section on "The fusion of cultural horizons: Cultural influences on the assessment of psychopathology in children and adolescents." *Applied Developmental Science, 1,* 108–112.

Iglehart, A. P. (1994). Kinship foster care: Placement service, and outcome issues. *Children and Youth Services Review, 16,* 107–122.

Jackson, J. F. (1986). Characteristics of Black infant attachment. *American Journal of Social Psychiatry, 6,* 32–35.

Jackson, J. F. (1993). Human behavioral genetics, Scarr's theory, and her view on interventions: A critical review and commentary on their implications. *Child Development, 64,* 1318–1332.

Joffe, J. M. & Albee, G. W. (Eds.). (1981). *Prevention through political action and social change.* Hanover, NH: University Press of New England, Vermont Conference on the Primary Prevention of Psychopathology.

Kelley, M. L., Power, T. G., & Wimbush, D. D. (1992). Determinants of disciplinary practices in low-income black mothers. *Child Development, 63,* 573–582.

Kelly, J. G. (1990). Changing contexts in the field of community psychology. *American Journal of Community Psychology, 18,* 769–792.

Kempe, C. H., Silverman, F. M., Steele, B. B., Drogemueller, W., & Silver, H. C. (1962). The battered child syndrome. *Journal of American Medical Association, 181,* 17–24.

Kennedy, J. H. & Bakeman, R. (1984). Real and ideal extended familism among Mexican Americans and Anglo Americans: On the meaning of "close family ties." *Human Organization, 43,* 65–70.

Kim, U. & Choi, S. (1994). Individualism, collectivism, and child development: A Korean perspective. In P. M. Greenfield & R. R. Cocking (Eds.), *Cross-cultural roots of minority child development.* Hillsdale, NJ: Lawrence Erlbaum Associates.

Kloos, B., McCoy, J., Stewart, E., Thomas, E., Wiley, A., Good, T., Hunt, G., Moore, T., & Rappaport, J. (1997). Bridging the gap: A community-based, open-systems approach to neighborhood and school consultation. *Journal of Educational and Psychological Consultation, 8,* 175–196.

Kusserow, R. P. (Inspector General). (1992). *State practices in using relatives for foster care.* Dallas, TX: Office of the Inspector General, Dallas Regional Office.

LaFrombroise, T., Hardin, L., Coleman, K., & Gerton, J. (1993). Psychological impact of biculturalism: Evidence and theory. *Psychological Bulletin, 114,* 395–412.

Leashore, B. R., McMurray, H. L., & Bailey, B. C. (1991). Reuniting and preserving African American families. In J. E. Everett, S. S. Chipungu, & B. R. Leashore (Eds.), *Child welfare: An Africentric perspective* (pp. 247–265). New Brunswick, NJ: Rutgers University Press.

Lerner, R. M. (1991). Changing organism-context relations as the basic process of development: A developmental-contextual perspective. *Developmental Psychology, 27,* 27–32.

Lerner, R. M. (1993). Early adolescence: Towards an agenda for the integration of research, policy, and intervention. In R. M. Lerner (Ed.), *Early adolescence: Perspectives on research, policy, and intervention* (pp. 1–13). Hillsdale, NJ: Erlbaum.

Levine, M. & Perkins, D. V. (1997). *Principles of community psychology* (2nd ed.). New York: Oxford University Press.

London, H. & Devore, W. (1988). Layers of understanding: Counseling ethnic minority families. *Family Relations, 37,* 310–314.

Loo, C., Fong, K. T., & Iwamasa, G. (1988). Ethnicity and cultural diversity: An analysis of work published in community psychology journals, 1965–1985. *Journal of Community Psychology, 16,* 332–349.

Luthar, S. S. (1999). *Poverty and children's adjustment.* Newbury Park, CA: Sage.

Luthar, S. S., Cicchetti, D., & Becker, B. (in press). The construct of resilience: A critical evaluation and guidelines for future work. *Child Development.*

Luthar, S. S. & Zigler, E. (1991). Vulnerability and competence: A review of research on resilience in childhood. *American Journal of Orthopsychiatry, 61,* 6–22.

Lykken, D. T. (1994). Predicting violence in the violent society. *Applied and Preventive Psychology, 2,* 13–20.

Main, M. & Hesse, E. (1990). Parents' unresolved traumatic experiences are related to infant disorganized attachment status: Is frightened and/or frightening parental behavior the linking mechanism? In M. T. Greenberg & D. Cicchetti (Eds.), *Attachment in the preschool years: Theory, research, and intervention. The John D. And Catherine T. MacArthur Foundation series on mental health and development* (pp. 161–182). Chicago: University of Chicago Press.

Main, M. & Solomon, J. (1990). Procedures for identifying infants as disorganized/disoriented during the Ainsworth Strange Situation. In M.T.

Greenberg, D. Cicchetti, & E.M. Cummings (Eds.), *Attachment in the preschool years: Theory, research and intervention* (pp. 121–160). Chicago: University of Chicago Press.

Markus, H. R. & Kitayama, S. (1991). Culture and the self: Implications for cognition, emotion, and motivation. *Psychological Review, 98,* 224–253.

Martinez, C., Jr. (1988). Clinical guidelines in cross-cultural mental health. In L. Comas-Diaz & E. E. Griffith (Eds.), *Wiley series in general and clinical psychiatry* (pp. 182–203). New York: Wiley.

Martinez, E. A. (1988). Child behavior in Mexican-American/Chicano families: Maternal teaching and childrearing practices. *Family Relations, 37,* 275–280.

Martinez, E. A. (1993). Parenting young children in Mexican American/Chicano families. In H. P. McAdoo (Ed.), *Family ethnicity: Strength in diversity* (pp. 184–192). Newbury Park, CA: Sage.

Masten, A., Best, K., & Garmezy, N. (1990). Resilience and development: Contribution from the study of children who overcome adversity. *Development and Psychopathology, 2,* 425–444.

Maton, K. I. & Salem, D. A. (1995). Organizational characteristics of empowering community settings: A multiple case study approach. *American Journal of Community Psychology, 23,* 631–656.

McAdoo, H. P. (1980). Black mothers and the extended family support network. In L. F. Rodgers-Rose (Ed.), *The Black woman* (pp. 125–144). Beverly Hills, CA: Sage.

McAdoo, H. P. (1993). *Family ethnicity: Strength in diversity.* Newbury Park, CA: Sage.

McAdoo, J. L. (1993). The roles of African American fathers: An ecological perspective. *Families in Society, 74,* 28–35.

McLoyd, V. C. (1990). Minority children: Introduction to the special issue. *Child Development, 61,* 263–266.

McLoyd, V. C. (1994). Research in the service of poor and ethnic/racial minority children: Fomenting change in models of scholarship. *Family and Consumer Sciences Research Journal, 23,* 56–66.

Melton, G. B. (1984). Development psychology and the law: The state of the art. *Journal of Family Law, 22,* 445–482.

Miller, P., Wiley, A., Fung, H., & Liang, C. (1997). Personal storytelling as a medium of socialization in Chinese and American families. *Child Development, 68,* 557–568.

Morrison, F. J., Lord, C., & Keating, D. P. (1984). Applied developmental psychology. In F. J. Morrison, C. Lord, & D. P. Keating (Eds.), *Applied developmental psychology* (Vol. 1) (pp. 4–20). New York: Academic Press.

National Center on Child Abuse and Neglect. (1988). *Study findings. Study of national incidence and prevalence of child abuse and neglect: 1988.* Washington, DC: Author.

National Clearinghouse on Child Abuse & Neglect. (1995). *What is child maltreatment? Publications: Fact Sheets.* [On-line]. Available: http// www.calib.com/nccanch/index.htm.

National Research Council. (1993). *Understanding child abuse and neglect.* Washington, DC: National Academy Press.

Padilla, A. M. (1995). *Hispanic psychology: Critical issues in theory and research.* Thousand Oaks, CA: Sage.

Panaccione, V. F. & Wahler, R. G. (1986). Child behavior, maternal depression, and social coercion as factors in the quality of child care. *Journal of Abnormal Child Psychology, 14,* 263 278.

Parke, R. D. & Collmer, C. W. (1975). Child abuse: An interdisciplinary analysis. In E. M. Hetherington (Ed.), *Review of child development research* (Vol. 5, pp. 509–590). Chicago: Chicago University Press.

Patterson, G. (1982). *Coercive family process.* Eugene, OR: Castalia.

Perkins, D. D. & Zimmerman, M. (1995). Empowerment theory, research and application. *American Journal of Community Psychology, 23,* 569–579.

Petit, M. R. & Curtis, P. A. (1997). *Child abuse and neglect: A look at the states.* Washington, DC: CWLA Press.

Phinney, J. S. (1990). Ethnic identity in adolescents and adults: Review of research. *Psychological Bulletin, 108,* 499–514.

Pianta, R. C., Egeland, B., & Erickson, M. F. (1989). The antecedents of maltreatment: Results of the Mother-Child Interaction Research Project. In D. Cicchette & V. Carlson (Eds.), *Child maltreatment* (pp. 203–253). New York: Cambridge University Press.

Rappaport, J. (1977). *Community psychology: Values, research and action.* New York: Holt, Rinehart & Winston.

Rappaport, J. (1981). In praise of paradox: A social policy of empowerment over prevention. *American Journal of Community Psychology, 9,* 1–25.

Rappaport, J. (1990). Research methods and the empowerment social agenda. In P. Tolan, C. Keys, F. Chertok, & L. Jason (Eds.), *Researching community psychology: Integrating theories and methodologies.* Washington, DC: American Psychological Association.

Rappaport, J. (1992). The death and resurrection of a community mental health movement. In M. Kessler, S. Goldston, & J. Joffe (Eds.), *The present and future of prevention: In Honor of George W. Albee* (pp. 78–98). Beverly Hills, CA: Sage.

Rappaport, J. (1994). Empowerment as a guide to doing research: Diversity as a positive value. In E. J. Trickett, R. Watts, & D. Birman (Eds.), *Human diversity: Perspectives on people in context* (pp. 359–382). San Francisco: Jossey-Bass.

Rappaport, J. (1995). Empowerment meets narrative: Listening to stories and creating settings. *American Journal of Community Psychology, 23,* 795–807.

Rappaport, J. (1998). The art of social change: Community narratives as resources for individual and collective identity. In X.B. Arriaga & S. Oskamp (Eds.), *Addressing community problems: Psychosocial research and intervention* (pp. 225–246). Thousand Oaks, CA: Sage.

Rappaport, J. & Seidman, E. (2000). *Handbook of community psychology.* New York: Klewer/Plenum.

Rappaport, J. & Stewart, E. (1997). A critical look at critical psychology: Elaborating the questions. In D. Fox & I. Prilleltensky (Eds.), *Critical psychology: An introductory handbook* (pp. 301–317). Thousand Oaks, CA: Sage.

Redhorse, J. G. (1980). Family structure and value orientation in American Indians. *Social Casework, 61,* 462–467.

Riger, S. (1993). What's wrong with empowerment. *American Journal of Community Psychology, 21,* 279–292.

Ringwalt, C. & Caye, J. (1989). The effect of demographic factors on perceptions of child neglect. *Children and Youth Services Review, 11,* 133–144.

Rogler, L. (1989). The meaning of culturally sensitive research in mental health. *American Journal of Psychiatry, 146,* 296–303.

Rutter, M. (1990). Psychosocial resilience and protective mechanisms. In J. Rolf, A. S. Masten, D. Cicchetti, K. H. Nuechterlein, & S. Weintraub (Eds.), *Risk and protective factors in the development of psychopathology* (pp. 181–214). New York: Cambridge University Press.

Rutter, M. & Garmezy, N. (1983). Developmental psychopathology. In E. M. Hetherington (Ed.), *Socialization, personality and social development* (pp. 775–911). New York: Wiley.

Saegert, S. & Winkel, G. (1996). Paths to community empowerment: Organizing at home. *American Journal of Community Psychology, 24,* 517–550.

Salzinger, S., Feldman, R. S., Hammer, M., & Rosario, M. (1993). The effects of physical abuse on children's social relationships. *Child Development, 64,* 169–187.

Sampson, E. E. (1993). Identity politics: Challenges to psychology's understanding. *American Psychologist, 48,* 1219–1230.

Sarason, S. B. (1986). The nature of social problem solving in social action. In E. Seidman, & J. Rappaport (Eds.), *Redefining social problems* (pp. 11–28). New York: Plenum.

Scarr, S. (1985). Constructing psychology: Making facts and fables for our times. *American Psychologist, 40,* 499–512.

Scholnick, E. K., Fisher, C. B., Brown, A., & Sigel, I. (1988, Spring). Report on applied developmental psychology. *APA Division 7 Newsletter,* 6–10.

Seidman, E. (1987). Toward a framework for primary prevention research. In J. Steinberg & M. Silverman (Eds.), *Preventing mental disorders: A research perspective.*

Seidman, E., Hughes, D., & Williams, N. (Eds.). (1993). Culturally anchored methodology [Special Issue]. *American Journal of Community Psychology, 21*(6).

Seidman, E. & Rappaport, J. (Eds.). (1986). *Redefining social problems.* New York: Plenum.

Shimkin, D. B., Louie, G. J., & Frate, D. A. (1978). The Black extended family: A basic rural institution and a mechanism of urban adaptation. In D. B. Shimkin, E. M. Shimkin, & D. A. Frate (Eds.), *The extended family in Black societies* (pp. 25–149). The Hague, Netherlands: Mouton.

Shore, M. F. (1998). Beyond self interest: Professional advocacy and the integration of theory, research, and practice. *American Psychologist, 53,* 474–479.

Sigel, I. & Cocking, R. R. (1980). Editors' message. *Journal of Applied Developmental Psychology, 1,* i–iii.

Sklar, H. (1995). *Chaos or community: Seeking solutions, not scapegoats for bad economics.* Boston: South End Press.

Spinetta, J. & Rigler, D. (1972). The child-abusing parent: A psychological review. *Psychological Bulletin, 77,* 296–304.

Sroufe, L. A. & Rutter, M. (1984). The domain of developmental psychopathology. *Child Development, 55,* 17–29.

Stack, C. B. (1974). *All our kin: Strategies for survival in a Black community.* New York: Harper and Row.

Stehno, S. M. (1982). Differential treatment of minority children in service systems. *Social Work, 27,* 39–45.

Stevenson, H. C. (1993). Validation of the scale of racial socialization for African American adolescents: A preliminary analysis. *Psychological Discourse, 24,* 12.

Stevenson, H. C. (1994). Validation of the scale of racial socialization for African American adolescents: Steps toward multidimensionality. *Journal of Black Psychology, 20,* 445–468.

Stevenson, H. C. (1995). Relationship of adolescent perceptions of racial socialization to racial identity. *Journal of Black Psychology, 21,* 49–70.

Sudarkrasa, N. (1988). Interpreting the African heritage in Afro-American family organization. In H. P. McAdoo (Ed.), *Black families* (2nd. ed.) (pp. 27–43). Newbury Park, CA: Sage.

Thomas, R. E. & Rappaport, J. (1996). Art as community narrative: A resource for social change. In M. B. Lykes, R. Liem, A. Banuazizi, & M. Morris (Eds.), *Myths about the powerless: Contesting social inequalities* (pp. 317–336). Philadelphia: Temple University Press.

Thompson, R. (1995). *Preventing child maltreatment through social support: A critical analysis.* Thousand Oaks, CA: Sage.

Tolan, P., Keys, C., Chertok, F., & Jason, L. (Eds.). (1990). *Researching community psychology: Integrating theories and methodologies.* Washington, DC: American Psychological Association.

Toth, S. L. & Cicchetti, D. (1999). Developmental psychopathology and child psychotherapy. In S. Russ & T. Ollendick (Eds.), *Handbook of psychotherapies with children and families* (pp. 15–44). New York: Plenum Press.

Triandis, H. C. (1989). Cross-cultural studies of individualism and collectivism. *Nebraska Symposium on Motivation, 37,* 41–133.

Trickett, E. J. (1996). A future for community psychology: The contexts of diversity and the diversity of contexts. *American Journal of Community Psychology, 24,* 209–229.

Trickett, E. J., Watts, R., & Birman, D. (Eds.). (1994). *Human diversity: Perspectives on people in context.* San Francisco: Jossey-Bass.

Turbett, P. & O'Toole, R. (1980). *Physicians' recognition of child abuse.* Presented to the American Sociological Association, New York.

Trickett, P. K., Aber, J. L., Carlson, V., & Cicchetti, D. (1991). Relationship of socioeconomic status to the etiology and developmental sequelae of physical child abuse. *Developmental Psychology, 27,* 148–158.

Turiel, E. (1994). Morality, authoritarianism, and personal agency in cultural contexts. In R. J. Sternberg & P. Ruzgis (Eds.), *Intelligence and personality* (pp. 271–299). Cambridge, UK: Cambridge University Press.

Van Ijzendoorn, M. H. & Kroonenberg, P. M. (1988). Cross cultural patterns of attachment: A meta analysis of the strange situation. *Child Development, 59,* 147–156.

Vega, W. A. (1990). Hispanic families in the 1980s: A decade of research. *Journal of Marriage and the Family, 52,* 1015–1024.

Waters, E., Vaughn, B. E., Posada, G., & Kondo-Ikemura, K. (1995). Caregiving, cultural, and cognitive perspectives on secure-base behavior and working models: New growing points of attachment theory and research. *Monographs of the Society for Research in Child Development, 60* (144, Nos. 2-3).

Werner, E. E. & Smith, R. (1982). *Vulnerable but invincible: A study of resilient children.* New York: McGraw-Hill.

Werner, E. E. & Smith, R. S. (Eds.). (1992). *Overcoming the odds: High risk children from birth to adulthood.* Ithaca, NY: Cornell University Press.

Wiley, A. R., Rose, A. J., Burger, L. K., & Miller, P. J. (1998). Constructing autonomous selves through narrative practices: A comparative study of working-class and middle-class families. *Child Development, 69,* 833–847.

Wulczyn, F. H. & Goerge, R. M. (1992). Foster care in New York and Illinois: The challenge of rapid change. *Social Service Review, 66,* 278–294.

Youniss, J. (1990). Cultural forces leading to scientific developmental psychology. In C. B. Fisher & W. W. Tryon (Eds.), *Ethics in applied developmental psychology: Emerging issues in an emerging field* (pp. 285–300). Norwood, NJ: Ablex.

Zeanah, C. H. Jr., Mammen, O. K., & Lieberman, A. F. (1993). Disorders of attachment. In C. H. Zeanah Jr. (Ed.), *Handbook of infant mental health* (pp. 332–349). New York, NY: Guilford.

Zigler, E. & Finn, M. (1984). Applied developmental psychology. In M. H. Bornstein & M. E. Lamb (Eds.), *Developmental psychology: An advanced textbook* (pp. 451–492). Hillsdale, NJ: Erlbaum.

Zuravin, S. & Greif, J. L. (1989). Normative and child-maltreating AFDC mothers. *Social Casework, 70,* 76–84.

# 4

# Wellness as an Ecological Enterprise

*James G. Kelly*

Emory Cowen has persistently and persuasively refocused prevention efforts away from illness, away from disorders, and beyond deficits. He has advocated for an understanding of the social conditions and personal qualities of health, of positive well-being, and of resilient coping. He has invited us to shift our ways of thinking and our ways of doing research. Martin Seligman's reference to psychology as a positive social science gives the Cowen treatise more visibility and more sanction [Seligman 1998].

The Wellness topic has significance for the analysis of risk and protective factors—currently of interest to prevention research investigators. The long-standing tradition of emphasizing epidemiological research for risk factors, such as abuses of substances, limited educational achievement, and the pernicious influences of various forms of social and racial discrimination, has established connections between the above factors and the expression of psychological maladies. However, this research tradition may not be as appropriate to examine protective factors. Devoting time and energy to the study of wellness is not simply a scrutiny of the absence of illness. Since the study of illness has been such a priority and so commanding of our attention for so long, it will take some doing to begin anew.

The following five ideas are presented to assist this shift in point of view. These five ideas reconceptualize how inquiries can be conceived and carried out. New criteria and new premises are employed; a different epistemology is invoked. This new enterprise could be referred to as the province of the Wellness scholar, a contextual scholar who focuses on situations and their impact on individuals. The Wellness scholar creates a pluralistic set of methods to examine the diversity of persons acting in a variety of situations.

These five ideas are:

1. Contextual thinking: an agenda for situated inquiry;

2. New disciplinary connections and pluralistic methods;

3. Learning with others rather than assessing others;

4. Learning about resilient and competent communities;

5. The analysis of variety and quality.

With these topics, the Wellness scholar embarks on an expedition to enlarge our understanding of the sources of healthy behavior. The five ideas underlying the paradigm of the Wellness scholar assert a different definition of what is "good" science.

## The First Idea: Contextual Thinking—An Agenda for Situated Inquiry

One resource in the search for knowledge is the increasing need to attend not only to the states or traits of individuals, but to the various extra influences that impact, impinge, and affect the expression of individual behavior. Some extra individual influences are: the local economy and the impact on the wage earner, particularly for child care; the presence of supportive employers who can work out staggered work schedules; the presence of friends, neighbors, and kin who can both contribute tangible aid and share rituals and ceremonies and traditions; the sense of public safety that enables the person to travel alone and at night; "user friendly" community service organizations that are accessible and responsive; the availability of mentors and/or more experienced persons who can provide help on coping with personal and organizational issues. Each of these topics represents constraints and/or resources that, when present, can aggravate or ease plights and close down or open up new opportunities. But these types of factors and forces are not usually within the purview of data collection. The range of topics for psychological investigation is often limited to just those factors that bear directly on the individual without considering that the individual is nested and situated in a milieu. These milieus are the sources of effects and influences that bear directly on the individual.

To shift paradigms is a challenge, for it requires the investigator to be involved with the individual informants long enough and deeply enough to become familiar with the less frequently examined ways in which local cultures define, limit, and/or promote the well-being of individuals. It is possible that new questions can be addressed: How do persons know when they are appreciated? How are persons in authority addressed without feeling the risk of recrimination? How do persons in a particular community express regard for others? How are differences of opinion addressed without anyone being stigmatized? How does a social setting foster creativity? How do groups become resources for their members? The answers to these questions not only arise from studying the qualities of individuals. The answers also derive from an analysis of the traditions, social norms, and expectations for behavior established within and across specific social settings. This is what is meant by the ecological enterprise: inquiry focuses on the person-environment fit of different individuals and varied settings [Kingry-Westergaard & Kelly 1990]. Understanding wellness is as much a topic of our contexts, our surroundings, as it is our personal qualities; an ecological enterprise is salient.

McLoyd, in an elegant review, focuses on the impact of poverty. "The link between socioeconomic disadvantage and children's socioemotional functioning appears to be mediated partly by harsh, inconsistent parenting and elevated exposure to acute and chronic stressors" [McLoyd 1998, 1985]. Most often, social scientists do not get close enough or listen attentively or seek out those who could inform us of the details of those circumstances and surroundings that limit skillful parenting or reduce various stressors in different communities. Contextual premises and thinking can point to the concrete and specific array of variables that may come into play. Most importantly, the ecological mission clarifies how different systemic factors come into play in different communities. To understand how "good parenting" may vary from community to community means acknowledging and defining how local customs and social norms contribute to the expression of behavior and the definitions of what behaviors are desirable. This realization of differences between people living in two different communities suggests that any reported differences may reflect variations in the very nature of the social structure of communities, so that what is being assessed is the lack of salience of any specific measure of good parenting. An ecological premise suggests that as communities differ, different conceptions of community are also salient for each of the different communities.

A challenge is to review our causal premises. To understand the expression of "good parenting" in a particular community means that the causal premises of the investigator as well as the informant must be considered. Some investigators may have as their causal premise "inconsistent parenting." Another investigator may focus on the "chronic stressors." McLoyd's point is that it is the combination of *both* factors that is essential, not simply one or the other.

Middle-class white investigators may operate on the belief that agency, efficacy, and the ability of the individual to rearrange environmental conditions is salient and feasible; their previous life experiences have validated their causal systems. Some other investigators may be more fatalistic, while still others may believe that a higher authority is a major causal force in their lives. Situated inquiry requires analyses of linguistic and cognitive styles and how these premises affect everyday constructions of topics that in turn affect the relationship of informant and investigator.

Situated inquiry gets at the linguistic and cognitive constructions that persons use in everyday acts. Such an inquiry can illuminate both the social constraints and the social resources within various milieus. How people define being "well" and being "sick," and how their immediate kin and confidants support or do not support these beliefs, can make the difference in whether prevention efforts are useful or fail. Situated inquiry focuses in on these micro-social processes [Seaburn et al. 1996].

Another defining feature of situated inquiry is the research relationship between the person inquiring and the person providing information. Situated research that is contextually based requires attending to the expression of trust in the research relationship.

Can people of a different social class trust a researcher who is different than they are? One community informant suggests that

African American citizens may respond to white investigators by saying what they think the investigator wants to know [Bagby 1996]. Dave Todd once described the research process as peeling an onion [Todd, personal communication, 1968]. It is a process of building levels of trust so that the informant is willing to not just fill out a questionnaire or even consent to an interview, but perhaps to disclose in that interview deeper reflections about themselves.

A recent report of persons responding to audio computer-assisted self-interviewing (audio-CASI) technology for measuring sensitive behaviors, such as male-male sex, injection drug use, and sexual contact with intravenous drug users reported these behaviors to be higher by factors of three or more. It is laudable and a significant methodological contribution that a more anonymous computer-assisted method can facilitate persons disclosing behavior that otherwise could be perceived as unacceptable. Yet, the availability of such technology may further erode researchers getting more closely and more personally in touch directly, without a computer interface, with the people and topics of interest. More effort is needed to assess the impact of persons participating in audio-CASI research, particularly on the informant's level of trust in the research process. [Bloom 1998; Turner et al. 1998]. Understanding concepts of informants' causal systems can also point to what is important to the participants in their social environments and whether responding to audio-CASI methods enhances or diminishes their level of trust.

One of the potential contributions of an ecological endeavor is that such inquiries may illuminate the factors that come into play for some individuals and not others, as pointed out in the implications of McLoyd's discussion of parenting. Maton and colleagues [1998], for example, have commented on understanding the variables contributing to the high educational achievement of African American males. They state: "Rearing academically successful African American sons requires the simultaneous presence of a constellation of promotive factors, encompassing socialization goals, parenting practices, parenting style, and community connectedness." If a study assesses one or two of these factors only, the lack of inclusion of the other critical factors may preclude strong findings from emerging. For instance, strict discipline and community connectedness without determined parental academic engagement, *or* educational engagement and community connectedness *without* nurturance and strict discipline, may not be sufficient in many cases to counteract the negative contextual factors facing black youth" [Maton 1993; Maton et al. 1998].

Persons who express a religious orientation may make the church and related church activities a source of inspiration and solace. Persons who are seeking social contact and are not churchgoers may turn to bookstores, bars, beauty parlors, exercise clubs, or a variety of other settings and activities as significant sources of stimulation and connection. It may be that in their preferred settings persons' causal beliefs become more ingrained through their social contacts and their personal relationships in these settings.

One of the features of social milieus is to solidify the meaning persons subscribe to everyday events. Understanding these personal and social meanings about life, and the views and beliefs about one's personal power to change negative factors, enhances or limits the desired effects of an imported prevention program.

Some of the connections between social context and the behavior of individuals have been established. For example, there is available information about how social environments impact our mood. George and Brief [1992] present a thesis for how organizational variables, for example, may influence behaviors like spontaneity. Spontaneity is defined as making constructive suggestions and spreading good will. Several decades of research in organizational psychology affirms that social environments *do* impact our behavior both within and outside of the work environment. The qualities of our everyday work environments impact our sense of optimism, our humanitarian acts, our civility, and our generative thinking in addition to our mood [Katz & Kahn 1978; Taylor et al. 1997].

Living in a community where there is dilapidated or boarded-up housing, poor illumination, or infrequent police visibility makes residents vigilant and fearful [Glidewell et al. 1998; Tandon et al. 1998]. The tradition of community organizing aims to affect a change in mood by making it possible for citizens who live in less attractive and decaying communities to address the systemic factors that are limiting the quality of life in the local community [Kahn 1982]. By direct action, they then can create the possibility that, through their actions, the members of the community will improve the conditions that are limiting their mood and the quality of their life. This is an essential point about an ecological thesis: people can influence the social conditions that are limiting their freedom, their dignity, and their opportunities for growth. They can also preserve the traditions and rituals that are health engendering. The Wellness scholar can play a potential role in being a resource for enhancing and preserving social systems.

Understanding the varieties of ways in which persons cope to change noxious physical or psychological environments is a salient topic. Knowledge from organizational and environmental psychology of how social environmental factors contribute to the expressions of health engendering behavior is beneficial intellectual resources [Katz & Kahn 1978; Stokols & Altman 1987; Stokols 1992]. Contextual thinking is clearly interdependent with intradisciplinary and interdisciplinary thinking. The validity of the Wellness scholar is dependent upon contextual understandings of people and their ties and relationships to their social settings.

## The Second Idea: New Disciplinary Connections and Pluralistic Methods

Situated knowledge is knowledge derived from appraisals of persons in terms of the specific locales, settings, and situations in which they are participants; the emphasis is on understanding the social dynamics of specific times and places and the impact of these temporal and community contexts on the individual.

*New* ways in which universities are organized, *new* ways in which doctoral students are educated, and *new* criteria for how research funds are allocated can ease the mission of the Wellness scholar. Wellness research, as situated research, depends upon thriving interconnections across disciplines.

For the past four years I have taught a doctoral level course on the history of community psychology [Kelly 1996]. The course reviews social science research, social movements, and policies that helped to create the field of community psychology.

The most stimulating and rewarding reading, as reported by students, is work conducted in a small village in Peru in the early 1950s by the anthropologist, Ed Wellin [Wellin 1955; Wellin 1998]. This work examined the micro-social structures of this community and pointed out the personal, small group and community factors that contributed to some persons boiling their water and others not doing so. Reasons *for* boiling and reasons for *not* boiling water were often the same. The power of this work attests to not only the subtlety of community structures, but also the complete insensitivity to these factors by the government physicians who were advocates for better health status for the residents. Wellin's work is a compelling example of the value of depth analyses of the communities in which preventive interventions are to be implanted. Wellin's work also attests to the value of psychologists working with persons in other disciplines.

Sources of health are expected to be learned and nourished and maintained in natural groupings of people as Wellin's work so graphically illustrates. Out of family traditions, ceremonies, and ritual occasions derive the opportunities for social bonds that give us our identities, sense of community, and our construction of our place in time and our history [Bell 1997]. These issues are also the province of other social scientists [Ochs & Capps 1996; Payne 1995]. While sociologists of science have affirmed that knowledge is situated, the commitment to carry out explicitly situated inquiry is still undeveloped [Geertz 1995; Lave & Wenger 1991; Neisser & Jopling 1997; Pollio et al. 1997; Shapin 1994]. This is even after the research and thinking of investigators such as Barker, Bronfenbrenner, Kelly, Maton, Moos, Trickett, and Raush [Barker 1965; Barker 1968; Bechtel 1990; Bronfenbrenner 1979; Kelly 1979; Moos 1973, 1976, 1979; Moos & Insel 1974; Raush et al. 1959; Raush et al. 1960; Schoggen & Fox 1989; Trickett 1984, 1989; Trickett et al. 1985].

Many scholars have advocated for some time the utility of pluralistic methods to address the issues of situational effects [Cronbach 1986]. Cronbach quoted Mary Hesse's challenge as she expressed it 20 years ago: "What progresses is the ability to use science to learn the environment" [Hesse 1978; Cronbach 1986, p. 4]. Cronbach has been a consistent voice in suggesting that inquiry is open-ended, and that the validity of measures is enhanced when there are multiple methods employed, and the research enterprise is conceived as a pluralistic process where a range of methods and data sources are invoked to enhance the understanding of phenomena [Cronbach 1986]. The topic of external validity is recast. To the extent that psychologists' theory of mind is embedded in a white culture, the psychologist getting ready to adopt ecological thinking examines the cultural premises under which he or she is working and then considers how these premises may be resources or constraints. Lillard describes these issues in detail [Lillard 1998].

The Wellness scholar is prepared to develop a working thesis to consider multiple causal systems when appraising behaviors such as socioemotional functioning. Ecological thinking focuses on the array of personal-social-historical factors that may impact on behavior in contrast to the direct nonreciprocal causal connections implied in some forms of psychological research. White presents a helpful treatise advocating for an analysis of the causal inferences put in use by the lay person [White 1990]. This is a potentially useful effort when the informants vary in race, ethnicity, gender, life style, sexual orientation, and social class.

Koch expressed alarm about the vitality of the dominant research tradition back in 1959 [Koch 1959]. His five points were recently summarized by Wertheimer and Robinson:

> First, the intervening variable paradigm for theory construction is deeply flawed; in short it does not work. Second, the range of potential generalization of the psychological "laws" that have been discovered to date is pitifully limited. Third, the link between theoretical constructs and operational definitions of these constructs usually is, at best, anemic and so loose as to be epistemologically unacceptable. Fourth, quantitative formulations of systematic relationships in empirical data are premature and often carried out to ludicrous degrees of presumed precision, when that degree of precision is totally unwarranted by the poor reliability and validity of the underlying measurements. Finally, the hypothetico-deductive model of scientific practice is incom-

plete, misleading, and ultimately not feasible. In short, it does not work either. [Wertheimer & Robinson 1998, p. 9]

So established are these emphases in psychology that Koch criticized, that the primary role of the researcher is still a distant, detached, objective observer. The controlled experiment, the questionnaire, the systematic sample survey, or the structured interview are cynosures. Such methods, while initially valid choices, soon, however, became commonplace and sacred conventions. The dominant use of these methods are self-defeating when the research mission is to be knowledgeable about what behaviors are health sustaining and how the qualities of social environments and social groupings nurture positive, prosocial behaviors.

The premises of the Wellness scholar shifts: topics now reside outside the traditional definitions of inquiry. It is certainly a challenge to realize an ecological expedition since research conventions seem so ingrained. What is needed are adventuresome investigators who chart new approaches and design new methods to fit the requirements of the situation rather than first choosing the statistical or research method and *then* finding a topic that matches the method. [Tolan et al. 1990].

To dig into the micro social systems that illustrate and define integrative and self-validating occasions requires that we attend to the everyday events and interactions of people and do so in concert with other disciplines. To understand why, in the above example, some people in a small Peruvian village boiled water and others did not, Wellin lived in the village for four years and, as a result, was able to understand the intricacies of water boiling because he developed a multifaceted understanding of the daily lives of the people and the cultural and group norms that were operating on individuals [Wellin 1998]. To fulfill the Wellness challenge, we increase our efforts to anchor communication, interaction, and collaboration with other investigators who are also invested in natural communities. Interdisciplinary and cross-disciplinary enterprises seem apt, and attractive.

While universities are not generally creating bridges across departmental structures that traditionally define disciplines and set boundaries on inquiry, there are exceptions. At the University of Illinois at Chicago (UIC), for example, The Office of Social Science

Research for the Social Sciences and the Great Cities Institute for the entire university are providing incentives for faculty in different departments to engage in research and to communicate about ideas that may over time create new ways of doing research.

Facilitating cross-disciplinary conversations is not easy or straight-forward [Jason et al. 1987]. John Gardiner, Director of the Office of Social Science Research at UIC comments:

> Bringing faculty together from different departments had mixed results. Some were so deeply nested in the vocabular-ies, funding systems, and publication outlets of their disci-plines that presentations based on other disciplines seemed unrelated to their own work. Others, however, seemed genuinely fascinated by the insights or alternative starting points and sought out advice on how to learn more, and some contacts led to joint projects using multiple ap-proaches..." [Gardiner 1998]

Wim Wievel, founder of the Great Cities Program at the University of Illinois at Chicago, states the potential of interdisciplinary thinking:

> Increasingly, universities engage in partnerships, in linkage with external organizations to pursue knowledge. For a business, a city government, or a community organization, problems are usually holistic. Working with them thus requires universities to be more holistic. While we need the deep expertise that specialization can bring, we also need people who can bridge across these specializations. It is amazing how excited faculty can get when they have an opportunity to get outside of their narrow field, and how creative they can be in discovering how the concepts of one field can be used in another.

> The Great Cities program takes the urban and metropolitan environment as its field, and thus draws on people from many disciplines. It encourages an interdisciplinary, not just a multidisciplinary approach: we have to do more than involve disciplines in their own ways, we have to get them to

talk to each other to let their insights be influenced and enriched by those of others. [Wievel, personal communication, June 1998]

NIH and other groups are encouraging ways to foster more interdisciplinary research [Azar 1998]. Norman B. Anderson, Director of NIH, Office of Behavioral and Social Science Research, supports the aphorism that, "Health problems do not organize themselves to be congruent with university departments" [Azar 1998, p. 18]. Knowledge domains may become more interdepartmental with the possibility of sharing current methods. As more and more ways are created to facilitate cross-disciplinary investigations, the promise of establishing situated knowledge may be realized.

The new opportunity for the Wellness scholar is to participate in the appraisal of methods and techniques that are developed by investigators representing different professions and with varying premises about scientific validity. This challenging opportunity depends on the local ecology of the participating investigators as they create their own social setting for interdisciplinary communication.

## The Third Idea: Listening with Others Rather than Assessing Others

Psychology's research tradition has been dominated by a commitment to rigorous and cumulative empirical investigations with tests and scales and experiments. To gain insight about the sources of everyday caring and respect as sources of wellness, new ways of doing our work are needed. This means that caring about the informants and creating trust to work with them emerges as a high priority. Feminist investigators have been paving the way for this type of work for several decades [Lieblich & Josselson 1994; Oakley 1981]. To appreciate the legacies of family, and peer contributions of social support and social networks, more detailed investigations of everyday life are essential. Anderson's ethnographic analyses of conjoining white and black cultures in a Philadelphia neighborhood is a revealing look at the everyday events that impact the lives of the residents in these two cultures [Anderson 1990].

The Wellness scholar changes not only research venues, but also portfolios of techniques and criteria for truth. The Wellness scholar adopts new directions and listens to the stories of persons as they describe the people, occasions, and events that have made it possible for them to become more socially developed, competent, and effective in their coping; the Wellness construct is enhanced by including narratives and oral histories.

Scholars interested in autobiography, oral histories, and narratives represent a variety of disciplines and perspectives including sociologists, anthropologists, cognitive psychologists, feminists, and linguists. Each of these investigators expresses a desire to understand the ways in which stories and personal tales illustrate major themes and topics in lives [Conway 1998; Denzin & Lincoln 1994; Ross 1991; Sarbin & Kitsuse 1994; Schwartz & Sudman 1994; Wolke 1997]. Even though these research activities may not represent a major thrust or paradigm within psychology, there is long tradition for this type of inquiry; [Buss 1985; Gergen 1993; Hatch & Wisniewski 1995; Linde 1993; McAdams 1996; Polkinghorne 1988]; more investigators are joining this tradition [Bruner 1990; Goldman 1996].

One consequence of this increased investment in an oral history/ storytelling tradition is that new questions are being raised about the relationship between the scientist and the informant. Literature is increasingly defining oral history as initiating a dialogue between informant and interviewer rather than as a unidirectional investigation [Barone 1995; Coles 1997].

The significance of oral histories as a legitimate form of inquiry makes explicit that there are in fact different ways to understand phenomena, an issue that has been difficult to recognize. The topic of validity expands to consider the relationship between the investigator and the informant and not simply the level of the correlation or the differences in reported means. In the ecological expedition, the heart of the matter *is* the context in which the work takes place.

Tyler, Pargament, and Gatz in 1983 presented a rationale for research to be undertaken where the investigator and the person providing the information are seen as reciprocally influencing each other in decisions about what to assess and how to assess it [Tyler et al. 1983]. Sarason and colleagues have invested in the same type of enterprise emphasizing the role of resource networks when generating community service programs [Sarason & Lorentz 1989, 1998].

The author has also invested in a collaborative process in documenting the development of African American community leaders [Glidewell et al. 1998; Kelly 1992a; Tandon et al. 1998]. When an inquiry is viewed as a reciprocal exchange between two people or two groups, the findings from such an inquiry become dependent upon the quality of the working relationship between the person stimulating the dialogue and the person who is relaying the information.

Engaging in this type of research emphasizes the personal values of the investigator. Too often, these topics are not considered when training research investigators. While personal qualities may vary with the community and the topic, some examples of those qualities that may facilitate collaborative inquiry are: openness to new experiences, investment in learning about new concepts, an ability to expend energy in the beginning of the working relationship; creating informal occasions where both parties can listen to each other; and creating social support groups for the investigator to help interpret unpredictable crises, etc. Certainly, such qualities as being a good listener define how well the obtained information will be salient, deep, and reflect the informants' stories; the present author has noted other generic qualities [Kelly 1971]. Here again the role of the distant, detached, objective observer is replaced by the investigator who expresses a genuine interest and care about the informant.

The topic of Wellness is elusive and subtle and cannot easily be grasped from a predesigned questionnaire. Yet more clarity about wellness can be derived from dialogue between investigator and informant. The Wellness scholar learns to converse rather than to just label or categorize. Listening includes a variety of discrete skills, as mentioned above, that can become a substantial resource to validate the person who is telling the story. Categorizing and labeling evolves, a conjoint process between the Wellness scholar and the informant, where the first priority is to understand the behavior of persons *in situ*. The listener can consolidate the storyteller's sense of self in these exchanges and relay back to the storyteller the listener's impressions for more reflection. The Wellness scholar is an attentive and well-prepared listener and learner.

This third idea specifically asserts that the Wellness scholar defines inquiry as a relationship; that without that working relationship of trust, the social intricacies that affect how innovations evolve or stagnate will not be clearly understood.

## The Fourth Idea: Learning About Resilient and Competent Communities

Listening to the reports of persons as they express their own health engendering experiences is also a rehearsal; a rehearsal to listen to the collective stories of resilient groups and communities. Some communities and groups engage each other and generate workable solutions for those social issues that confront them [Iscoe 1974]. At this larger level of analysis, insights can be gained about the social norms and traditions of how groups and communities organize their personal, organizational, and community resources to create a culture that affirms such core values as participation, justice, and dignity.

Decades ago, the topic of community studies was a significant part of sociological and anthropological research. A premise for this tradition was that communities were essential to social life and influenced the behavior of individuals. The works of W. Lloyd Warner [1949]; William Foote Whyte [1943]; Floyd Hunter [1953]; Robert Dahl and C. E. Lindblom [1953]; and Herbert Gans [1962, 1967] are reference points for this tradition [Clausen 1956]. Working on the Wellness Concept is an opportunity to reinitiate such activities. If the role of community structures and processes in affecting wellness behavior can be clarified, then the underlying social fabric can be illuminated as potential positive sources of health engendering behavior. The climate of communities can either enable or diminish opportunities for individuals to feel engaged and active and purposeful and validated. The mediating roles of the small group, organizational, and community structures in facilitating wellness behavior can then be addressed.

When research data is collected from field experiments on participant democracy, the results are not always consistently positive [Feder 1998]. As with all "real" system innovations, some things work, others do not. But the legacy of such efforts is to give representatives from different levels of an organization an opportunity to reinvest their talents and energies. This is one criteria to ascertain whether a collaborative or participative enterprise is judged to be worthwhile: "Would representatives from all levels of the organization or community do it again?" When such participative projects are productive and a reservoir of social norms are established, communities may establish conditions of trust and cohesiveness. Such conditions may in turn promote standards for the expression of wellness behavior. It is thought that when cohesiveness and trust are operative, there are more opportunities to discuss what matters and to then establish norms that enable the desired behavior to be expressed. The topic of community capacity has been a focus of the research of Wandersman and colleagues, as well as the community development work of McKnight [Fetterman 1996; Wandersman & Florin 1990; McKnight 1995]. The Centers for Disease Control and Prevention convened a symposium in December 1995 to examine this topic. Social and organizational networks and a sense of community emerged as two of the nine topics that participants recommended for further study [Goodman et al. 1998]. The Project on Human Development in Chicago Neighborhoods has employed the concept of collective efficacy that describes the informal controls that are potentially operable in local communities. These include such activities as "monitoring of spontaneous play groups among children, a willingness to intervene to prevent acts such as truancy and street-corner "hanging" by teenage peer groups, and the confrontation of persons who are exploiting or disturbing public space" [Sampson et al. 1997, p. 918]. Locating these activities and behaviors in specific communities requires attentive listening, dialoguing, and reconnaissance. The various listening skills acquired and tried out with individuals can be expanded to multiple levels of analysis at the community level [Kelly et al. 1988]. Campbell and Ahrens created a multiple case study using qualitative interviews with rape victims, rape victim advocates, and workers from the human service organizations to assess at different levels and from different perspectives how to change the community response to rape. This is an excellent example of multiple levels analyses [Campbell & Ahrens 1998].

Two concepts from social psychology and organizational psychology can nourish these tasks: *social norms* and *boundary spanning*. These venerable terms have immediate appeal. Knowledge of social norms can clarify the shared values and informal standards of behavior that affect how wellness behavior can be promoted, honored, and maintained in specific communities.

Murray Levine addressed the topic of social norms in terms of initiating prevention programs. Levine pointed out that if we understand the process of establishing norms, we have a basis to understand the processes to establish a sense of community. Rather than viewing preventive interventions as a technique of inoculation, he advocated, "Prevention efforts change norms ... an effective preventive intervention will go beyond affecting individuals" [Levine 1998].

Social norms reflect the guiding standards that in turn affect the expressions of behavior in that community.

Opp has provided three criteria to investigate the significance of social norms: (1) The communication opportunities between people in a social group that make it possible to pass the norm to others; (2) The cohesiveness of the group and the extent to which shared or uniform behavior is valued; (3) The importance of the norm for the group [Opp 1982]. A situated understanding of how these criteria are expressed can contribute to the analysis of specific micro factors that operate to facilitate the norms being shared. This is particularly so when understanding the descriptive norms of what people actually do in any given situation [Cialdini & Trost 1998]. These authors have pointed out: "Recent meta-analyses indicate that the most successful prevention programs for adolescents not only teach resistance skills, but also modify the social proof for using drugs: the programs change the descriptive norms about the prevalence of use among students and are delivered and reinforced by similar others, their peers (Tobler 1986, 1995)" [Cialdini & Trost 1998, p. 157]. A recently published example of the power of social norms is the work of Miller, Klotz, and Eckholdt [1998]. In an intervention with gay male prostitutes, the effectiveness of the intervention was enhanced because it directly and specifically targeted key leaders and respected friends to spread the word about HIV prevention, thereby changing the social norms from unprotected to protected sex. Approval by others is a powerful source for norm creation.

What is often missing is to "hunker down" into the daily lives of people to understand and appreciate the subtle ways in which the social norms set the tone, if not the basis, for the criteria for approval. Finding out who is most important to an individual and assessing how the informant thinks that these important people prefer him or her to behave points to the potential power of situated knowledge. The empirical literature on the emergence and transmission of norms is small, as Cialdini and Trost point out [Cialdini & Trost 1998]. However, the significance of norms for understanding wellness behavior seems apt, timely, and long overdue.

The concept of boundary spanning can lead to understandings of how the community or group makes contact and encourages reciprocal connections to other groups and organizations. Boundary spanning is a construct most identified with organizational psychology [At-Twaijri & Montanari 1987; Katz & Kahn 1978]. The notion is that the boundary of an organization is a key location between an organization and its surrounding environment [Dollinger 1984; Jemison 1984]. Persons who function in roles that influence communication between the host organization and other organizations are considered to be in boundary roles and are referred to as boundary spanners [Kelly et al. 2000]. If information and the exchange of resources can contribute to the health or efficacy of a group or organization, then the active nature of boundary spanning and the status of the person who activates these roles are of some significance. If the concept of Wellness can be conceptualized as a process to identify and exchange personal, organizational, and community resources, then boundary spanning activities are salient. Laumann et al. [1977] have stated that exchanges of communication and information is necessary in community decision making if local issues are to be resolved [Azelton 1994]. This makes boundary spanning a particularly appropriate concept to understand the group or organization's ability to adapt.

A topic for future investigation is whether the various ways in which interdependence can develop between groups and organizations increase the vitality of these organizations. Vitality—reserve energy for coping with crises, for example—may impact the positive socialization processes for future leadership behavior and further promote the capacity of members of organizations to carry out activities that promote wellness behavior, such as norms for sharing information and commitments to establish organizational values to increase trust and dignity. Emphasizing such concepts may expand options so that the study of wellness will not be restricted to the study of individuals! The point of emphasis is that the study of wellness is an interdisciplinary and multidisciplinary enterprise; an ecological expedition for Wellness depends upon the contributions of multiple research traditions.

The concepts of social norms and boundary spanning applied to the analysis of resilient communities can test the notion of whether personal growth and development can be enhanced when the places in which we live and work have linkages to other groups and organizations. An ecological premise is that the adaptive capacity of individuals and organizations can be enhanced when exchanges of information and resources between two organizations are a part of the everyday life of participants. The Wellness scholar works to understand how groups and communities identify whether personal and organizational resources do or do not facilitate institutional forms of coping.

## The Fifth Idea: The Analysis of Variety and Diversity

Null hypothesis significance testing (NHST) has limited our understanding of research topics [Cohen 1994]. The reverence for the analysis of differences between individuals and groups has been ritualized.

There are other options. In 1962 John Tukey emphasized "detective work" as the metaphor for statistical analysis rather than "sanctification" [Tukey 1962]. He later detailed this thesis in his classic book *Exploratory Data Analysis* [Tukey 1977]. More recent sources for these ideas are represented in the work of Behrens and Loftus [Behrens 1997; Loftus 1996]. Cortina and Dunlap have summarized their review of NHST with the following comment: "the abuses of NHST have come about largely because of a lack of judgment or education with respect to those using the procedure. The cure lies in improving education and, consequently judgment, not in abolishing the method" [Cortina & Dunlop 1997].

The limitations of null hypothesis testing has been acknowledged as timely and needed by the APA Board of Scientific Affairs, with the creation in 1996 of the Task Force on Statistical Inference [Board of Scientific Affairs, APA 1997].

To quote from the interim report of the task force:

> It is the view of the task force that there are many ways of using statistical methods to help us understand the phenomena we are studying (e.g., Bayesian methods, graphical and exploratory data analysis methods, hypothesis testing strategies). We endorse a policy of inclusiveness that allows any procedure that appropriately sheds light on the phenomenon of interest to be included in the arsenal of the research scientist. [Board of Scientific Affairs, APA 1996]

Adopting Tukey's detective metaphor and applying it to Wellness investigations enhances the possibilities of finding diverse patterns of Wellness. It seems that what is more informative is seeing how many *different* patterns of wellness are prevalent in any community in contrast to focusing on what are the modal patterns of wellness.

Rapkin and Luke expressed this issue directly for community psychologists:

> Quantitative methods focus on central tendencies; means, main effects, regression lines, discriminant functions, structural models. These techniques yield the best results when all cases conform to a given model and literally fall in line. However, models that emphasize uniformity seem inconsistent with the appreciation for diversity that community psychologists value [Rapkin & Luke 1993, p. 249].

They continue with a detailed exposition of the uses of cluster analysis to describe diversity in a sample.

Linear lines of concordance in traditional analyses can communicate that "outliers" are deviants rather than sources of potential feedback for further "detective" work. Other visual displays of data, by the use of Box Plots and Scatter plots, can communicate the arrays of responses [Tufte 1983, 1998]. Campbell, in an analysis of the rape victim's experiences with a state legal, medical, and mental health system, used cluster analysis to clarify the experiences of rape victims with these large social systems. Using cluster analytic techniques, she discovered that there is no monolithic experience; there are only diverse experiences that vary by race and social class [Campbell 1998].

Premature celebration of modal patterns of wellness behavior can inadvertently communicate a monolithic, unintended preferred standard for behavior rather than expressing the variety of potentially valid wellness behaviors. This is particularly so when the persons providing the data are from different social classes or ethnic groups and do not represent the usual reference point of college students as informants for psychological inquiry.

This fifth idea has additional meaning. It has long been observed that persons at the margin often are the sources of innovation and have the motivation for constructive change [Katz & Kahn 1978]. The marginal person, whose behavior deviates from the norm, may be a valid resource of generative action [Kelly 1992b]. Persons at the margin become potential sources for revitalizing groups and communities [Angelique & Campbell 1998]. Increasing consciousness about differences and variety, accompanied by methods of analysis that reflect patterns of variety, is a potentially useful approach to reduce any premature promulgation of a preference standard for desirable wellness behavior [Trickett et al. 1994].

Examining patterns of diversity in wellness behavior can be a constructive force to limit the reification of the Wellness concept. In employing this fifth idea, individuals are not considered as a part of a homogeneous group but rather as a set of individuals who share qualities that they may not share with others. Not all people are considered equally well for all conditions or situations. An ecological perspective views some persons as "well" for one particular situation or setting, but not another. Exploratory data analysis techniques are particularly apt for understanding patterns of behavior as they are expressed on "the ground," where there may not be an apparent prior theoretical rationale or basis for predictions. Since interpretations of variance are sometimes conceived as "noise" or "error" rather than as a source of information, patterns of variability can provide an alternative frame of reference.

One implication of focusing on the variety of responses is that multiple types of interventions for varied forms of wellness can be created. This is in contrast to the dominant intervention protocol that assumes that any one intervention is universally applicable.

## Conclusion

Emory Cowen has been a major exponent for redefining the focus for psychological inquiry, particularly inquiry that involves designing prevention research or evaluating preventive interventions. Emory's manifold examples have helped to redirect research to topics of positive sources of interpersonal and social relationships. I am pleased to offer some ideas that were stimulated from his original and continuing impetus.

I am suggesting that one point of view for generating Wellness inquiry is to create an ecological expedition. Five ideas were offered to begin the expedition that could potentially establish a new domain, that of the Wellness scholar.

The five ideas are heuristic topics of how ecological thinking can influence the type of information to be sought and found. These ideas were presented under the following five headings: Contextual Thinking: An Agenda for Situated Inquiry, New Disciplinary Connections, and Pluralistic Methods; Listening with Others Rather than Assessing Others; Learning about Resilient and Competent Communities; The Analysis of Variety and Diversity.

The framing premise for these five ideas is that knowledge about Wellness is a process of inquiry that is cross-disciplinary and is a process that defines research as a personal relationship. This is so because to understand Wellness means understanding the varied ways in which persons construct meaning, create social ties, and establish a workable culture. In this sense, the Wellness scholar also has the potential to be a resource for healing when understanding the various sources of social cohesion.

## References

Anderson, E. (1990). *Street wise: Race, class and change in an urban community.* Chicago: University of Chicago Press.

Angelique, H. & Campbell, R. (1998). Diversity among women: The need for visibility, dangerous dialogue and action. *The Community Psychologist, 31* (1), 30–32.

At-Twaijri, M. I. & Montanari, J. R. (1987). The impact of context and choice on the boundary-spanning process: An empirical extension. *Human Relations, 40*, 781–798.

Azar, B. (1998, May). Federal agencies encourage more cross-disciplinary work. *APA Monitor, 18*, 18.

Azelton, L. S. (1994). Boundary spanning and community leadership. Unpublished manuscript. University of Illinois at Chicago.

Bagby, M. (1996). *Documenting community leadership.* Videotape recording. University of Illinois at Chicago, Department of Psychology.

Barker, R. G. (1965). Explorations in ecological psychology. *American Psychologist, 20*, 1–14.

Barker, R. G. (1968). *Ecological psychology: Concepts and methods for studying the environment of human behavior.* Stanford, CA: Stanford University Press.

Barone, T. (1995). Persuasive writings, vigilant readings, and reconstructed characters: The paradox of trust in educational storysharing. In J. Hatch & R. Wisniewski (Eds.), *Life, history and narrative* (pp. 63–74). London: Falmer Press.

Bechtel, R. (Ed.). (1990). The Midwest Psychological Field Station: A celebration of its founding. *Environment and Behavior, 22* (4). New York: Sage Publications.

Behrens, J. (1997). Principles and procedures of exploratory data analysis. *Psychological Methods, 2*(2), 131–160.

Bell, C. (1997). *Ritual perspectives and dimensions.* New York: Oxford Press.

Bloom, D. E. (1998, May). Technology, experimentation, and the quality of survey data. *Science, 280*, 789–968.

Board of Scientific Affairs, American Psychological Association. (1996, December 14–15). Task force on statistical inference initial report (draft). Available [on-line] at: http://www.apa.org/science/tfsi.html.

Board of Scientific Affairs, American Psychological Association. (1997, March/ April.) Task force on statistical inference identifies charge and produces report. *Psychological Science Agenda*, 9–10.

Bronfenbrenner, U. (1979). *The Ecology of Human Development.* Cambridge, MA: Harvard University Press.

Bruner, J. (1990). *Acts of meaning*. Cambridge, MA: Harvard University Press.

Buss, F. L. (1985). *Dignity: Lower income women tell of their lives and struggles*. Ann Arbor: University of Michigan Press.

Campbell, R. (1998). The community response to rape: Victims' experiences with the legal, medical, and mental health systems. *American Journal of Community Psychology, 26*, 355–379..

Campbell, R. & Ahrens, C. (1998). Innovative community services for rape victims: An application of multiple case study methodology. *American Journal of Community Psychology, 26*, 537–572.

Cialdini, R. & Trost, M. (1998). Social influence: Social norms, conformity, and compliance. In D. Gilbert, S. Fiske, & G. Lindzey (Eds.), *The handbook of social psychology* (pp. 151–192). New York: McGraw Hill.

Clausen, J. A. (1956). *Sociology and the field of mental health*. New York: Sage.

Cohen, J. (1994). The earth is round (p < .05). *American Psychologist, 49* (12), 997–1003.

Coles, R. (1997). *Doing documentary work*. New York: Oxford.

Conway, J. K. (1998, April). *When memory speaks: Reflections on autobiography*. New York: Knopf.

Cortina, J. & Dunlap, W. P. (1997). On the logic and purpose of significance testing. *Psychological Methods, 2*(2), 161–172.

Cronbach, L. J. (1986). Social inquiry by and for earthlings. In D. W. Fiske & R. A. Shweder (Eds.), *Metatheory in social science* (pp. 83–107). Chicago: University of Chicago Press.

Dahl, R. & Lindblom, C. E. (1953). *Politics, economics and welfare: Planning and politico-economic systems resolved into basic social processes*. New York: Harper & Row.

Davis, A., Gardner, B., & Gardner, M. R. (1941). *Deep south: A social anthropological study of caste and class*. Chicago: University of Chicago Press.

Denzin, N. K. & Lincoln, Y. S. (Eds.). (1994). *Handbook of qualitative research*. Thousand Oaks, CA: Sage.

Dollinger, M. (1984). Environmental boundary spanning and information process on organizational performance. *Academy of Management Journal, 27*, 351–368.

Feder, B. (1998, February 21). The little project that couldn't: Others learn from a failed test in worker democracy. *The New York Times, Business Day*, B1–B3.

Fetterman, D. M., Kaftarian, S. J., & Wandersman, A. (Eds.). (1996). *Empowerment evaluation: Knowledge and tools for self-assessment and accountability*. Thousand Oaks, CA: Sage.

Gans, H. J. (1962). *The urban villagers: Group and class in the life of Italian-Americans*. New York: Free Press.

Gans, H. (1967). *The Livittowners: Ways of life and politics in a new suburban community*. New York: Columbia University Press.

Geertz, C. (1995). *After the fact: Two countries, four decades, one anthropologist*. Cambridge, MA: Harvard University Press.

George, J. M. & Brief, A. P. (1992). Feeling good—doing good: A conceptual analysis of the mood at work—organizational spontaneity relationship. *Psychological Bulletin, 112*, 310–329.

Gergan, K. J. (Ed.). (1993). *Refiguring self and psychology*. Hants, UK: Dartmouth Publishing.

Glidewell, J. C., Kelly, J. G., Bagby, M., & Dickerson, A. (1998). Natural development of community leadership. In R. Scott Tindale, L. Heath, J. Edwards, E. J. Posavac, F. B. Bryant, Y. Suarez-Balcazar, E. Henderson-King, & J. Myers (Eds.), *Social psychological applications to social issues: Theory and research on small groups,* (Vol. 4) (pp. 61–86). New York: Plenum.

Goldman, A. E. (1996). *Take my word*. Berkeley: University of California Press.

Goodman, R. M., Speers, M. A., McLeroy, K., Fawcett, S., Kegler, M., Smith, P. R., Sterling, T. D., & Wallerstein, N. (1998). Identifying and refining the dimensions of community capacity to provide a basis for measurement. *Health Education and Behavior, 25*, 258–278.

Hatch, J. A. & Wisniewski, R. (Eds.). (1995). *Life history and narrative*. London: Falmer Press.

Hesse, M. (1978). Theory and value in the social sciences. In C. Hookway & P. Pettit (Eds.), *Action and interpretation: Studies in the philosophy of the social sciences*. Cambridge, UK: Cambridge University Press.

Hunter, F. (1953). *Community power structure: A study of decision makers*. Chapel Hill: University of North Carolina Press.

Iscoe, I. (1974). Community psychology and the competent community. *American Psychologist, 29*, 607–613.

Jason, L. A., Hess, R. E., Felner, R. D., & Moritsugu, J. N. (1987). *Prevention in human services: Volume 5. Prevention: Toward a multidisciplinary approach*. New York: Haworth.

Jemison, D. (1984). The importance of boundary spanning roles in strategic decision-making. *Journal of Management Studies, 21*(2), 131–152.

Kahn, S. (1982). *A guide for grassroots leaders: Organizing.* New York: McGraw.

Katz, D. & Kahn, R. (1978). *The social psychology of organizations* (2nd ed.). New York: Wiley.

Kelly, J. G. (1971). Qualities for the community psychologist. *American Psychologist, 26,* 897–903.

Kelly, J. G. (Ed.). (1979). *Adolescent boys in high school: A psychological study of coping and adaptation.* Hillsdale, NJ: Lawrence Erlbaum.

Kelly, J. G. (1992a). *Ecological inquiry and a collaborative enterprise: A commentary on "The Chicago Experience."* Unpublished manuscript, University of Illinois at Chicago.

Kelly, J. G. (1992b). Gerald Caplan's paradigm: Bridging psychotherapy and public health practice. In W. P. Erchul (Ed.), *Consultation in community, school and organizational practice: Gerald Caplan's contributions to professional psychology* (pp. 75–85). Washington, DC: Hemisphere Publishing Corp.

Kelly, J. G. (1996). The history and varied epistemologies of community psychology: Describing the UIC course. *The Community Psychologist, 29*(1), 14–17.

Kelly, J. G., Dassoff, N., Levin, I., Schreckengost, J., Stelzner, S., & Altman, B. (1988). *A guide to conducting prevention research in the community: First steps.* Binghamton, NY: Haworth.

Kelly, J. G., Altman, B. E., Ryan, A. M., & Stelzner, S. (2000). Understanding and changing social systems. In J. Rapapport & E. Seidman (Eds.), *The handbook of community psychology* (pp. 133–159). New York: Plenum.

Kingry-Westergaard, C. & Kelly, J. G. (1990). A contextualist epistemology for ecological research. In P. Tolan, C. Keys, F. Chertok, & L. Jason (Eds.), *Researching community psychology: Issues of theory and methods* (pp. 23–31). Washington, DC: APA.

Koch, S. (Ed.). (1959). *Formulations of the person and the social context.* New York: McGraw-Hill.

Laumann, E., Marsden, P., & Galaskiewicz, J. (1977). Community-elite influence structures: Extension of a network approach. *American Journal of Sociology, 83,* 595–631.

Lave, J. & Wenger, E. (1991). *Situated learning: Legitimate peripheral participation.* Cambridge, UK: Cambridge University Press.

Levine, M. (1998). Prevention and community. *American Journal of Community Psychology, 26*(2), 189–206.

Lieblich, A. & Josselson, R. (Eds.). (1994). *Exploring identity and gender: The narrative study of lives* (Vol. 2). Thousand Oaks, CA: Sage Publications.

Lillard, A. (1998). Ethnopsychologies: Cultural variations in theories of mind. *Psychological Bulletin, 123*(1), 3–32.

Linde, C. (1993). *Life stories: The creation of coherence.* New York: Oxford University Press.

Loftus, G. R. (1996). Psychology will be a much better science when we change the way we analyze data. *American Psychological Society,* 161–171.

Maton, K. I. (1993). Moving beyond the individual level of analysis in mutual help group research: An ecological paradigm. *Journal of Applied Behavioral Science, 29,* 272–286.

Maton, K., Hrabowski III, F., & Grelf, G. L. (1998). Preparing the way: A qualitative study of high achieving African American males and the role of the family. *American Journal of Community Psychology, 26,* 639–668

McAdams, D. P. (1996). Personality, modernity, and the storied self: A contemporary framework for studying persons. *Psychological Inquiry, 7*(4), 295–321.

McLoyd, V. (1998). Socioeconomic disadvantage and child development. *American Psychologist, 53*(2), 185–204.

McKnight, John. (1995). *The careless society.* New York: Basic Books.

Miller, R., Klotz, D., & Eckholdt, H. (1998). HIV prevention with male prostitutes and patrons of hustler bars: Replication of an HIV preventive intervention. *American Journal of Community Psychology, 26*(1), 97–131.

Moos, R. H. (1973). Conceptualizations of human environments. *American Psychologist, 28,* 652–665.

Moos, R. H. & Insel, P. (1974). *Issues in social ecology.* Palo Alto, CA: National Press Books.

Moos, R. H. (1976). *The human context: Environmental determinants of behavior.* New York: Wiley.

Moos, R. H. (1979). Social climate measurement and feedback. In R. Muñoz, L. Snowden, & J. Kelly (Eds.), *Social and psychological research in community settings* (pp. 145–182). San Francisco: Jossey-Bass.

Neisser, U. & Jopling, D. A. (Eds.). (1997). *The conceptual self in context: Culture, experience, self-understanding* (pp. 3–285). Cambridge, UK: Cambridge University Press.

Oakley, A. (1981). Interviewing women: A contradiction in terms. In H. Roberts (Ed.), *Doing feminist research* (pp. 30–61). London: Routledge.

Ochs, E. & Capps, L. (1996). Narrating the self. *Annual Review of Anthropology, 25*, 19–43.

Opp, K. D. (1982). The evolutionary emergence of norms. *British Journal of Social Psychology, 21,* 139–149.

Payne, C. M. (1995). *I've got the light of freedom: The organizing tradition and the Mississippi freedom struggle.* Berkeley: University of California Press, Ltd.

Polkinghorne, D. E. (1988). *Narrative knowing and the human sciences.* Albany, NY: SUNY Press.

Pollio, H. R., Henley, T., & Thompson, C. B. (1997). *The phenomenology of everyday life.* Cambridge, UK: Cambridge University Press.

Rapkin, B. & Luke, D. (1993). Cluster analysis in community research: Epistemology and practice. *American Journal of Community Psychology, 21*(2), 247–277.

Raush, H. L., Dittmann, A. T., & Taylor, T. J. (1959). The interpersonal behavior of children in residential treatment. *Journal of Abnormal and Social Psychology, 58,* 9–26.

Raush, H. L., Farbman, L., & Llewellyn, L. G. (1960). Person, setting and change in social interaction: II. A normal-control study. *Human Relations, 13,* 305–333.

Ross, B. M. (1991). *Remembering the personal past: Descriptions of autobiographical memory.* New York: Oxford University Press.

Sampson, R. J., Raudenbush, S. W., & Earls, F. (1997). Neighborhoods and violent crime: A multilevel study of collective efficacy. *Science, 277,* 918–924.

Sarason, S. B. & Lorentz, E. (1989). *The challenge of the resource exchange network.* Cambridge, MA: Brookline Books.

Sarason, S. B. & Lorentz, E. (1998). *Crossing boundaries: Collaboration, coordination, and the redefinition of resources.* San Francisco: Jossey-Bass Publishers.

Sarbin, T. R. & Kitsuse, J. I. (Eds.). (1994). *Constructing the social.* London: Sage.

Schoggen, P. & Fox, K. (1989). *Behavior settings: A revision and extension of Roger G. Barker's "Ecological Psychology."* Stanford, CA: Stanford University Press.

Schwarz, N. & Sudman, S. (Eds.). *Autobiographical memory and the validity of retrospective reports.* New York: Springer-Verlag.

Seaburn, D. B., Lorenz, A. D., Gunn, W. B. Jr., Gawinski, B. A., & Mauksch, L. B. (1994). *Models of collaboration* (pp. 3–350). Oakland, CA: New Harbinger Publishing.

Seligman, M. E. P. (1998). President's column. *APA Monitor, 29,* 2–5.

Shapin, S. (1994). *A social history of truth.* Chicago: University of Chicago Press.

Stokols, D. (1992). Establishing and maintaining healthy environments: Toward a social ecology of health promotion. *American Psychologist, 47,* 6–22.

Stokols, D. & Altman, I. (Eds.). (1987). *Handbook of environmental psychology, Volume 1.* New York: Wiley.

Tandon, S. D., Azelton, L. S., Kelly, J. G., & Strickland, A. (1998). Constructing a tree for community leaders: Contexts and processes in collaborative inquiry. *American Journal of Community Psychology, 26*(4), 669–696.

Taylor, S. E., Repetti, R. L., & Seeman, T. (1997). Health psychology. What is an unhealthy environment and how does it get under the skin? *Annual Review of Psychology, 48,* 411–47.

Tobler, N. S. (1986). Meta-analysis of 143 adolescent drug prevention programs: Quantitative outcome results of program participants compared to a control or comparison group. *Journal of Drug Issues, 16,* 537–568.

Tobler, N. S. (1995, June). *Interactive programs are successful: A new meta-analysis findings.* Paper presented at the Society for Prevention Research Meeting, Scottsdale, AZ.

Tolan, P., Keys, C., Chertok, F., & Jason, L. (Eds.). (1990). *Researching community psychology.* Washington DC: APA.

Trickett, E. J. (1984). Towards a distinctive community psychology: An ecological metaphor for training and the conduct of research. *American Journal of Community Psychology, 12,* 261–279.

Trickett, E. J. (1989). Taking ecology seriously: A community development approach to individually based interventions. In L. Bond & B. Compas (Eds.), *Primary prevention in the schools* (pp. 361–390). Hanover, NH: University of New England Press.

Trickett, E. J., Kelly, J. G., & Vincent, T. A. (1985). The spirit of ecological inquiry in community research. In E. Susskind & D. Klein (Eds.), *Community research: Methods, paradigms, and applications* (pp. 331–406). New York: Praeger.

Trickett, E. J., Watts, R. J., & Birman, D. (Eds.). (1994). *Human diversity: Perspectives on People in Context.* San Francisco: Jossey-Bass.

Tufte, E. R. (1983). *The visual display of quantitative information.* Cheshire, CT: Graphics Press.

Tufte, E. R. (1998). *Visual explanations: Images and quantities, evidence and narrative.* Cheshire, CT: Graphics Press.

Tukey, J. (1962). Analyzing data: Sanctification or detective work? *American Psychologist, 24,* 83–91.

Tukey, J. (1977). *Exploratory data analysis.* Reading, MA: Addison-Wesley.

Turner, C. F., Ku, L., Rogers, S. M., Lindberg, L. D., Pleck, J. H., & Sonenstein, F. L. (1998, May). Adolescent sexual behavior, drug use, and violence: Increased reporting with computer survey technology. *Science, 280,* 867–873.

Tyler, F., Pargament, K., & Gatz, M. (1983). The resource collaborator role: A model for interactions involving psychologists. *American Psychologist,* 388–397.

Wandersman, A. & Florin, P. (1990). Citizen participation, voluntary organizations and community development: Insights for empowerment and research [Special issue]. *American Journal of Community Psychology, 18*(1).

Warner, W. L. (1949). *Democracy in Jonesville.* New York: Harper.

Wellin, E. (1955). Water boiling in a Peruvian town. In B. D. Paul & W. B. Miller (Eds.), *Health, culture, and community* (pp. 71–103). New York: Sage.

Wellin, E. (1998). *Exemplars of community psychology* (Video). Chicago: University of Illinois at Chicago.

Wertheimer, M. & Robinson, D. (1998). Two views of psychology: A study of a science. *Contemporary Psychology, 43*(1) 7–12.

White, P. (1990). Ideas about causation in philosophy and psychology. *Psychological Bulletin, 108*(1), 3–18.

Whyte, W. F. (1943). *Street corner society.* Chicago: University of Chicago Press.

Wolke, B., Gershkovich, I., & Polo, M. (1997, August). *Examining the complexity of most memorable autobiographical experiences.* Paper submitted to the American Psychological Association, Chicago, IL.

## Acknowledgments

The following persons read drafts of the chapter and/or offered useful substantive and editorial suggestions. I have appreciated their comments on this chapter: Becki Campbell, Paul Dolinko, Caroline Leopold, Robin Miller, Tony Orum, and Julian Rappaport.

# 5

# Resilience as Cumulative Competence Promotion and Stress Protection: Theory and Intervention[1]

*Peter A. Wyman, Irwin Sandler, Sharlene Wolchik, and Kathleen Nelson*[2]

This chapter is concerned with understanding processes that foster resilience and with the development of programs to promote resilience in children and adolescents. Resilience is defined as a child's achievement of positive developmental outcomes and avoidance of maladaptive outcomes, under significantly adverse conditions [Wyman, Cowen et al. 1999]. Resilience has been conceptualized as an important component within a broader concept of wellness [Cowen 1994]. Children's resilience has been investigated within several distinct research perspectives. A primary goal of this chapter is the integration of knowledge about resilience that comes from two of those research domains: (a) studies of multiple risk factors and resilience, and (b) studies focusing on processes of stress and coping in the context of specific life stressors.

Current perspectives on resilience reflect knowledge accrued from a number of research domains, some going back several decades [see Cicchetti & Garmezy 1993]. The early roots of research on resilience include studies of psychopathological conditions in childhood [Garmezy 1970; Garmezy & Streitman 1974], children reared in poverty [Elder 1974; Festinger 1983; Pavenstedt 1965], and children exposed to trauma [Epstein 1979; Moskovitz 1983]. In studies of children within each of these contexts, investigators noted examples of children manifesting competent development. Such unexpected positive outcomes challenged the current dominant theoretical views of development, which tended to view adjustive outcomes as highly determined by early adverse experiences. Growing recognition that manifestations of competence under adversity were not aberrant created the impetus for a number of investigators to better understand the variability in children's adaptation to life adversity [e.g., Garmezy & Rutter 1983].

Importantly, the study of mastery and adaptation has come to be viewed as a valid domain of inquiry in its own right. Over the last few decades, a number of research programs have sought to enhance understanding of children who manifest sound development in the context of multiple life stressors and adversities [e.g., Cowen et al. 1990; Garmezy et al. 1984; Luthar 1991; Rutter, Cox, et al. 1975; Rutter, Yule, et al. 1975; Sameroff et al. 1987; Werner & Smith 1982; Wyman et al. 1991]. The major contributions of these studies of risk and resilience have been to: (a) identify resources across children's developmental contexts that predict successful adjustment for children exposed to multiple life adversities; and (b) clarify models of how these resources relate to adaptation (e.g., identifying proximal versus distal variables and compensatory versus protective variables). Although this research focus on children exposed to multiple adversities is a valid reflection of the fact that children often experience many, co-occurring life stressors, this approach has not illuminated the characteristic challenges or adaptive tasks posed by the specific stressful situations, or the processes by which children adapt to those situations.

Parallel to studies of multiple risk and resilience, another research approach focused on children's coping with specific adverse life situations. Research in this tradition grew from the social psychological literature on stress and coping [Lazarus & Folkman 1984] and from the sociological literature on the social origins of mental and physical health problems [e.g., Avison & Gotlib 1994; Brown & Harris 1989]. This literature has focused intensively on issues of defining the nature of stressful situations [e.g., Coddington 1972; Compas 1987; Felner et al. 1988; Gersten et al. 1977], and on conceptualizing and studying coping and other processes of adaptation to stressors [Ayers et al. 1998]. Studies from a stress and coping perspective have been applied to a diverse range of specific stressful situations such as parent depression [Hammen 1997], physical illness [Worsham et al. 1997], divorce [Sandler et al. 1994], death of a parent [Lutzke et al. 1997], and academic stressors [Skinner & Wellborne 1997]. This literature has contributed to our understanding of the stressors encountered in specific adverse situations [e.g., Wolchik et al. 1986] and of children's coping responses that contribute to better outcomes in these situations [e.g., Sandler et al. 1994]. Two primary goals of this chapter are: (1) integration of the complementary knowledge about children's resilience that comes from the two preceding research areas, and (2) description of an approach for enhancing wellness among children who face adversity, drawn from knowledge accrued by studies of children's adaptation to multiple and discrete adverse processes.

## Resilience and Wellness

There are two primary reasons why wellness promotion should focus on children who experience adverse environmental conditions. First, children who experience high psychosocial adversity are a naturally defined population for whom the goals of wellness promotion are highly relevant. Many children in the United States encounter serious adversities that can have a considerable impact on their development. At this time in the United States, approximately 22% of children live in poverty [McLoyd 1998]; 40% experience parental divorce before they reach age 16 [Cherlin 1992]; between 1.5% and 5% experience sexual abuse, physical abuse, or neglect each year [Emery & Laumann-Billings 1998]; 19% experience chronic illness or physical disability[3] [Newacheck & Stoddard 1994]; 3.4% experience the death of a parent [U. S. Bureau of the Census 1990]; and 6.6 million children live with an alcoholic parent [Russell et al. 1985]. Children exposed to adverse environments are more likely to evidence maladjustment (e.g., high rates of problems in mental health, substance use, and physical health), and are less likely to attain positive developmental outcomes such as competence in academics and peer relations, positive sense of self, and realistic sense of control [Wolchik & Sandler 1997].

The second primary reason that the study of children in adversity is relevant to the goals of wellness promotion is the heuristic value in understanding adaptation to a wide range of conditions. Even in highly adverse conditions where the likelihood of dysfunction is great, children manifest significant variability in adjustment, including some who demonstrate highly competent functioning [Masten et al. 1990]. The latter positive outcomes are related to the presence of protective resources and "self-righting" processes. Clarifying such positive development for children, where it is least expected, offers an important window to understanding both normal and abnormal developmental processes [Cicchetti & Garmezy 1993]. For example, understanding how some children who experience highly adverse conditions maintain beliefs in their own efficacy, while others develop beliefs that presage helplessness, deepens our knowledge of how these beliefs develop as a function of child-environment interactions.

Our discussion of resilience is framed within the broader concept of wellness articulated by Cowen [1991, 1994, 1998]. An assumption of a wellness framework is that the development of healthy personal and environmental systems leads both to promotion of positive well-being and to reduction in dysfunction, because the two are outcomes of interrelated developmental processes. A wellness framework also emphasizes the embeddedness of children's development within systems (e.g., parent-child relationships, peer groups, classrooms). The development of well-being occurs in complex person-environment interacting systems that change with age, vary according to cultural and socioeconomic context, and thus may occur via a number of different pathways.

Two aspects of the wellness framework require special comment. First, the framework of wellness promotion provides a valuable counterpoint to the mental health field's dominant paradigm: a focus on understanding and ameliorating dysfunction. While a wellness perspective does include the reduction of dysfunction and pathology as a goal, its mandate is broader in that it emphasizes the promotion of those functions (behavioral, psychological, and biological) that comprise health and well-being for children.

Second, the wellness framework emphasizes the close association between the generation of knowledge about wellness promoting processes and the implementation of such knowledge in programs to improve children's well-being. This framework has three primary emphases:

- Program development and implementation should systematically apply findings from generative research, and evaluation of such programs should contribute further to our understanding of the developmental processes. The mutually reinforcing cycle of research and application, utilizing rigorous methodology, can lead to advances in both theory and intervention programs.

- Programs for enhancing children's well-being should occur early. The efficacy of such interventions will be greater if they occur as individual competencies and social structures that promote well-being are developing, rather than later, when competencies may be lacking and dysfunction may be more deeply rooted.

- Programs should be actively disseminated to reach children within their real-world settings (e.g., schools), and to enhance the systems (i.e., family relationships, classroom environments) within which children develop.

This chapter discusses theoretical and intervention issues in resilience in five sections. As a necessary precursor to discussing resilience, the first section discusses the characteristics of environmental adversities. The second section discusses the concept of resilience, emphasizing two key processes that underlie resilience within an organizational developmental framework. The next two sections apply these concepts to enhance understanding of resilience and efforts to promote resilience for children who experience adversities that are often conceptualized differently: a) chronic, multiple adversities; and b) specific adverse situations such as parental divorce, that begin as acute changes and that may lead to chronic adverse conditions. Finally, we discuss some implications for future research on the promotion of resilience.

## Quality and Ecology of Adversity in Development

Studying the processes by which children under adversity develop problems or competencies requires, initially, a careful conceptualization of the qualitative and ecological characteristics of life adversity. Qualitative characteristics of adversities refer to aspects of the relationship between the individual child and the environment that either induce stress or that interfere with accomplishment of developmental tasks. Stress has been defined as a "relationship between the person and the environment that is appraised as taxing or exceeding his or her resources and endangering his or her well-being" [Lazarus & Folkman 1984]. Children (and their social networks) actively adapt to stressful conditions, resulting in changes at the biological, psychological, and social-environmental levels. These adaptations affect the course of development, leading either to increased competence and well-being or to the development of physical or emotional and behavioral disorder. A second way in which environmental conditions can be adverse is that they may not provide the conditions necessary to foster competence in accomplishing normative developmental tasks. For example, a child's family, school, and neighborhood may lack the environmental "scaffolds" that "enable the child to function at the growing edge of his or her capabilities" [Masten & Coatsworth 1998]. The ecological properties of adversities refer to their timing, the domains in which they occur, and their dynamic relations to other adversities. A moderate amount of research has focused on identifying important qualitative and ecological characteristics of adversities, and on testing their relations to different developmental outcomes.

## Qualitative Dimensions of Adversity

What qualities of environmental conditions make them stressful to children? Early life stress research [Coddington 1972] defined stress in terms of changes from a steady state that required adjustment to reestablish a homeostatic balance. It was posited that excessive change would require readjustment that exceeds the individual's adaptive capacity, and would lead to health and mental health problems. Considerable empirical research found, however, that physical and psychological health problems were primarily related to negative, but not positive, changes. Positive changes, in contrast, are associated with indices of well-being (e.g., self-esteem, positive affect) [Reich & Zautra 1988; Sandler et al. 1991].

Subsequent research has focused on identifying more specific qualities of negative events according to objective raters and children themselves. Objective ratings of the negative qualities of events include global judgments by objective raters of the likely negative impact of an event in the context of the child's life [Goodyer 1990; Adrian & Hammen 1993]. More specific ways in which negative events can be classified include the microsystem in which the event occurs, such as family, peer group, or school [Seidman et al. 1995]. Alternatively, other researchers have identified experiential qualities of events such as losses, entrances, disappointments, and conflicts, using either rater judgments [Goodyer et al. 1997; Sandler, Reynolds et al. 1992] or empirical approaches [Sandler & Ramsay 1980] to identify underlying dimensions.

The stress-inducing qualities of events can also be conceptualized theoretically by describing the variety of ways in which needs or goals are not satisfied or are threatened as children interact with their environments over time [Lazarus & Folkman 1984]. Lazarus [1991] views stressful events as those that are appraised as threatening or harming one's commitments, such as self- and social-esteem, moral values, and life goals. Drawing on this theoretical perspective of stressors, Sheets, Sandler, and West [1996], for example, used confirmatory factor analysis to identify three dimensions (threat to self, other-related threat, and material loss) that accounted for the stressful event appraisals of children of divorce.

Conceptualization of stressful life circumstances can also be based on a theoretical model of human motivation. Skinner and Wellborn [1994], for example, identify adversities as environmental conditions that "threaten or damage ... three basic psychological needs" [p. 107]: relatedness, competence, and autonomy. According to the motivational model they employ [Connell & Wellborne 1991; Deci & Ryan 1985], behavior is organized and directed to satisfy these three basic needs, and the social context can either support or impede the satisfaction of each of these needs. Conditions that impede satisfaction of these needs include neglect, chaos, and coercion. Neglect impedes satisfaction of the need for relatedness, through insufficient positive involvement from important social partners, including a lack of positive affective attention, time, and interest.

Chaos impedes satisfaction of the need for competence, through a lack of structure and information about how to reach desired outcomes. Coercion impedes satisfaction of the need for autonomy and involves minimal choice, respect, and freedom of expression for the child.

Adversities can also be evaluated in terms of interference with accomplishing stage-appropriate developmental tasks. Masten and Coatsworth [1998] have described normative tasks across developmental periods (and within cultures) and the problems of successful accomplishment of those tasks under unfavorable environmental conditions. An adversity might impede a child's accomplishment of developmental tasks by: (1) blocking appropriate mastery opportunities, (2) distracting the child from engaging in the tasks, or (3) presenting demands that exceed the child's capacity to succeed at the tasks. For example, during middle childhood, interference with academic achievement might arise from the lack of an engaging school or classroom that makes appropriate demands relative to the child's ability, or from the presence of salient competing events such as family or community violence.

Although many conditions that interfere with developmental tasks are the same as those that are experienced as stressful or that impede satisfying motivational needs, this is not always the case. For example, a child's association with deviant peers might satisfy immediate needs and increase a sense of relatedness and control. Therefore, association with deviant peers would not be experienced as stressful. However, these relationships may lead to longer-term problems, such as later failures in academic competence or conduct that leads to problems with the law [Tolan et al. 1997; Rutter et al. 1995], and thus channel children toward increased exposure to other stressors such as violence, unemployment, and imprisonment.

## Ecological Properties of Adversity

The ecology of adversity refers to the duration and intensity of adverse conditions, domains of role functioning and settings in which adversities occur, and the interrelatedness of adversities. For example, events with a relatively short duration are considered acute, and those with a longer duration are considered chronic. Acute events might be large or small in degree of intensity, ranging from those that seriously threaten valued goals and arouse a great deal of negative affect over a prolonged period, or they may be minor hassles that arouse short-term distress. Chronic adversities include those enduring conditions that last over a prolonged period of time and that may not have a distinct point of onset or offset, such as living in poverty or in a dangerous neighborhood, or living in a family with a high level of conflict.

Some investigators have proposed that chronic adverse conditions, rather than acute events, account for the development of mental health problems [Gersten et al. 1977]. However, adverse events and conditions are best thought of as being dynamically linked in a chain of mutual causation, rather than as independent influences on development [Rutter & Sandberg 1992]. Acute events often initiate chronic ongoing adverse conditions. For example, Felner, Terre, and Rowlison [1988] described a transitional events model of parental divorce, in which divorce leads to a range of stressful conditions as the family restructures, such as children's loss of time with one or both parents, economic difficulties, and interparental conflict. Likewise, chronic adverse conditions may lead to the occurrence of major negative events. As a case in point, divorce is more likely to occur among parents who have a history of antisocial personality problems, low income, criminal offenses, substance abuse problems, or prior family transitions [Lahey et al. 1988; Robins 1986; Capaldi & Patterson 1991]. Finally, some major adversities involve a web of chronic and acute adversities. Spacarelli [1994], for example, disaggregated child sexual abuse to identify events involved in the abuse itself, those related to negative processes in the family, and those that follow public disclosure.

Another ecological aspect of adversity concerns the co-occurrence of adverse conditions [Goodyer 1994]. Some families may be particularly susceptible to the occurrence of negative life events, either because of the characteristics of specific family members (e.g., mental disorder in a parent leads to multiple negative events for children), or because of the chain reactions of some conditions leading to a string of other adverse events (e.g., poverty leading to exposure to neighborhood violence). The co-occurrence of adverse conditions is particularly significant because of evidence that the effects of adverse conditions are cumulative, either in an additive or multiplicative fashion [Goodyer 1994].

## Psychosocial Resources and Processes of Resilience

In this section, we shift focus from the nature of adversity to address three questions about resilience:

1. Which child and environmental resources help to offset the effects of serious adversity and favor positive development rather than pathology? We conceptualize resources as relatively stable characteristics of children (e.g., intelligence) or of their environments (e.g., parenting style).

2. How do these resources influence processes that enhance successful adaptation? We conceptualize two primary types of processes: (a) protection from negative effects of stressors, and (b) enhancement of developmental objectives.

3. Finally, how do these resources and processes fit into a broader organizational-developmental model for understanding resilience across development?

Studies of children facing a variety of different adverse conditions underscore the differences in how children adapt [Cicchetti & Garmezy 1993; Luthar & Zigler 1991; Masten 1990; Rutter, Cox, et al. 1975; Wyman et al. 1991, 1992]. Although some traumatic experiences (e.g., catastrophic abuse) can overwhelm the adaptive capacity of virtually all children, there is wide variation in the quality of children's adaptations to most adverse conditions. Although early conceptualizations about variability in adaptation to adversity emphasized the putative role of exceptional characteristics of "invulnerable" children [Garmezy & Neuchterlein 1972] and atypical adaptation [Baldwin et al. 1993]. More recently investigators have focused on general developmental processes to explain adaptation [Masten & Coatsworth 1998; Wyman, Cowen, et al. 1999].

## Levels of Resources and Processes of Resilience

Resources linked to positive adaptation for children in adversity can be conceptualized in three relatively stable systems within an ecological framework: (1) Child-centered (ontogenic-developmental) characteristics, including components of regulatory style (e.g., temperament) [Eisenberg et al.1997], intelligence [Luthar & Zigler 1992], and self-system variables such as beliefs about self-worth, control, or future expectations [Cowen et al. 1992; Kim et al. 1997; Parker et al. 1990; Wyman et al. 1993]. (2) Structural and relational characteristics of a child's family or other intimate (micro-) systems in which children develop. These characteristics include continuity and quality of key caregiving relationships [Masten et al. 1990; Werner & Smith 1982, 1992; Wyman, Cowen, et al. 1991, 1999], as well as more distal factors such as parent education, health, and well-being [Baldwin et al. 1993; Wyman et al. 1999]. (3) Community, or macro-system resources, which include characteristics of neighborhoods and schools, such as the level of organization, social support, or availability of positive models and mentors [Sampson et al. 1997; Werner & Smith 1982].

These resources are conceptualized as facilitating the occurrence of two processes that bring about positive adaptation to adversity. One process is to protect children from the stressful cognitive and emotional effects of adverse environmental conditions. A second process is to facilitate positive mastery of normative developmental challenges (i.e., stage-salient tasks) under adverse conditions.

*Stress-protective function of resources.* Life adversities occur in dynamic interactions with the child and with the systems that comprise the child's developmental context. These dynamic interactions affect how the child interprets an adversity, how the child responds to it, and whether the adversity is resolved, recurs, or leads to further adversities over time.

Rutter [1990] describes several processes that can reduce the negative impact of an adversity. First, the child's exposure to or involvement with an adversity may be reduced. For example, a parent may shield a child from exposure to an adversity or ensure that the adversity does not escalate to lead to other negative experiences for the child. Second, a child's experience of an adversity may be altered in a way that the negative effects are minimized.

We propose that the negative effects of adversities may be minimized cognitively, emotionally, and behaviorally. Cognitively, the internal representation of an adverse experience may be altered in a way that maintains a child's positive evaluation of self, sense of competence and control, and relatedness to others [Skinner & Wellborn 1994; Sandler et al. 1989]. Emotionally, a child may be helped to regulate the negative affect associated with the experience, and to minimize the occurrence of any debilitating negative affect in other, similar situations [Eisenberg et al. 1997]. Behaviorally, a child's response to the situation may be altered so that the child continues to be positively engaged with developmentally important goals such as relating well to peers and family, and adapting well to school.

For example, children respond cognitively, behaviorally, and emotionally to the problem of being bullied by other children at school. Some children might tolerate the distress of engaging with the problem by seeking assistance from a responsive parent or adult, or by asserting the right not to be bullied. They might be successful in stopping the bullying, which reduces their negative affect, and helps children see themselves as more competent. Other children might reduce their arousal by avoiding thinking or telling others about the problem. They might refuse to go to school, which may lead to further interpersonal problems and to a diminished sense of self-efficacy. Thus, children's resources (i.e., personal characteristics, family relations, and community) influence the processes they engage in to adapt to the adversities as well as the outcomes of their transactions with the adversity. For example, a child with a positive sense of self-worth and a sense of efficacy in dealing with problems, who has attentive parents and who is embedded in a supportive community context, is more likely to engage in processes that lead to successful resolution of stressors than a child with fewer resources.

Effective adaptation to adverse life circumstances often involves a careful balancing act between alternative goals. For children experiencing uncontrollable events such as interparental conflict, for example, an optimal balance might simultaneously involve: recognizing that they would like the conflict to end because they care about their parents and feel distressed, but accepting that they are not responsible for or capable of bringing about this change, and that they need to reduce their distress by limiting their exposure to the conflict and focusing instead on their normative developmental tasks [Rossman & Rosenberg 1992; Jenkins et al. 1988].

*Development-enhancing function of resources.* A second function of resources associated with resilience is to facilitate accomplishment of normative stage-salient developmental tasks [Sroufe 1979]. Stage-salient tasks describe the phase-specific growth and development objectives in physiological, affective, cognitive, and behavioral systems. In early infancy, for example, these tasks are concentrated on a child's ability to establish physiological and affective regulation [Carlson & Sroufe 1995]. Effective regulation in those areas, in turn, relates to a young child's ability to maintain organized behavior and interaction with caregivers [Brazelton et al. 1974]. The age-salient tasks for children in later childhood reflect the need for increasing self-regulation of behavior and functioning in a wider range of domains. Competence at each developmental phase reflects a child's successful mastery of the age-related objectives that define well-being for a child in his or her social and cultural context [Masten & Coatsworth 1998]. Disordered behavior, conversely, involves a series of deviations from adaptive resolutions of these normative developmental tasks [Carlson & Sroufe 1995; Sroufe 1990].

Emotional regulation during infancy, for example, depends on both the infant's capacities and the resources present in the infant's caregiving system. Infant capacities that facilitate regulation include the ability to attend to human facial features and to initiate and withdraw from interactions [Emde 1989; Tronick 1989]. Infant capacities alone, however, are not sufficient to ensure adequate self-regulation. Flexible and adaptive regulation also depends on the ability of children's principal caregivers to coordinate mutually regulating interactions [Tronick 1989; Gianino & Tronick 1988].

## An Organizational-Developmental Perspective

An organizational-developmental framework [Egeland et al. 1993; Teo et al. 1996; Waters & Sroufe 1983] focuses on the processes of organization and reorganization of a child's behavior that occur in response to phase-specific developmental issues. It views development as characterized by a process of increasing hierarchical differentiation and organization. A central construct within this perspective is adaptation. Adaptation describes an active process by which a child strives to meet these age-salient objectives by drawing on both internal and external resources. Thus, the organizational perspective emphasizes adaptive outcomes at each phase of development as reflecting a transactional process between child and environment. Although this transactional process continues throughout development, the role and function of child, caregiving, and extrafamilial resources change across developmental periods.

An organizational-developmental model also provides a framework for viewing patterns of continuity vs. discontinuity in adaptation across developmental periods. Specifically, the form of a child's current adaptation influences how a child approaches future developmental tasks. In that sense, there is coherence and continuity in a child's adaptation [Sroufe 1979; Teo et al. 1996]. At the same time, other mechanisms and processes can initiate discontinuity (either enhancement or erosion) in adaptation. Potential sources of discontinuity include: (a) exposure to new adversity or improvement in prior adverse conditions; (b) changes in quality of caregiving; (c) new opportunities embedded in developmental shifts (e.g., new relationships); and (d) a child's acquisition of or failure to acquire age-appropriate capacities [Wyman, Cowen et al. 1999].

An organizational perspective consists of a set of heuristic tools that can be applied to understanding development across the continuum from disorder to competence [Cicchetti & Sroufe 1978; Sroufe 1979]. Within this perspective, both maladjustment and competence are viewed as processes that extend over time, not as fixed "outcomes." Those processes are shaped by a developmental context of change and growth.

Cicchetti and Schneider-Rosen [1986], for example, applied an organizational approach to illustrate how the initiation and manifestation of depression in children may be linked to developmental changes in self cognitions during childhood. Prior to 7 to 8 years of age, children's conceptions of self are conceived primarily in physicalistic terms [Selman 1980]. That is, young children define themselves based on material and active characteristics, such as possessions, typical activities, and bodily features. Moreover, young children's self-evaluations tend to be based on absolute standards, rather than on comparisons with other children. Beginning around age 7 or 8, self-cognitions undergo several qualitative transformations associated with the transition from preoperational to operational thought [White 1965]. During that transition, self-views are based increasingly on psychological self-understanding (e.g., stable traits or attributes); comparative self-evaluation (contrasting one's own performance with the performance of other children); and competency, rather than action-based, standards.

The preceding changes in self-cognitions affect the stability, form, and content of children's attributions about self and thus the capacity to manifest a stable affective and cognitive state, both of which are characteristic of depression in adults [Abramson et al. 1978]. For example, the transition from physicalistic to psychological conceptions of self is related to children's capacity to make stable attributions about self. Because physicalistic and action-based attributes are relatively transitory, self-attributions prior to age 7 or 8 would tend to be unstable. As children's self-attributions become based increasingly on enduring internal qualities, the attributions that older children make about themselves become more stable. Stable, negative attributions about self are associated with enduring depressive symptomology. Thus, in response to certain experiences (e.g., noncontingency, failure), older children can make attributions about self that can predispose depression. In sum, organization and change within one developmental system (i.e., cognitive) affects children's interpretations of their interactions with their environments (i.e., attributions regarding self), which can affect other systems (e.g., affective responses), and, potentially, enable the development of depression as a consequence of adverse experiences [Cicchetti & Schneider-Rosen 1986].

Resilience, conversely, describes processes whereby children utilize self-righting capacities that enable them to traverse a pathway of adaptation [Cicchetti & Rogosch 1997] in the context of adverse experiences. Resources and attributes relevant to resilience are those that enable children to maintain cognitive, affective, and behavioral well-being and to master developmental objectives. Whereas certain attributions to adversities may, for example, initiate depression or other disorder [Cicchetti & Schneider-Rosen 1986], other attributions may enhance resilience. For example, children who attribute negative events to external, specific, and unstable causes (rather than to internal, stable causes) may be protected from the negative effects of stressors on self-worth and sense of efficacy. A wellness perspective, moreover, suggests that well-being should be conceptualized not merely as the absence of pathology, or disorder, but as the presence of attributes that comprise competence for children of a given age, in a given cultural context.

## Organizational-Developmental Model for Resilience

Within an organizational-developmental framework, resilience describes children's capacity to master age-salient objectives, or to demonstrate improvement in adaptation, under conditions of significant adversity [Waters & Sroufe 1983; Wyman, Cowen, et al. 1999]. Although adaptive capacity for successful mastery of challenges can become incorporated into a child's functioning, the resources and processes that contribute to resilient adaptations may operate at the individual, family, or community levels. The organizational perspective provides a framework for outlining how the salience and role of these resources changes across development.

Figure 1 outlines hypothesized processes in children's resilient adaptations. The figure shows that environmental adversities threaten children's positive well-being and interfere with children attaining developmentally appropriate competencies. Resources enhance adaptation processes to support children's mastery of developmental objectives and to maintain their cognitive-affective well-being under conditions of adversity. Adaptation can involve internal processes such as children's perceptions of competence and efficacy, appraisals of adversities, or transactions between children and external resources, such as those that create a regulated parent-child relationship. At each developmental phase, the quality of adaptation depends on the availability of sufficient resources for mastering objectives [Masten & Coatsworth 1998], and the capacity of these resources to moderate the cognitive and affective consequences of adversities.

**Figure 1. Process Model of Resilience**

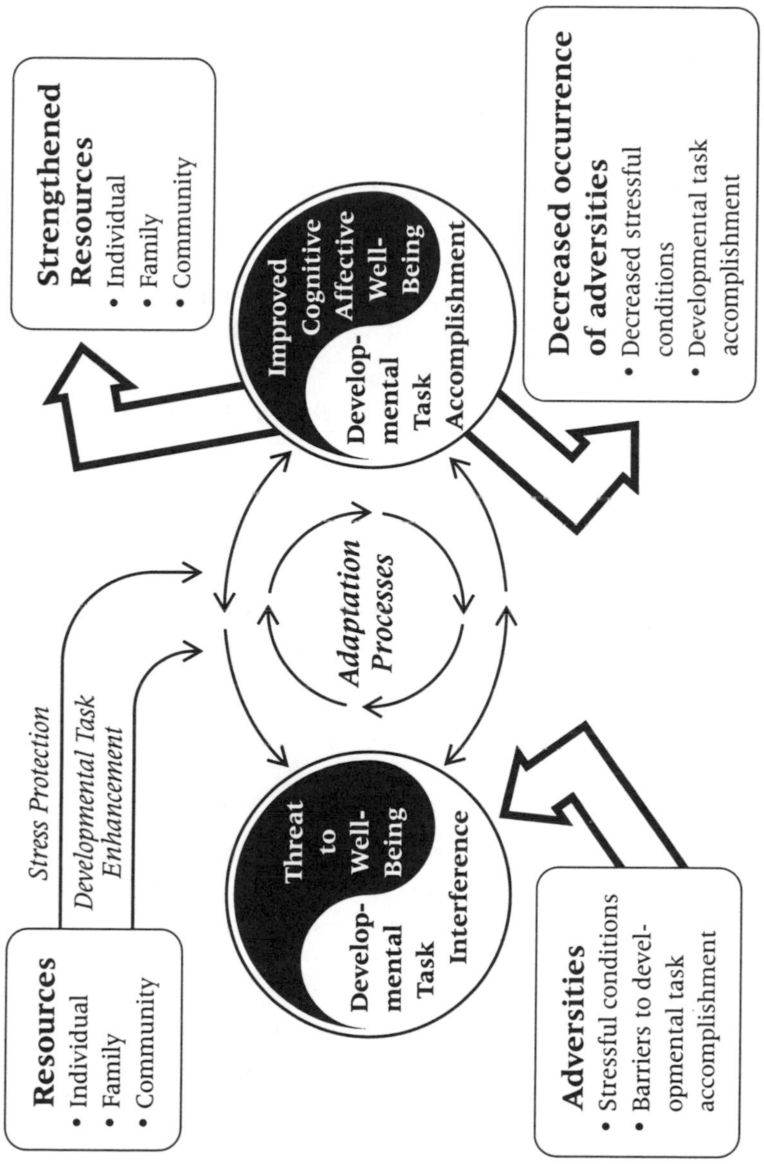

The model also describes how successful adaptation strengthens individual and social resources and decreases the occurrence of adversity over time. Successful adaptation may lead children to acquire greater competencies and to hold more positive beliefs in their efficacy. Likewise, positive changes at the family and community level may occur as a function of successful adaptation to adversities. Over time, successful adaptation may also lead to increased opportunities for children to accomplish future developmental tasks, and to a decrease in the likely occurrence of adverse conditions. We will now apply these concepts and consider the intervention implications that derive from them for two types of adverse conditions: chronic and multiple stressful conditions and parental divorce.

## Multiple and Chronic Adversities: Resilience and Interventions

Stressors in children's lives rarely occur in isolation. For many, childhood is marked by multiple, often co-occurring adversities. The sections to follow discuss: (a) the interrelations among adversities, and relations between chronic adversity and maladjustment; (b) how individual, family, and community resources may promote children's positive adjustment in the context of chronic life stress; and (c) how prevention programs can profitably use this knowledge to enhance wellness.

### Multiple, Chronic Adversity and Children's Development

Although some adversities have their primary impact at an individual, family, or community level, they often have rippling effects to create additional adverse conditions across these systems. For example, whereas 22% of American children currently live in poverty, the rate of poverty is over 50% for children who live in a single-parent home [Durlak 1997]. Children who live in poverty, in turn, are more likely to have problems in cognitive-developmental, physical health, academic achievement, and social-emotional domains in early childhood [McLoyd 1998]. As another example, parental psychological problems can lead to inconsistent parenting and child conduct problems, which reciprocally increase parental distress and stress in the family [Capaldi & Patterson 1991]. The point for emphasis here is that adverse conditions may foster other adversities at the child, family, and community levels, and may become chronic and persistent over time. As the number and chronicity of adversities increase, multiple systems of children's developmental context are negatively affected.

A recent study of 1,179 urban children by Kilmer et al. [1998] well illustrates the multiple, interrelated life adversities faced by many poor children. Drawn from 20 school sites, their sample was comprised of 6- to 12-year-old children and was 69% minority. Parents reported an average of 6 out of 30 potential adverse life circumstances or events during their children's lifetime. Adversities clustered into five factors: (1) family turmoil, (2) poverty, (3) family dissolution, (4) illness/injury, and (5) neighborhood violence. The most common adversities among the sample were those reflecting family turmoil (e.g., 40% parental divorce; 25% had a family member with a substance use problem). Consistent with other findings on the high incidence of violence in the lives of urban youth, 25% of the parents described their neighborhood as unsafe, and 10% of the children had seen someone get badly hurt.

Several studies find that chronically and multiply stressed children face formidable challenges to adaptation. For example, one study found that rates of maladjustment were approximately 10 times higher for children exposed to four or more adverse conditions (e.g., parental discord, paternal criminality, maternal psychiatric disorder) versus zero or one [Rutter 1979]. Goodyer [1994] found that children who experienced three adverse conditions were nearly 100 times more likely to be at a diagnostically classifiable level of depression than were children who had experienced none of the adversities. Similarly sharp increases in likelihood of maladjustment have been found among sociodemographically diverse community samples of children [Williams 1990; Sterling et al. 1985], and in samples with distinct hardship, such as children with a psychiatrically disabled parent [Sameroff et al. 1987].

## Child Resources for Children Experiencing Multiple and Chronic Adversities

Child characteristics may enhance resilience in adverse conditions because they foster mastery of key developmental tasks, moderate potentially negative effects of adversities, prevent adversities from escalating, or enable children to obtain other key resources. For example, sound bio-behavioral organization and positive disposition in infancy and early childhood may strongly favor positive adaptation to adverse conditions in multiple ways. In several studies of high-risk groups of children, a parent's perception of his or her young child as easy to engage [Werner & Smith 1982] or as well-regulated and positive in mood [Wyman, Cowen, et al. 1991, 1999] predicted healthy subsequent adaptation for children. The preceding individual differences, which may in part reflect inherited temperament [Rothbart & Ahadi 1994], can influence how parents and others interact with children. For example, several studies have found that parents interact less positively and more punitively with temperamentally difficult children than with their siblings who are perceived as less difficult [Lee & Bates 1985; Rutter & Quinton 1984]. Findings from a recent prospective study suggest that temperament may affect children's susceptibility to adverse rearing experiences, which are particularly likely for families living in adversity. Specifically, among a sample of infant boys, those who were high in negative emotionality were more adversely affected by poor parenting, compared to boys lower in negative emotionality [Belsky et al. 1998].

For older children, a number of child qualities are linked to enhanced adaptation for children in adversity. These attributes reflect the increasing differentiation and organization of behavior with age. Several of these resources appear both to promote attainment of developmental objectives and to protect from exposure and escalation of life stressors. These resources include: intelligence and evidence of good intellectual function [Kandel et al. 1988; Masten & Coatsworth 1998]; social competence, including effective interpersonal problem-solving skills and sensitivity to others' experiences [Cowen et al. 1992; Parker et al. 1990]; internal and realistic attributions of control about life adversities [Cowen et al. 1992; Wannon 1990]; and sound self-system functioning as reflected by positive self-efficacy, self-worth, and positive expectations for the future [Cicchetti et al. 1993; Wyman et al. 1993].

Intelligence appears to enhance numerous adaptation processes. Children with good intellectual functioning, for example, are more likely to succeed in school, which not only enhances attainment of key developmental objectives (i.e., educational, social), but also can promote efficacy and associations with other high-achieving children [Masten & Coatsworth 1998]. The important role of sound cognitive functioning in adaptation may also be due to the role of cognitive processes that mediate children's experience of specific life adversities. A child's attribution of personal control regarding life stressors is one such process. In studies of urban children exposed to multiple adversities, well-adjusted children reported less control over stressors deemed uncontrollable (e.g., parental divorce or alcohol use) and more control over stressors deemed controllable (e.g., interpersonal conflicts) [Cowen et al. 1992; Wannon 1990]. The ability to accurately perceive problems that they can and cannot control may facilitate children's disengagement from ongoing negative processes and promote children's engagement in age-appropriate tasks.

Other aspects of children's organization of self-experience are important in adaptation to environmental challenges. For example, Wyman, Kilmer, et al. [1999] identified a cluster of child self-rated characteristics among 7- to 9-year-old urban children that reflected self-system competence (e.g., perceptions of competence, self-worth, and positive future expectations). Positive self-system competence, above and beyond the effects of parenting competence, distinguished well-adjusted from sociodemographically comparable, maladjusted children who shared the common risk of chronic life stress. There is some evidence that aspects of the self-system can have protective effects. In an earlier study with highly stressed 9- to 12-year-old urban children, Wyman et al. [1993] found that positive future expectations predicted enhanced school adjustment over a 3-year period, and that positive expectations attenuated the negative effects of high adversity on perceptions of competence.

## Familial and Extrafamilial Resources

Findings from first generation studies of childhood resilience demonstrated that the quality and continuity of caregiving children experienced significantly predicted differences in their adaptation to adversity [Masten et al. 1990; Rutter, Cox, et al. 1975; Rutter, Yule, et al. 1975; Werner & Smith 1982, 1992]. Many life adversities involve a negative effect on the caregiving system. For example, they may lead to separation from caregivers (e.g., death of a parent, family dissolution), or impairment of caregivers (e.g., substance abuse, psychiatric disorder). These early studies suggested that the continued satisfaction of basic relational needs in the face of these disrupting adversities is a central factor accounting for successful adaptation [Masten 1994; Masten & Coatsworth 1998].

More recent studies have sought to identify salient dimensions within the caregiving system that enhance adaptation at different ages and to clarify the processes involved. For example, Wyman, Cowen, et al. [1999] identified parents' nurturant involvement with their children during preschool and school age periods, more positive expectations, consistent discipline practices, appropriate developmental expectations, and emotionally responsive parenting attitudes, as predictors of positive adaptation among 7- to 9-year-old urban children exposed to multiple, chronic life adversity. An additional finding was that competent, responsive caregiving was a direct, proximal predictor of children's positive adjustment, and a mediator of contextual resources such as parent education and health.

Other studies indicate that children's caregiving systems can be protective by preventing the exacerbation of ongoing adversities, or by preventing new ones from occurring. In a study examining change in conduct problems, Gest et al. [1993] found evidence for such a protective process during the period across middle childhood to adolescence. Specifically, children who experienced more competent parenting in middle childhood were less likely to report adversity in adolescence, which in turn was associated with a modest decrease in conduct problems. Similarly, several studies have found that strict parental supervision and control can play a highly protective function for youth in neighborhoods where violence and delinquency rates are high [Baldwin et al. 1990; Patterson & Stouthamer-Loeber 1984].

A principal focus of our approach to understanding resilience has been to identify how changes that occur with development can open up opportunities for enhanced adaptation. One such significant change across development is that children interact in an increasingly broader social context (i.e., in schools, peer groups). New relational opportunities within those settings have been shown to provide new, important resources with the potential for altering developmental trajectories [Werner & Smith 1982; 1992]. As one case in point, studies of both inner-city youth and youth raised in institutions found that those who attained a positive, cohabiting partner were more likely to show positive adjustive changes, including, for some, a switch out of conduct disorder toward more prosocial behavior [Quinton et al. 1993; Pickles & Rutter 1991].

One intriguing implication of the preceding findings is that children, as they develop, can draw on a broader range of resources to adapt to adversity. Early developmental realities dictate that salient resources will be in children's caregiving and self-systems. With increasing age, however, children can draw on more complex and differentiated combinations of resources such as peers, adults outside the family, and competencies in a range of roles across different settings. The specific resources that children draw on, however, may depend on their prior life experience and development. One study found that a history of early neglect or abuse influenced the types of resources children were likely to draw on for enhancing adaptation. Specifically, positive adjustment over time for children with histories of parental neglect or abuse was more likely to be associated with enhancements in personal mastery and competence. In contrast, relational resources figured prominently in positive adaptation for nonabused or nonneglected children [Cicchetti & Rogosch 1997].

## Cumulative Competence Promotion and Stress Protection

There are many challenges for interventions to enhance wellness for children facing chronic and multiple adversities. Interventions that focus on a child's adaptation to one adversity, for example, may not address other concurrent life stressors or prepare children for adaptation to future adversities. Moreover, achievement of wellness outcomes also depends on a child's access to resources that may be unavailable in their social context [Wyman, Cowen, et al. 1999].

Cumulative protection [Coie et al. 1993; Masten & Coatsworth 1998; Masten & Wright 1998] describes a promising intervention strategy designed to address ongoing challenges to adaptation. The intent of cumulative protection is the promotion of multiple resources and amelioration of multiple risks. Through enhancement of resources across levels of children's developmental systems, a cumulative protection approach seeks to establish a foundation upon which children successfully negotiate challenges across childhood and adolescence [Masten & Coatsworth 1998].

We propose the term *"cumulative competence promotion and stress protection"* to describe how interventions can be enhanced by attention to the two primary processes of adaptation outlined in the organizational-developmental model of resilience. These processes are: (a) enhancing protection from the negative effects (emotional, cognitive, behavioral) of adverse experiences and conditions; and (b) facilitating positive mastery of normative developmental objectives. The likelihood that these goals will facilitate enduring positive adaptation appears greater if two conditions are met. First, resources should be enhanced across different systems of the child's developmental context (child, familial, and community). Second, the effects of interventions may be more enduring if they promote the organization of resources across levels (including children's self-regulation) linking competencies between and among systems.

There are many protective processes [Rutter 1990] that interventions can seek to enhance. For illustrative purposes, we highlight two such processes. The first involves creating environments that minimize a child's exposure to adversities. During infancy and early childhood, for example, exposure to adversities is largely a function of a small number of dyadic, caregiver-child relationships. Enhancing the caregiver's own functioning and resources is a principal means of decreasing young children's exposure to adverse conditions. With increasing age, children's protection involves monitoring children's activities, keeping them from adverse environments, and providing children access to environments that nurture healthy development (e.g., preschool settings, prosocial peers).

The second protective process involves preventing escalation of adversities. Despite the best efforts at protection, children will experience multiple adverse events. Children will develop serious illnesses, family disruptions will occur, and children will experience problems with friends and in school. Child and family responses to adversities can either escalate the adversities, by transforming discrete events into chronic negative conditions, or responses can facilitate successful resolution of an adversities and create new stable structures for positive development. For example, children with difficult tempera-

ments react to changes and adversities in ways that elicit noncon-
structive parental responses [Rutter & Quinton 1984]. Similarly,
parental distress in adverse conditions can lead to ineffective parenting
and increased child behavior problems [Simons et al. 1993]. Children's
increased behavior problems may, in turn, lead to increasing parental
distress. However, enhancement of a child's biobehavioral organization during infancy and early childhood may prevent the escalation of
adversities in the family. Further, interventions that improve parents'
functioning and decrease their distress (e.g., parenting skills, education, employment) may decrease children's exposure to ongoing
family adversity.

Figure 2 illustrates several intervention objectives for infancy and
early childhood that draw on the goals of cumulative competence
promotion and stress protection. The model illustrates enhancement
of resources in multiple systems within a child's developmental
context that incorporates the twin goals of increasing developmental
task enhancement and decreasing the occurrence and negative effects
of adversities. Enhancement of child health and emotionally responsive caregiving, for example, promotes a regulated caregiver-child
relationship, within which children master many primary developmental objectives (e.g., affect regulation, attachment) [Carlson &
Sroufe 1995]. Likewise, enhancement of parental resources can decrease familial adversities and prevent escalation of existing problems. The figure shows how intervention effects can be incorporated
into the child's self-system, the parental caregiving system, and the
extra-familial support system through developmental reorganization. These strengthened systems become resources that children can
draw on for subsequent adaptative challenges.

Two types of intervention models have demonstrated effectiveness in enhancing wellness outcomes for children experiencing multiple and chronic adversities. Their success illustrates the potential for
interventions that can achieve the goals of cumulative competence
promotion and stress protection. The first models discussed below are
comprehensive home visitation programs [Hardy & Street 1989; Olds
et al. 1986; Olds & Kitzman 1993] that have targeted children and
their principal caregivers from the prenatal period into early childhood. Similarly, successful preschool enrichment programs [Campbell
& Ramey 1995; Horacek et al. 1987; Schweinhart & Weikart 1988]

# Figure 2. Intervention Model for Cumulative Competence Promotion and Stress Protection

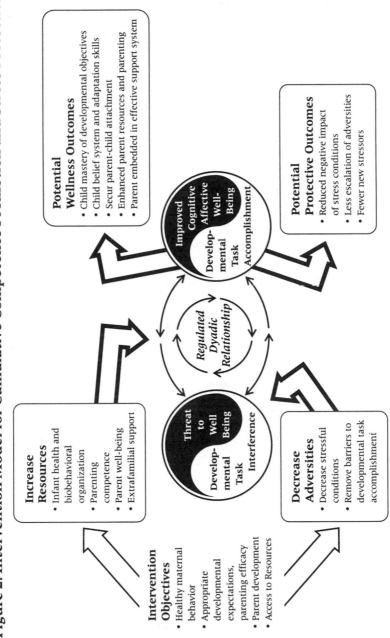

emphasize a comprehensive intervention strategy to enhance parenting competence, family support, and family access to psychosocial resources, and to increase cognitive, social, and emotional stimulation for children.

The home visitation program developed by Olds and colleagues exemplifies an early life intervention that promotes multiple competence-enhancing and protective processes [Olds et al. 1986]. In brief overview, this program targeted first-time mothers, who had one or more of several risk criteria (i.e., poverty, single parent status, or young age). Home visitations by community health nurses, which began during pregnancy, occurred for up to two years and focused on: a) the mother's behavior and knowledge about how to promote infant health and development, and b) the mother's own use of formal and informal support services.

Benefits of the program have been most strongly evident for groups who have received longer (i.e., two years) home visitation. Participating mothers demonstrated healthier behavior during pregnancy, had fewer birth complications, and had fewer low birthweight children compared to mothers who did not receive the intervention. After the two-year program, mothers were providing more age-appropriate stimulation and involvement to their children. Longer-term benefits were evident for both children and mothers. For example, children in the program, compared to controls, demonstrated more positive cognitive development and fewer adverse medical conditions. Mothers had better educational and work records, which improved the environment for both child and mother and is an important example of a long-term protective process. Importantly, several initial program outcomes (e.g., lower rates of child maltreatment, more positive developmental outcomes among children) were found to endure for up to 15 years [Olds et al. 1997].

## Children Experiencing Parental Divorce: Resilience and Intervention

This section will discuss resilience and interventions to promote resilience for children who have experienced divorce. Divorce is one of the most prevalent major stressors, experienced by over 40% of children in the United States before they become adults [Cherlin 1992]. Negative consequences of divorce include increased mental health and substance use problems [Chase-Lansdale et al.1995; Zill et al. 1993; Needle et al. 1990] and decreased competence in areas such as academic achievement [Guidabaldi & Perry 1985] and beliefs about positive self-worth [Parish & Wigle 1985]. However, negative outcomes are not inevitable, and research has identified sources of resilience for children who experience parental divorce and interventions that promote positive outcomes.

## Divorce and Multiple Adversities

Although divorce is almost universally experienced as an aversive event by children, marked by the separation of the parents, its most important effects on children are attributable to the multiple changes that follow. The process of transition in the family structure involving multiple changes can often lead to additional adversities [Felner et al. 1988]. Divorce-related adversities, such as interparental conflict, children's loss of time with parents, moves, economic problems, and parental distress, may occur over a prolonged period of time. Many postdivorce stressors occur in the domain of family relations, involve interpersonal losses and conflict, and are often not easily controllable by children [Sandler et al. 1988]. Children who experience more postdivorce stressors manifest more mental health problems [Sandler et al. 1991], and resilience research seeks to identify the process by which this occurs so those processes can be altered. For example, interparental conflict may lead to increased problems by threatening emotional security, decreasing effective parenting, and distracting children from accomplishing stage-appropriate developmental tasks [Cummings & Davies 1994]. The challenge for resilience research is to identify factors that affect the level of adversities that occur following divorce, to explain how children are protected from the effects of divorce-related adversities, and to identify how interventions might build resilience where it does not naturally occur.

## Child Characteristics as Sources of Resilience Following Parental Divorce

Because children cannot control the occurrence of many divorce-related stressors, their individual resources that moderate their experience of divorce stressors may be most helpful in protecting them from the negative effects of these stressors. We distinguish children's relatively stable traits or belief systems from the specific actions and processes by which they adapt to divorce stressors.

Empirical studies have identified four stable child resources as being related to the quality of children's adjustment following divorce: (1) control beliefs [Kim et al. 1997]; (2) positive and negative cognitive biases in interpreting divorce stressors [Mazur et al. 1992; Mazur et al. 1999]; (3) interpersonal understanding [Kurdek et al. 1981]; and (4) temperament [Lengua et al. 1998]. These relatively stable child characteristics may facilitate healthy postdivorce adjustment because they enable children to adapt to specific divorce-related stressors in ways that protect their emotional well-being and enable them to accomplish developmental tasks.

Research has begun to identify the processes by which children adapt to divorce stressors and to identify those that may be more protective. Three aspects of adaptation processes can be conceptualized. These are: (1) children's appraisal of postdivorce stressors; (2) the strategies children use to cope with stressors; and (3) children's perceptions of their coping efficacy.

Appraisals of threat involve children's subjective evaluations of the degree to which needs such as goals, commitments, and relationships are threatened by the stressor. For example, interparental conflicts are seen as more threatening to children who believe that they have played a role in originating the conflict or that they may be physically harmed. Sheets et al. [1996] studied children's appraisals of negative events that occurred following parental divorce and found that more negative appraisals of divorce stressors predicted greater mental health problems over and above the reported occurrence of divorce events. Appraisals that enable children to evaluate stressors as less personally threatening may help protect them from the negative effects of divorce events.

Coping is defined as what children think or do to adapt in stressful situations. Sandler, Tein, and West [1994] studied the relations between coping and children's postdivorce adjustment problems. They found that active coping (a combination of problem solving and positive thinking) predicted lower depression, prospectively, and buffered the effects of stress on conduct problems in a cross-sectional model. Each of the two aspects of active coping may be protective for different types of divorce stressors. For events that are more easily controlled by children, problem solving coping may be more adaptive, while for less controllable events, children may benefit from cognitively reframing them in ways that promote reassurance and optimism. On the other hand, avoidant coping related to higher internalizing and externalizing problems cross-sectionally, but did not predict adjustment problems in prospective analyses. Avoidant coping may be maladaptive because it keeps children from dealing with stressors in ways that allow them to either resolve the problems or to obtain a positive, more reassuring interpretation of the problem.

Coping efficacy is defined as children's evaluations of the success of their coping efforts to meet the demands of stressful situations [Lazarus & Folkman 1984]. Sandler, Tein, Mehta, Wolchik, and Ayers [in press] assessed perceptions of coping efficacy in a sample of children of divorce. They found consistent support, in both cross-sectional and prospective longitudinal analyses, for coping efficacy as a mediator of the relations between active coping and internalizing problems. Active coping related to higher perceived coping efficacy, which in turn accounted for the relations between active coping and fewer psychological problems. This study provides evidence that the protective effects of coping may be mediated by increasing children's perceptions that they can effectively deal with the problems in their lives.

Several studies have begun to investigate links between stable child resources and the processes children engage in to adapt to divorce [Lengua et al. 1999]. Kim-Bae, Sandler, and MacKinnon [1998], for example, found that negative appraisals of divorce stress mediated the relations between locus of control beliefs and symptoms. Theoretically, there is an iterative process that occurs over time, whereby children's control beliefs affect their appraisals of divorce stressors, which feed back to affect development of their control beliefs and the processes they engage in to adapt to future stressors.

## Social Environmental Relations as Sources of Resilience

Parental divorce affects key caregiving relationships as well as other systems that comprise the child's developmental context. Divorce can fundamentally alter both the continuity and quality of relationships with parents. For many children of divorce, the quality and amount of contact with parents decrease markedly as divorce-induced stress and "task overload" lead to parental distress and distraction from the parenting role. Disruptions in other microsystem-level relationships also occur. For example, relocation disrupts peer social networks and requires adjustment to new school environments, and the frequency and nature of contact with grandparents and other relatives are altered. In addition, divorce is often followed by other transitions in family composition as parents develop new intimate relations and children acquire new stepfamily relations. The number of marital transitions children experience has been related to significant increases in children's mental health problems [Capaldi & Patterson 1991]. Children's social relationships may promote resilience by preventing the occurrence of some of these adverse changes or by protecting children from their negative impact. In addition, key social relations may facilitate children's successful involvement in accomplishing stage-salient developmental tasks. Below we discuss how resilience is promoted by the three most well-studied microsystems: the mother-child relationship, the father-child relationship, and relationships with peers.

Children and adolescents whose mothers, following divorce, provide high levels of warmth, affection, and effective, consistent discipline experience fewer behavior problems, higher self-esteem, and better academic performance than children with low-quality mother-child relationships [e.g., Capaldi & Patterson 1991; Emery & Forehand 1994; Forehand et al. 1990; Guidubaldi et al. 1983; Hess & Camara 1979; Hetherington et al. 1992; Peterson & Zill, 1986; Wolchik, West, et al. 1993]. There is also evidence that high-quality mother-child relationships mitigate the negative effects of divorce stressors on psychological adjustment and competencies for children, although such evidence has not been found for adolescents [Camara & Resnick 1987; Hetherington et al. 1982; Wolchik et al. 1998; Summers et al. 1998].

Mother-child relationships may protect children from the negative effects of divorce by influencing how children appraise and cope with divorce stress. High-quality relationships may: (1) reduce fears of abandonment, which partially mediate the relation between negative divorce events and adjustment problems [Tein et al. 1996]; (2) promote children's sense of belonging, which may reduce the threat of divorce stressors [Kliewer et al. 1994]; and (3) convey the notion that support or assistance is available [Kliewer et al. 1994], which may lead to enhanced efficacy beliefs or more adaptive coping strategies. Additionally, mothers who have high-quality relationships with their children may actively shield them from exposure to divorce-related stressors, such as interparental conflict and financial concerns. It is also possible that warm, affectionate, and consistent caregiving mothers may facilitate the mastery of stage-salient developmental tasks by supporting the child's engagement in stage-salient activities such as schoolwork and social activities.

Although there is mixed support for the positive impact of frequency of child-father (noncustodial parent) contact on children's postdivorce adjustment [see Amato 1993], recent research suggests that factors such as interparental conflict and the noncustodial parent's psychological adjustment may moderate the relationship between contact and adaptation [Healy et al. 1990; Kline et al. 1991]. Further, the few studies that have examined the quality, versus quantity, of this relationship fairly consistently indicate that higher quality relationships are associated with better postdivorce adjustment [e.g., Clarke-Stewart & Hayward 1996; Simons et al. 1994; Tschann et al. 1989]. Similar to mother-child relationships, high-quality father-child relationships may promote positive adaptation by providing developmentally-enhancing interactions and opportunities, strengthening individual resources or processes of adaptation, or reducing children's exposure to divorce stressors in the father-child relationship, such as paternal depression or derogation of the ex-spouse. Furthermore, high-quality father-child relationships may be associated with increased monetary support by fathers, thereby reducing the occurrence of financial difficulties in the family. Finally, high-quality father-child relations may reduce task overload experienced by the custodial mother, which may in turn increase the quality of the mother-child relationship.

The limited research on the role of peer networks suggests that high-quality, supportive relationships promote positive adaptation

[Cowen, Pedro-Carroll, et al. 1990; Lustig et al. 1992]. The protective effects of these relationships may occur because they keep children engaged in mastering developmentally appropriate activities that promote competencies. Alternatively, these relationships may provide emotional support and advice that alter children's internal representations of divorce stressors by enhancing perceptions of self-worth or facilitating effective coping.

## Interventions for Children of Divorce

Preventive interventions for children of divorce have been designed to promote one of two primary goals: (a) enhance children's ability to adapt to divorce stress, or (b) facilitate effective parenting after divorce. Although interventions for children of divorce are widespread, less than a dozen have been evaluated in an experimental or quasi-experimental fashion. Of those that have been evaluated, results have generally been positive, indicating that these programs promote increases in competencies and decreases in symptomatology among participating children. Although there has been little research on the mediating mechanisms by which these programs work, the organizational-developmental framework of resilience is useful for conceptualizing these mechanisms.

Interventions that work directly with children are designed primarily to modify their emotional and cognitive responses so that they are protected from the negative effects of divorce stress. Grych and Fincham [1997] note that child-focused interventions generally seek to accomplish three tasks: (1) provide a supportive environment composed of peers experiencing similar adversities; (2) increase accuracy of children's understanding of divorce; and (3) teach skills for coping with divorce stressors. In the Children of Divorce Intervention Project (CODIP) [Pedro-Carroll & Cowen 1985], for example, the most widely evaluated child-focused intervention to date, a supportive group environment is fostered within the first few sessions by having children share common divorce-related experiences and feelings. Like most child-focused interventions, the majority of substantive material in CODIP is geared toward improving children's understanding of divorce and their coping skills. To improve children's cognitive understanding of divorce, information about the divorce process is provided and common misconceptions, such as blame and unrealistic control beliefs, are corrected. Adaptive coping efforts are encouraged through instruction in problem-solving, communication, and anger management skills [Pedro-Carroll & Cowen, 1985; Pedro-Carroll et al. 1992]. Controlled evaluations with diverse groups of children have shown that children who participate in CODIP, relative to children from intact and divorced homes who do not, show fewer misconceptions about divorce and improvements in problem-solving and communication skills [Alpert-Gillis et al. 1989; Pedro-Carroll & Alpert-Gillis 1997; Pedro-Carroll et al. 1992; Pedro-Carroll & Cowen 1985; Pedro-Carroll et al. 1986].

According to the organizational-developmental framework, one would expect that these enhanced adaptation processes would strengthen children's competencies and adjustment. Indeed, several studies show that CODIP participants show gains in quality of adjustment in both the home and school settings [Alpert-Gillis et al. 1989; Pedro-Carroll & Alpert-Gillis 1997; Pedro-Carroll et al. 1992; Pedro-Carroll & Cowen 1985; Pedro-Carroll et al. 1986], with some effects maintained up to two years postintervention [Pedro-Carroll et al. 1999]. However, mediational analyses to determine specific links between changes in children's cognition and coping skills and changes in their long-term well-being have not yet been done in this or other child-focused programs [Grych & Fincham 1992, 1997].

A second category of intervention for children of divorce focuses on custodial parents, to enhance their postdivorce parenting behavior. The New Beginnings Project, developed by Wolchik and colleagues, is a parent-focused intervention for custodial mothers that teaches effective discipline strategies and parenting practices to strengthen mother-child relationships. These practices include positive family activities, use of listening skills, and the use of positive reinforcement [Wolchik et al. 1993, 1999]. Another parent-focused intervention, developed by Forgatch and DeGarmo [1999], emphasizes the use of noncoercive discipline practices. Controlled evaluations of these parenting-focused programs have demonstrated program efficacy in improving parenting and reducing adjustment problems. Moreover, mediational analyses have found that improvements in mother-child relationship quality and discipline [Wolchik et al. 1999] account for improvements in child adjustment. The extent to which these improvements in child adjustment are stable changes, which might influence future efforts at adaptation to adversity, is unknown. However, Wolchik et al. [1999] report that improvements in children's adjustment problems are maintained among children of participating mothers at least six months postintervention.

The organizational developmental model we have presented suggests that the stability of positive effects of these programs will be a function of how well interventions create individual and family systems that promote children's success in developmental tasks, reduce the occurrence of future stressors, and protect children from negative changes that occur as the family restructures. For example, children with positive coping efficacy beliefs and with good communication skills should have enhanced ability to adapt effectively to future adversities [Sandler et al., in press] and to prevent acute stressors from becoming chronic. Likewise, more effective parents may create home environments with fewer adversities, such as family distress and conflict, and in which acute adversities do not escalate to become chronic conditions for children and families.

Thus, the stability of positive benefits of these programs may depend on whether enhancement of specific developmental competencies or risk/protective processes have radiating positive benefits throughout the individual and family systems. There is some early evidence that this may occur. For example, although both the Wolchik and Forgatch parenting programs were designed to affect parenting and did not directly address the parents' own mental health, parents in both programs showed a decrease in psychological symptoms. These positive changes, if maintained over time, can be expected to reduce the occurrence of stressors that impact the child.

Theoretically, the greatest long-term benefit would be derived from cumulative competence promotion and stress protection programs that improve the multiple child and family sources of resilience for children of divorce. However, such comprehensive interventions have yet to demonstrate their efficacy. For example, the additive effects of programs that simultaneously enhance parenting and children's coping have not yet been demonstrated. Three empirical studies have tested additive protective intervention models that combined child and parent interventions [Stolberg & Garrison 1985; Stolberg & Mahler 1994; Wolchik et al. 1998], and none of them have demonstrated significant additive effects of the interventions. More research is needed on how to design optimal interventions to promote multiple complementary paths to resilience in this population.

## Summary and Conclusion

In order to conceptualize interventions that promote resilience, this chapter first considered several basic theoretical issues. These issues included a conceptualization of adverse conditions, sources of resilience resources, and the mediating processes of adaptation that lead to healthy outcomes under conditions of adversity. We believe that the articulation of these conceptual processes will be fruitful in organizing and guiding future theoretical research on resilience, in conceptualizing future interventions, and in evaluating the mechanisms by which interventions work to promote resilience. By systematically testing the effects of strengthening resilience resources, we believe that a great deal will be learned about human resilience and, indeed, about society's ability to improve the wellness of children living in conditions of adversity.

We have outlined broad elements of an intervention strategy, cumulative competence promotion and stress protection, which incorporates knowledge from the resilience and the stress and coping research traditions. Findings from both research traditions support promoting multiple resources to enhance children's resilience. Furthermore, evaluation of such interventions needs to adopt a broad perspective, with the expectation that the effects of a successful intervention may reverberate through multiple systems, including the individual child, family, and, when delivered on a community or school-wide basis, on macrosystems as well. Although one effect of a successful intervention may be to decrease the occurrence of future adverse conditions, it is expected that negative events will continue to occur and that effective coping with prior events should strengthen skills to cope adaptively with later events. Effective coping in turn should facilitate children's efficacy and positive expectations, which will enable them to engage successfully with age-appropriate developmental tasks under adverse conditions. Similarly, effective parenting under adverse conditions should strengthen parenting skills, which will be an important resource helping the family adapt to later stressors.

The resilience literature has focused on identifying resources that lead to successful accomplishment of age-appropriate developmental tasks under conditions of adversity [Masten & Coatsworth 1998]. Mastery of age-appropriate tasks may have the long-term effect of helping children build the skills necessary for successfully meeting later developmental tasks. Success in earlier developmental tasks may also channel children into environmental conditions where later adversities are less likely to occur, and to build resources (e.g., positive self-system) that enable them to adapt more successfully when adversities do occur. Thus, concepts from the stress and coping literature and from the resilience literature are complementary in conceptualizing interventions to promote resilience.

## Notes

1. The preparation of this chapter was supported, in part, by the William T. Grant Foundation.

2. The first two authors contributed equally to the writing of this chapter.

3. Although these are conditions that primarily affect the individual, they also create problematic relationships between the individual child and the environment.

## References

Abramson, L. Y., Seligman, M. E. P., & Teasdale, J. D. (1978). Learned helplessness in humans: Critique and reformulation. *Journal of Abnormal Psychology, 87*, 49–74.

Adrian, C. & Hammen, C. (1993). Stress exposure and stress generation in children of depressed mothers. *Journal of Consulting and Clinical Psychology, 61*, 354–359.

Alpert-Gillis, L. J., Pedro-Carroll, J. L., & Cowen, E. L. (1989). The Children of Divorce Intervention Program: Development, implementation, and evaluation of a program for young urban children. *Journal of Consulting and Clinical Psychology, 57,* 583–589.

Amato, P. R. (1993). Children's adjustment to divorce: Theories, hypotheses, and empirical support. *Journal of Marriage and the Family, 55,* 23–38.

Avison, W. R. & Gotlib, I. H. (1994). Introduction and overview. In W. R. Avison & I. H. Gotlib (Eds.), *Stress and mental health: Contemporary issues and prospects for the future* (pp. 3–15). New York: Plenum.

Ayers, T., S., Sandler, I. N., & Twohey, J. (1998). Conceptualization and measurement of coping in children and adolescents. In T. H. Ollendick & R. J. Prinz (Eds.), *Advances in clinical child psychology* (Vol. 20) (pp. 243–301). New York: Plenum Press.

Baldwin, A. L., Baldwin, C., & Cole, R. E. (1990). Stress-resistant families and stress-resistant children. In J. Rolf, A. S. Masten, D. Cicchetti, K. H. Nuechterlein, & S. Weintraub (Eds.), *Risk and protective factors in the development of psychopathology* (pp. 257–280). New York: Cambridge University Press.

Baldwin, A. L., Baldwin, C. P., Kasser, T., Zax, M., Sameroff, A., & Seifer, R. (1993). Contextual risk and resiliency during late adolescence. *Development and Psychopathology, 5,* 741–761.

Belsky, J., Hsieh, K., & Crnic, K. (1998). Mothering, fathering, and infant negativity as antecedents of boys' externalizing problems and inhibition at age 3 years: Differential susceptibility to rearing experience? *Development and Psychopathology, 10,* 301–319.

Brazelton, T. B., Koslowski, B., & Main, M. (1974). The origins of reciprocity: The early mother-infant interaction. In M. Lewis & L. Rosenblum (Eds.), *The effect of the infant on its caregiver* (pp. 49–76). New York: Wiley.

Brown, G. W. & Harris, T. O. (1989). *Life events and illness.* New York: Guilford Press.

Camara, K. A. & Resnick, G. (1987). Marital and parental subsystems in mother-custody, father-custody and two-parent households: Effects on children's social development. In J. Vincent (Ed.), *Advances in family assessment, intervention and research* (Vol. 4) (pp. 165–196). Greenwich, CT: JAI.

Campbell, F. A. & Ramey, C. T. (1995). Cognitive and school outcomes for high-risk African-American students at middle adolescence: Positive effects of early intervention. *American Educational Research Journal, 32,* 743–772.

Capaldi, D. M. & Patterson, G.R. (1991). Relation of parental transitions to boys' adjustment problems: I. A linear hypothesis. II. Mothers at risk for transitions and unskilled parenting. *Developmental Psychology, 27(3)*, 489–504.

Carlson, E. A. & Sroufe, L. A. (1995). Contributions of attachment theory to developmental psychopathology. In D. Cicchetti & D. J. Cohen (Eds.), *Developmental psychopathology: Theory and methods* (Vol. 1) (pp. 581–617). New York: John Wiley & Sons.

Chase-Lansdale, P. L., Cherlin, A. J., & Kiernan, K. E. (1995). The long-term effects of parental divorce on the mental health of young adults: A developmental perspective. *Child Development, 66*, 1614–1634.

Cherlin, A. J. (1992). *Marriage, divorce and remarriage.* Cambridge, MA: Harvard University Press.

Cicchetti, D. & Garmezy, N. (1993). Prospects and promises in the study of resilience. *Development and Psychopathology, 5*, 497–502.

Cicchetti, D. & Rogosch, F. A. (1997). The role of self-organization in the promotion of resilience in maltreated children. *Development and Psychopathology, 9*, 797–815.

Cicchetti, D., Rogosch, F. A., Lynch, M., & Holt, K. D. (1993). Resilience in maltreated children: Processes leading to adaptive outcomes. *Development and Psychopathology, 5*, 629–648.

Cicchetti, D. & Schneider-Rosen, K. (1986). An organizational approach to childhood depression. In M. Rutter, C. Izard, & P. Read (Eds.), *Depression in young people: Clinical and developmental perspectives* (pp. 71–134). New York: Guilford Press.

Cicchetti, D. & Sroufe, L. A. (1978). An organization view of affect: Illustration from the study of Down's syndrome infants. In M. Lewis & L. Rosenblum (Eds.), *The development of affect* (pp. 309–350). New York: Plenum Press.

Clarke-Stewart, K. A. & Hayward, C. (1996). Advantages of father custody and contact for the psychological well-being of school-age children. *Journal of Applied Developmental Psychology, 17*, 239–270.

Coddington, R. D. (1972). The significance of life events as etiologic factors in the diseases of children: II. A study of a normal population. *Journal of Psychosomatic Research, 1b*, 205–213.

Coie, J. D., Watt, N. F., West, S. G., Hawkins, J. D., Asarnow, J. R., Markman, H. J., Ramey, S. L., Shure, M. B., & Long, B. (1993). The science of prevention: A conceptual framework and some directions for a national research program. *American Psychologist, 48,* 1013–1022.

Compas, B. E. (1987). Stress and life events during childhood and adolescence. *Clinical Psychology Review, 7,* 275–302.

Connell, J. P. & Wellborn, J. G. (1991). Competence, autonomy and relatedness: A motivational analysis of self-system processes. In M. Gunnar & L. A. Sroufe (Eds.), *Minnesota Symposium on Child Psychology* (Vol. 23) (pp. 43–77). Chicago: University of Chicago Press.

Cowen, E. L., Pedro-Carroll, J. L., & Alpert-Gillis, L. J. (1990). Relationships between support and adjustment among children of divorce. *Journal of Child Psychology and Psychiatry, 31,* 727–735.

Cowen, E. L., Work, W. C., Wyman, P. A., Parker, G. R., Wannon, M., & Gribble, P. A. (1992). Test comparisons among stress-affected, stress-resilient and nonclassified fourth through sixth grade urban children. *Journal of Community Psychology, 20,* 200–214.

Cowen, E. L., Wyman, P. A., Work, W. C., & Parker, G. R. (1990). The Rochester Child Resilience Project (RCRP): Overview and summary of first year findings. *Development and Psychopathology, 2,* 193–212.

Cowen, E. L. (1991). In pursuit of wellness. *American Psychologist, 46,* 404–408.

Cowen, E. L. (1994). The enhancement of psychological wellness: Challenges and opportunities. *American Journal of Community Psychology, 22,* 149–179.

Cowen, E. L. (1998). In sickness and in health: Primary prevention's vows revisited. In D. Cicchetti & S. L. Toth (Eds.), *Rochester Symposium on Developmental Psychopathology: Vol. 10. Developmental approaches to prevention and intervention* (pp. 1–24). Rochester, NY: University of Rochester Press.

Cummings, E. M. & Davies, P. T. (1994). *Children and marital conflict.* New York: Guilford.

Deci, E. L. & Ryan, R. M. (1985). *Intrinsic motivation and self-determination in human behavior.* New York: Plenum Press.

Durlak, J. A. (1997). *Successful prevention programs for children and adolescents.* New York: Plenum.

Egeland, B., Carlson, E. A., & Sroufe, L. A. (1993). Resilience as process. *Development and Psychopathology, 5,* 517–528.

Eisenberg, N., Fabes, R., & Guthrie, I. K. (1997). Coping with stress: The roles of regulation and development. In S. A. Wolchik & I. N. Sandler (Eds.),

*Handbook of children's coping: Linking theory and intervention.* (pp. 41–73). New York: Plenum.

Elder, G. H., Jr. (1974). *Children of the Great Depression.* Chicago: University of Chicago Press.

Emde, R. (1989). The infant's relationship experience: Developmental and affective aspects. In A. Sameroff & R. Emde (Eds.), *Relationship disturbances in early childhood* (pp. 33–51). New York: Basic Books.

Emery, R. E. & Laumann-Billings, L. (1998). An overview of the nature, causes, and consequences of abusive family relationships: Toward differentiating maltreatment and violence. *American Psychologist, 53,* 121–135.

Emery, R. E. & Forehand, R. (1994). Parental divorce and children's well-being: A focus on resilience. In R. J. Haggerty, M. Rutter & L. Sherrod (Eds.), *Risk and resilience in children.* London: Cambridge University Press.

Epstein, H. (1979). *Children of the Holocaust.* New York: Penguin Books.

Felner, R. D., Terre, L., & Rowlison, R. (1988). A life transition framework for understanding marital dissolution and family reorganization. In S. Wolchik & P. Karoly (Eds.), *Children of divorce: Empirical perspective on adjustment* (pp. 35–66). New York: Gardner Press.

Festinger, T. (1983). *No one ever asked us.* New York: Columbia University Press.

Fogas, B. S., Wolchik, S. A., & Braver, S. L. (1987, August). *Parenting behavior and psychopathology in children of divorce: Buffering effects.* Paper presented at the American Psychological Association Convention, New York, NY.

Forehand, R., McCombs, A. T., Wierson, M., Brody, G., & Fauber, R. (1990). The role of maternal functioning and parenting skills in adolescent functioning following parental divorce. *Journal of Abnormal Psychology, 99,* 278–283.

Forgatch, M. S. & DeGarmo, D. S. (1999). Parenting through change: An effective prevention program for single mothers. *Journal of Consulting and Clinical Psychology, 67,* 711–724.

Garmezy, N. (1970). Process and reactive schizophrenia: Some conceptions and issues. *Schizophrenia Bulletin, 2,* 30–74.

Garmezy, N., Masten, A. S., & Tellegen, A. (1984). The study of stress and competence in children: A building block for developmental psychopathology. *Child Development, 55,* 97–111.

Garmezy, N. & Nuechterlein, K. (1972). Invulnerable children: The fact and fiction of competence and disadvantage. *American Journal of Orthopsychiatry, 42*, 328–329.

Garmezy N. & Rutter, M. (1983). *Stress, coping, and development in children.* New York: McGraw-Hill.

Garmezy, N. & Streitman, S. (1974). Children at risk: The search for antecedents to schizophrenia. Part I: Conceptual models and research methods. *Schizophrenia Bulletin, 8*, 14–90.

Gersten, J. C., Langner, T. S., Eisenberg, T. G., & Simcha-Fagan, O. (1977). An evaluation of the etiologic role of stressful life-change events in psychological disorders. *Journal of Health and Social Behavior, 18*, 228–244.

Gest, S. D., Neeman, J., Hubbard, J. J., Masten, A. S., & Tellegen, A. (1993). Parenting quality, adversity and conduct problems in adolescence: Testing process oriented models of resilience. *Development and Psychopathology, 5*, 663–682.

Gianino, A. & Tronick, E. Z. (1988). The mutual regulation model: The infant's self and interactive regulation coping and defense. In T. Field, P. McCabe, & N. Schneiderman (Eds.), *Stress and coping* (pp. 47–68). Hillsdale, NJ: Erlbaum.

Goodyer, I. M. (1990). Annotation: Recent life events and psychiatric disorder in school age children. *Journal of Child Psychology and Psychiatry, 31*, 839–848.

Goodyer, I. M. (1994). Developmental psychopathology: The impact of recent life events in anxious and depressed school-age children. *Journal of the Royal Society of Medicine, 87*, 327–329.

Goodyer, I. M., Herbert, J., Tamplin, A., Secher, S. M., & Pearson, J. (1997). Short-term outcome of major depression: II. Life events, family dysfunction, and friendship difficulties as predictors of persistent disorder. *Journal of the American Academy of Child and Adolescent Psychiatry, 36*, 474–480.

Grych, J. H. & Fincham, F. D. (1997). Children's adaptation to divorce: From description to explanation. In S. A. Wolchik & I. N. Sandler (Eds.), *Handbook of children's coping: Linking theory and intervention.* New York: Plenum.

Grych, J. H. & Fincham, F. D. (1992). Interventions for children of divorce: Toward greater integration of research and action. *Psychological Bulletin, 111*(3), 434–454.

Guidubaldi, J., Cleminshaw, H., Perry, J., & Kehle, T. J. (1983, August). *Factors affecting the adjustment of children from divorced families.* Paper presented at the Annual Meeting of the American Psychological Association, Anaheim, CA.

Guidabaldi, J. & Perry, J. D. (1985). Divorce and mental health sequelae for children: A two-year follow-up of a nationwide sample. *Journal of the American Academy of Child Psychiatry, 24*, 531–537.

Hammen, C. (1997). Children of depressed parents: The stress context. In S. A. Wolchik & I. N. Sandler (Eds.), *Handbook of children's coping: Linking theory and intervention* (pp. 131–159). New York: Plenum Press.

Hardy, J. B. & Street, R. (1989). Family support and parenting education in the home: An effective extension of clinic-based preventive health care services for poor children. *Pediatrics, 115*, 927–931.

Healy, J. M., Malley, J. E., & Stewart, A. J. (1990). Children and their fathers after parental separation. *American Journal of Orthopsychiatry, 60*, 531–543.

Hess, R. D. & Camara, K. (1979). Post-divorce family relationships as mediating factors in the consequence of divorce for children. *Journal of Social Issues, 25*, 79–96.

Hetherington, E. M. & Camara, K. A. (1984). Families in transition: The process of dissolution and reconstitution. In R. Parks (Ed.), *Review of child development research* (Vol. 7) (pp. 398–439). Chicago: University of Chicago Press.

Hetherington, E. M., Clingempeel, W. G., Anderson, E. R., Deal, J. E., Stanley-Hagan, M., Hollier, E. A., & Lindner, M. S. (1992). Coping with marital transitions: A family systems perspective. *Monographs of the Society for Research in Child Development, 57* (2–3, Serial No. 227).

Hetherington, E. M., Cox, M., & Cox, R. (1982). Effects of divorce on parents and children. In M. Lamb (Ed.), *Nontraditional families* (pp. 233–288). Hillsdale, NJ: Erlbaum.

Horacek, H. J., Ramey, C. T., Campbell, F. A., Hoffmann, K. P., & Fletcher, R. H. (1987). Predicting school failure and assessing early intervention with high-risk children. *Journal of the American Academy of Child and Adolescent Psychiatry, 26*, 758–763.

Jenkins, J. M., Smith, M. A., & Graham, P. J. (1988). Coping with parental quarrels. *Journal of the American Academy of Child and Adolescent Psychiatry, 28*, 182–189.

Kandel, E., Mednick, S. A., Kirkegaard-Sorenson, L., Hutchings, B., Knop, J., Rosenberg, R., & Schulsinger. F. (1988). IQ as protective factor for subjects at high risk for antisocial behavior. *Journal of Consulting and Clinical Psychology, 56*, 224–226.

Kilmer, R. P., Cowen, E. L., Wyman, P. A., Work, W. C., & Magnus, K. B. (1998). Differences in stressors experienced by urban African-American, White and Hispanic children. *Journal of Community Psychology, 26,* 415–428.

Kim, L. S., Sandler, I. N., & Tein, J.-Y. (1997), Locus of control as a stress moderator and mediator in children of divorce. *Journal of Abnormal Child Psychology, 25,* 145–155.

Kim-Bae, L. S., Sandler, I. N., & MacKinnon, D. (1998). *Coping and negative appraisal as mediators between locus of control and psychological symptoms.* Manuscript submitted for publication.

Kliewer, W., Sandler, I. N., & Wolchik, S. A. (1994). Family socialization of threat appraisal and coping: Coaching, modeling, and family context. In K. Hurrelmann & F. Nestmann (Eds.), *Social networks and social support in childhood and adolescence* (pp. 271–291). Berlin: Walter de Gruyter.

Kline, M., Johnston, J. R., & Tschann, J. M. (1991). The long shadow of marital conflict: A model of children's post-divorce adjustment. *Journal of Marriage and the Family, 53,* 297–309.

Kurdek, L. A., Blisk, D., & Siesky, A. E. (1981). Correlates of children's long-term adjustment to their parents' divorce. *Developmental Psychology, 17,* 565–579.

Lahey, B. B., Hartdagen, S. E., Frick, P. J., McBurnett, K., Connor, R., & Hynd, G. W. (1988). Conduct disorder: Parsing the confounded relation of parental divorce and antisocial personality. *Journal of Abnormal Psychology, 97,* 334–337.

Lazarus, R. S. (1991). *Emotion and adaptation.* New York: Oxford University Press.

Lazarus, R. S. & Folkman, S. (1984). *Stress, appraisal and coping.* New York: Springer.

Lee, C. L. & Bates, J. E. (1985). Mother-child interaction at age two years and perceived difficult temperament. *Child Development, 56,* 1314–1325.

Lengua, L., Sandler, I. N., West, S. G., Wolchik, S. A., & Curran, P. J. (1999). Emotionality and self-regulation, threat appraisal and coping in children of divorce. *Development and Psychopathology, 11,* 15–39.

Lengua, L. J., West, S. G., & Sandler, I. N. (1998). Temperament as a predictor of symptomatology in children: Addressing contamination of measures. *Child Development, 69,* 164–182.

Lustig, J. L., Wolchik, S. A., & Braver, S. L. (1992). Social support in chumships and children's adjustment to divorce. *American Journal of Community Psychology, 20,* 393–399.

Luthar, S. & Zigler, E. (1992). Intelligence and social competence among high-risk adolescents. *Development and psychopathology, 4*, 287–301.

Luthar, S. S. (1991). Vulnerability and resilience: A study of high-risk adolescents. *Child Development, 62*, 600–616.

Luthar, S. S. & Zigler, E. (1991). Vulnerability and competence: A review of research on resilience in childhood. *American Journal of Orthopsychiatry, 61*, 6–22.

Lutzke, J. R., Ayers, T. S., Sandler, I. N., & Barr, A. (1999). Risks and interventions for the parentally bereaved child. In S. A. Wolchik & I. N. Sandler (Eds.), *Handbook of children's coping: Linking theory and intervention* (pp. 215–245). New York: Plenum Press.

Masten, A. S. (1994). Resilience in individual development: Successful adaptation despite risk and adversity. In M. Wang & E. Gordon (Eds.), *Risk and resilience in inner city America: Challenges and prospects* (pp. 3–25). Hillsdale, NJ: Erlbaum.

Masten, A. S., Best, K. M., & Garmezy, N. (1990). Resilience and development: Contributions from the study of children who overcome adversity. *Development and Psychopathology, 2*, 425–444.

Masten, A. S. & Coatsworth, J. D. (1995). Competence, resilience and psychopathology. In D. Cicchetti & D. J. Cohen (Eds.), *Developmental psychopathology: Risk, disorder and adaptation* (Vol. 2) (pp. 715–752). New York: Wiley.

Masten, A. S. & Coatsworth, J. D. (1998). The development of competence in favorable and unfavorable environments: Lessons from research on successful children. *American Psychologist, 53*, 205–220.

Masten, A. S. & Wright, M. (1998). Cumulative risk and protection models of child maltreatment. In B. B. R. Rossman & M. S. Rosenberg (Eds.), *Multiple victimization of children: Conceptual, developmental, research and treatment issues* (pp. 7–30). Binghamton, NY: Haworth.

Mazur, E., Wolchik, S., & Sandler, I. N. (1992). Negative cognitive errors and positive illusions for stressful divorce-related events: Predictors of children's psychological adjustment. *Journal of Abnormal Child Psychology, 20*, 523–542.

Mazur, E., Wolchik, S. A., Virdin, L., Sandler, I. N., & West, S. G. (1999). Cognitive mediators of children's adjustment to stressful divorce events: The role of negative cognitive errors and positive illusions. *Child Development, 70*, 231–246.

McLoyd, V. (1998). Socioeconomic disadvantage and child development. *American Psychologist, 53*, 185–204.

Moskovitz, S. (1983). *Love despite hate.* New York: Schocken Books.

Needle, R. H., Su, S., & Doherty, W. J. (1990). Divorce, remarriage, and adolescent substance use: A prospective longitudinal study. *Journal of Marriage and the Family, 52*, 157–169.

Newacheck, P. A. & Stoddard, J. J. (1994). Prevalence and impact of multiple childhood chronic illnesses. *Journal of Pediatrics, 124*, 40–48.

Olds, D., Eckenrode, J., Henderson, C. R. Jr., Kitzman, H., Powers, J., Cole, R., Sidora, K., Morris, P., Pettitt, L. M., & Luckey, D. (1997). Long-term effects of home visitation on maternal life course and child abuse and neglect: 15-year follow-up of a randomized trial. *Journal of the American Medical Association, 278*, 637–643.

Olds, D. L., Henderson, C. R. Jr., Chamberlin, R., & Tatelbaum, R. (1986). Preventing child abuse and neglect: A randomized trial of nurse home visitation. *Pediatrics, 78*, 65–78.

Olds, D. L. & Kitzman, H. (1993). Review of research on home visiting for pregnant women and parents of young children. *The Future of Children, 3*, 53–92.

Parish, T. S. & Wigle, S. E. (1985). A longitudinal study of the impact of parental divorce on adolescents' evaluations of self and parents. *Adolescence, 20*, 239–245.

Parker, G. R., Cowen, E. L., Work, W. C., & Wyman, P. A. (1990). Test correlates of stress resilience among urban school children. *Journal of Primary Prevention, 11*, 19–35.

Patterson, G. R. & Stouthamer-Loeber, M. (1984). The correlation of family management practices and delinquency. *Child Development, 55*, 1299–1307.

Pavenstedt, E. (1965). A comparison of the childrearing environment of upper-lower and very low-lower class families. *American Journal of Orthopsychiatry, 35*, 89–98.

Pedro-Carroll, J. L. & Alpert-Gillis, L. J. (1997). Preventive interventions for children of divorce: A developmental model for 5 and 6 year old children. *The Journal of Primary Prevention, 18*, 5–23.

Pedro-Carroll, J. L., Alpert-Gillis, L. J., & Cowen, E. L. (1992). An evaluation of the efficacy of a preventive intervention for 4th-6th grade urban children of divorce. *The Journal of Primary Prevention, 13*, 115–130.

Pedro-Carroll, J. L. & Cowen, E. L. (1985). The Children of Divorce Intervention Program: An investigation of the efficacy of a school-based prevention program. *Journal of Consulting and Clinical Psychology, 53*, 603–611.

Pedro-Carroll, J. L., Cowen, E. L., Hightower, D., & Guare, J. C. (1986). Preventive intervention with latency-aged children of divorce: A replication study. *American Journal of Community Psychology, 14*(3), 277–290.

Pedro-Carroll, J. L., Sutton, S. E., & Wyman, P. A. (1999). A two-year follow-up evaluation of a preventive intervention for young children of divorce. *School Psychology Review, 28*, 467–476.

Peterson, J. L. & Zill, N. (1986). Marital disruption, parent-child relationships, and behavior problems in children. *Journal of Marriage and the Family, 48*, 295–307.

Pickles, A. & Rutter, M. (1991). Statistical and conceptual models of "turning points" in developmental processes. In D. Magnusson, L. Bergman, G. Rudinger, & B. Torestad (Eds.), *Problems and methods in longitudinal research: Stability and change* (pp. 131–165). Cambridge, UK: Cambridge University Press.

Quinton, D., Pickles, A., Maughan, B., & Rutter, M. (1993). Partners, peers, and pathways: Assortative pairing and continuities in conduct disorder. *Development and Psychopathology, 5*, 763–783.

Reich, J. W. & Zautra, A. J. (1988). Direct and stress-moderating effects of positive life experiences. In L. H. Cohen (Ed.), *Life events and psychological functioning: Theoretical and methodological issues* (pp. 149–180). Newbury Park: Sage.

Robins, L. (1986). The consequences of conduct disorder in girls. In D. Olweus, J. Block, & M. Radke-Yarrow (Eds.), *Development of antisocial and prosocial behavior: Research, theories and issues* (pp. 385–408). San Diego, CA: Academic Press.

Rossman, B. B. R. & Rosenberg, M. S. (1992). Family stress and functioning in children: The moderating effects of children's beliefs about their control over parental conflict. *Journal of Child Psychology and Psychiatry, 33*, 699–715.

Rothbart, M. K. & Ahadi, S. A. (1994). Temperament and the development of personality. *Journal of Abnormal Psychology, 103*, 55–66.

Russell, M., Henderson, C., & Blume, S. (1985). *Children of alcoholics: A review of the literature*. New York: Children of Alcoholics Foundation.

Rutter, M. (1979). Protective factors in children's responses to stress and disadvantage. In M. W. Kent & J. E. Rolf (Eds.), *Primary prevention of psychopathology: Social competence in children* (Vol. 3) (pp. 49–74). Hanover, NH: University Press of New England.

Rutter, M. (1990). Psychosocial resilience and protective mechanisms. In J. Rolf, A. S. Masten, D. Cicchetti, K. H. Nuechterlein, & S. Weintraub (Eds.), *Risk and protective factors in the development of psychopathology* (pp. 181–1214). New York: Cambridge University Press.

Rutter, M., Champion, L., Quinton, D., Maughan, B., & Pickles, A. (1995). Understanding individual differences in environmental risk exposure. In P. Moen, G. H. Elder, & K. Luscher (Eds.), *Examining lives in context: Perspectives on the ecology of human development* (pp. 61–93). Washington, DC: American Psychological Association.

Rutter, M., Cox, A., Tupling, C., Berger, M., & Yule, W. (1975). Attainment and adjustment in two geographical areas: I. The prevalence of psychiatric disorder. *British Journal of Psychiatry, 126,* 493–509.

Rutter, M., Yule, B., Quinton, D., Rowlands, O., Yule, W., & Berger, M. (1975). Attainment and adjustment in two geographical areas: III. Some factors accounting for area differences. *British Journal of Psychiatry, 126,* 520–533.

Rutter, M. & Quinton, D. (1984). Long-term follow-up of women institutionalized in childhood: Factors promoting good functioning in adult life. *British Journal of Developmental Psychology, 18,* 225–234.

Rutter, M. & Sandberg, S. (1992). Psychosocial stressors: Concepts, causes and effects. *European Child and Adolescent Psychiatry, 1,* 3–13.

Sameroff, A. J., Seifer, R., Zax, M., & Barocas, R. (1987). Early indicators of developmental risk: The Rochester Longitudinal Study. *Schizophrenia Bulletin, 13,* 383–394.

Sampson, R. J., Raudenbush, S. W., & Earls, F. (1997). Neighborhoods and violent crime: A multilevel study of collective efficacy. *Science, 277,* 918–924.

Sandler, I. N., Miller, P., Short, J., & Wolchik, S. A. (1989). Social support as a protective factor for children in stress. In D. Belle (Ed.), *Children's social networks and social supports* (pp. 277–307). New York: Wiley.

Sandler, I. N., Wolchik, S. A., Braver, S., & Fogas, B. (1991). Stability and quality of life events and psychological symptomatology in children of divorce. *American Journal of Community Psychology, 19,* 501–520.

Sandler, I. N. & Ramsay, T. B. (1980). Dimensional analysis of children's stressful life events. *American Journal of Community Psychology, 8,* 285–302.

Sandler, I. N., Reynolds, K., Kliewer, W., & Ramirez, R. (1992). Specificity of the relation between life events and psychological symptomatology. *Journal of Clinical Child Psychology, 21,* 240–248.

Sandler, I. N., Tein, J., & West, S. G. (1994). Coping, stress and psychological symptoms of children of divorce: A cross-sectional and longitudinal study. *Child Development, 65,* 1744–1763.

Sandler, I. N., Tein, J.-Y., Mehta, P., Wolchik, S., & Ayers, T. (in press). Coping efficacy and psychological problems of children of divorce. *Child Development.*

Sandler, I. N., Wolchik, S. A., & Braver, S. L. (1988). The stressors of children's postdivorce environments. In S. Wolchik & P. Karoly (Eds.), *Children of divorce: Empirical perspective on adjustment* (pp. 111–145). New York: Gardner Press.

Schweinhart, L. J. & Weikart, D. P. (1988). The High Scope/Perry Preschool Program. In R. H. Price, E. L. Cowen, R. P. Lorion, & J. Ramos-McKay (Eds.), *14 ounces of prevention: A casebook for practitioners* (pp. 53–65). Washington, DC: American Psychological Association.

Seidman, E., Allen, L., Aber, J. L., Mitchell, C., Feinman, J., Yoshikawa, H., Comtois, K. A., Golz, J., Miller, R. L., Ortiz-Torres, B., & Roper, G. C. (1995). Development and validation of adolescent-perceived microsystem scales: Social support, daily hassles, and involvement. *American Journal of Community Psychology, 23,* 335–389.

Selman, R. (1980). *The growth of interpersonal understanding.* New York: Academic Press.

Seltzer, J. A. (1994) Consequences of marital dissolution for children. *Annual Review of Sociology, 20,* 235–266.

Sheets, V., Sandler, I. N., & West, S. (1996). Appraisals of negative events by preadolescent children of divorce. *Child Development, 67,* 2166–2182.

Simons, R. L., Lorenz, F. O., Wu, C.-I., Conger, R. D. (1993). Social network and marital support as mediators and moderators of the impact of stress and depression on parental behavior. *Developmental Psychology, 29,* 368–381.

Simons, R. L., Whitbeck, L. B., Beaman, J., & Conger, R. D. (1994) The impact of mothers' parenting, involvement by nonresidential fathers, and parental conflict on the adjustment of adolescent children. *Journal of Marriage and the Family, 56,* 356–374.

Skinner, E. A. & Wellborn, J. G. (1994). Coping during childhood and adolescence: A motivational perspective. In D. R. Lerner & M. Perlmutter

(Eds.), *Life-span development and behavior* (pp. 91–123). Hillsdale, NJ: Erlbaum.

Skinner, E. A., & Wellborn, J. G. (1997). Children's coping in the academic domain. In S. A. Wolchik & I. N. Sandler (Eds.), *Handbook of children's coping: Linking theory and intervention.* (pp. 387–423). New York: Plenum Press.

Spacarelli, S. (1994). Stress, appraisal and coping in child sexual abuse: A theoretical and empirical review. *Psychological Bulletin, 116*, 340–362.

Sroufe, L. A. (1979). The coherence of individual development: Early care, attachment, and subsequent developmental issues. *American Psychologist, 34*, 834–841.

Sroufe, L. A. (1990). An organizational perspective on the self. In D. Cicchetti & M. Beeghly (Eds.), *The self in transition: Infancy to childhood (*pp. 281–307). Chicago: University of Chicago Press.

Sterling, S., Cowen, E. L., Weissberg, R. P., Lotyczewski, B. S., & Boike, M. (1985). Recent stressful life events and young children's school adjustment. *American Journal of Community Psychology, 13*, 87–98.

Stolberg, A. L. & Garrison, K. M. (1985). Evaluating a primary prevention program for children of divorce. *American Journal of Community Psychology, 13*(2), 111–124.

Stolberg, A. L. & Mahler, J. (1994). Enhancing treatment gains in a school-based intervention for children of divorce through skill training, parental involvement, and transfer procedures. *Journal of Consulting and Clinical Psychology, 63*(1), 147–156.

Summers, P., Forehand, R., & Armistead, L. (1998). Parental divorce during early adolescence in Caucasian families: The role of family process variables in predicting the long-term consequences for early adult psychological adjustment. *Journal of Consulting and Clinical Psychology, 66*, 327–336.

Tein, J. Y., Wolchik, S. A., Wilcox, K. L., & Sandler, I. N. (1996, August). *Mediational role of fear of abandonment for children of divorce.* Paper presented at the 104th Annual Convention of the American Psychological Association, Toronto, Canada.

Teo, A., Carlson, E., Mathieu, P. J., Egeland, B., & Sroufe, L. A. (1996). A prospective longitudinal study of psychosocial predictors of achievement. *Journal of School Psychology, 34*, 285–306.

Tolan, P. H., Guerra, N. G., & Montaini-Klovdahl, L. R. (1997). Staying out of harm's way: Coping and the development of inner-city children. In S. A.

Wolchik & I. N. Sandler (Eds.), *Handbook of children's coping: Linking theory and intervention.* (pp. 453–481). New York: Plenum.

Tronick, E. Z. (1989). Emotions and emotional communication in infants. *American Psychologist, 44,* 112–119.

Tschann, J. M., Johnston, J. R., Kline, M., & Wallerstein, J. S. (1989). Family process and children's functioning during divorce. *Journal of Marriage and the Family, 51,* 431–444.

U. S. Bureau of the Census. (1990). *Statistical abstracts of the U.S., 1990* (110th ed.). Washington, DC: U.S. Government Printing Office.

Wannon, M. (1990). *Children's control beliefs about controllable and uncontrollable events: Their relationship to stress resilience and psychosocial adjustment.* Unpublished Ph.D. dissertation, University of Rochester, NY.

Waters, E. & Sroufe, L. A. (1983). Social competence as developmental construct. *Developmental Review, 3,* 79–97.

Werner, E. E. & Smith, R. S. (1982). *Vulnerable but invincible: A study of resilient children.* New York: McGraw-Hill.

Werner, E. E. & Smith, R. S. (1992). *Overcoming the odds: High risk children from birth to adulthood.* Ithaca, NY: Cornell University Press.

White, S. H. (1965). Evidence for a hierarchical arrangement of learning processes. In L. Lipsett & C. Spiker (Eds.), *Advances in child development and behavior* (Vol. 2). New York: Academic Press.

Williams, S., Anderson, J., McGee, R., & Silva, P.A. (1990). Risk factors for behavioral and emotional disorder in preadolescent children. *Journal of the American Academy of Child and Adolescent Psychiatry, 29,* 413–419.

Wolchik, S. A. & Sandler, I. N. (1997). *Handbook of children's coping: Linking theory and intervention.* New York: Plenum Press.

Wolchik, S. A., Sandler, I. N., Braver, S. L., & Fogas, B. S. (1986). Events of parental divorce: Stressfulness ratings by children, parents, and clinicians. *American Journal of Community Psychology, 14,* 59–75.

Wolchik, S. A., West, S. G., Sandler, I. N., Tein, J.-Y., Coatsworth, D., Lengua, L., Weiss, L., Anderson, E., Greene, S., & Griffin, W. (1999). *The New Beginnings program for divorced families: An experimental evaluation of theory-based single-component and dual-component programs.* Manuscript submitted for publication.

Wolchik, S. A., West, S. G., Westover, S., Sandler, I. N., Martin, A., Lustig, J., Tein, J.-Y., & Fisher, J. (1993). The Children of Divorce Parenting

Intervention: Outcome evaluation of an empirically based program. *American Journal of Community Psychology, 21*(3), 293–331.

Wolchik, S. A., Wilcox, K., Tein, J.-Y. & Sandler, I. N. (1998). *Does high quality parenting buffer the effects of negative divorce events on children's postdivorce psychological problems?* Unpublished manuscript, Arizona State University.

Worsham, N. L., Compas, B. E., & Ey, S. (1997). Children's coping with parental illness. In S. A. Wolchik & I. N. Sandler (Eds.), *Handbook of children's coping: Linking theory and intervention* (pp. 195–215). New York: Plenum Press.

Wyman, P. A., Cowen, E. L., Work, W. C., Hoyt-Meyers, L. A., Magnus, K. B., & Fagen, D. B. (1999). Caregiving and developmental factors differentiating young at-risk urban children showing resilient versus stress-affected outcomes: A replication and extension. *Child Development, 70,* 645–659.

Wyman, P. A., Cowen, E. L., Work, W. C., & Kerley, J. H. (1993). The role of children's future expectations in self-system functioning and adjustment to life-stress. *Development and Psychopathology, 5,* 649–661.

Wyman, P. A., Cowen, E. L., Work, W. C., & Parker, G. R. (1991). Developmental and family milieu interview correlates of resilience in urban children who have experienced major life-stress. *American Journal of Community Psychology, 19,* 405–426.

Wyman, P. A., Cowen, E. L., Work, W. C., Raoof, A., Gribble, P. A., Parker, G. R., & Wannon, M. (1992). Interviews with children who experienced major life stress: Family and child attributes that predict resilient outcomes. *Journal of the American Academy of Child and Adolescent Psychiatry, 31,* 904–910.

Wyman, P. A., Kilmer, R. P., Cowen, E. L., & Lotyczweski, B. S. (1999). *Resilience among urban children experiencing nonoptimal caregiving: Risk and protective effects.* Manuscript submitted for publication.

Zill, N., Morrison, D. R., & Coiro, M. J. (1993). Long-term effects of parental divorce on parent-child relationships, adjustment, and achievement in young adulthood. *Journal of Family Psychology, 7,* 91–103.

# 6

## Suggestions for the Investigation of Psychological Wellness in the Neighborhood Context: Toward a Pluralistic Neighborhood Theory

*Mark S. Aber and Martin Nieto*

### Introduction

Cowen [1994] argued that if we are to enhance psychological wellness, we need to identify the features of influential social environments that support its development. In this chapter, we take up Cowen's challenge by exploring how neighborhood structures and processes might influence psychological wellness. Toward this aim, we review aspects of the pioneering theories of the Chicago School Sociologists [Burgess 1925; Park 1936; Shaw & McKay 1942]. Since the early parts of this century, the community social organization theories of the Chicago School have guided scientific and policy approaches to neighborhood crime and poverty. Because these theories have been and are so influential, continuing to provide the conceptual foundation for most contemporary neighborhood research, efforts to study psychological wellness in the neighborhood context will have to reckon with both their theoretical claims and the empirical findings purported to support them.

While the Chicago School tradition has much to offer the study of neighborhoods and wellness, both conceptually and methodologically, there is much to be cautious about as well. Imbedded in much of this work are questionable assumptions that must be articulated and examined, blind spots where theory and research must be developed, and weaknesses that must be shored up if we are to integrate Cowen's vision of a psychology of wellness into neighborhood work. Here, due to space limitations, we focus on the weaknesses of community social organization theories for the study of wellness. We argue that a wellness-oriented neighborhood research agenda cannot rest securely on the problem-focused, ethnocentric assumptions of these theories. We offer suggestions upon which a more useful Pluralistic Neighborhood Theory might be built.

Like community organization theories, Pluralistic Neighborhood Theory posits that the effects of neighborhood structure and social processes on psychological wellness must be understood within their broader historical, social, political, and economic contexts. However, pluralistic neighborhood theory deliberately seeks to provide a counterbalance to the prescriptive ideals and ethnocentrism inherent in most community organization theories. To do so, pluralistic neighborhood theory recognizes multiple standards of health and wellness at both the individual and neighborhood level. In keeping with recent advances in understanding the role of social contexts in development and psychopathology [Cicchetti & Aber 1998], it grants a central place to people's own views of their neighborhoods [see e.g., Seidman et al. 1998] and argues that these are critical for understanding neighborhood effects on wellness. In addition, pluralistic neighborhood theory argues for the study of variation within neighborhood groups categorized on factors that have traditionally been thought to determine neighborhood social processes from a community social organization perspective—factors such as socioeconomic and racial composition [Duncan & Aber 1997; Korbin et al. 1998; Sampson et al. 1997]. It is anticipated that research conducted from the perspective of pluralistic neighborhood theory might illuminate the transactional relations between neighborhood structure and social processes that are grounded in the lived experience of neighborhood residents.

In the Chicago School framework, neighborhoods and communities link macroeconomic, political, and social structure and change to the life experiences of city residents. A well-known example of work from this perspective is that of William Julius Wilson [1987, 1996]. It documents how the loss of manufacturing jobs devastated the work f inner-city American communities during the 1970s and 80s. Similarly, work by Sampson, Raudenbush & Earls [1997] is illustrative of a growing body of literature which builds on the classic theory and research of Shaw and McKay [1942] and demonstrates effects of neighborhood poverty, immigrant concentration, and residential mobility on community organization, collective efficacy, and crime. Increasingly, outcomes such as teen childbearing, academic achievement, educational attainment, and mental health are being studied within the same general framework [e.g., Aber et al. 1997; Brooks-Gunn et al. 1993; Crane 1991; Dornbusch et al. 1991; Duncan 1994; Garner & Raudenbush 1991].

While contemporary efforts to understand neighborhoods as contexts for human development and social change have generated important extensions and integration of Chicago School theory, they have maintained the problem focus of this earlier work. Virtually no explicit attention has been devoted to the implications of neighborhoods for psychological wellness. In much the same way, mental health scholarship and professional activity have focused on pathology—its genesis and treatment. Initial sociological analyses of neighborhoods and now their multidisciplinary progeny have attended primarily to the socially and psychologically toxic elements of neighborhoods, all but completely ignoring wellness at both the individual and neighborhood levels. Instead, the study of neighborhoods has dwelled on how the life chances of urban residents, particularly those in low-income neighborhoods, are compromised by the harsh conditions there. Pluralistic neighborhood theory promises to fill this void.

We begin this chapter by considering the definition of neighborhood. Both for our purposes here and for the longer-term project of examining wellness in the neighborhood context, attention to the definition and measurement of the neighborhood construct is called for. We argue that in order for it to be useful, the definition(s) of neighborhood given by pluralistic neighborhood theory ultimately must be informed by the goals and agenda of the wellness orientation. Next, we compare the concepts of neighborhood and community. Pluralistic neighborhood theory, if it intends to build on prior neighborhood and community theory and research, must distinguish the multiple and only sometimes overlapping meanings assigned to these constructs in the literature. We then examine several aspects of Shaw and McKay's [1942] social disorganization theory. Originally developed to account for the distribution of crime and delinquency across the city of Chicago, social disorganization theory has become among the growing number of psychologists interested in neighborhood effects, the most influential of the community social organization theories. As such, it is a particularly useful place to begin exploring the implications of neighborhood for the study of psychological wellness. Our interest here is not to evaluate the quality and extent of empirical support for the theory, but rather to examine how this theory, as a representative of other deficit-focused community social organization theories, has influenced the direction and assumptions of neighborhood work, and what it implies for work directed toward wellness. Consequently, in what follows, we use social disorganization theory to illustrate issues that typically apply to community social organization theory more generally.

## Defining Neighborhood

Despite nearly a hundred years of scholarly interest in neighborhoods, the question of what precisely constitutes a neighborhood remains unresolved and largely unexamined. Prior to the mid-1800s, when the city was viewed as an undifferentiated center of commerce and culture, the concept of neighborhood did not exist [Miller 1981]. The neighborhood construct emerged in American sociology around the turn of the century when notions of semiautonomous neighborhoods, zones, and sectors were created to explain the growth and functioning of urban areas [see e.g., Burgess 1925; Park 1915; Hoyt 1939]. Park [1915], writing about the development of neighborhoods in early 20th century American cities, suggested that where private ownership of land prevails, city populations become segregated and classified not so much by centralized design or control as by individuals' pursuit of "personal tastes and convenience, vocational and economic interests" [p. 579]. He argued these processes give rise to neighborhoods.

> In the course of time every section and quarter of the city takes on something of the character and qualities of its inhabitants. Each separate part of the city is inevitably

stained with the peculiar sentiments of its population. The effect of this is to convert what was at first a mere geographical expression into a neighborhood, that is to say, a locality with sentiments, traditions, and a history of its own. Within this neighborhood the continuity of the historical processes is somehow maintained. The past imposes itself upon the present and the life of every locality moves on with a certain momentum of its own, more or less independent of the larger circle of life and interests about it. . . . Proximity and neighborly contact are the basis for the simplest and most elementary form of association with which we have to do in the organization of city life. Local interests and associations breed local sentiment, and, under a system which makes residence the basis for participation in the government, the neighborhood becomes the basis of political control. In the social and political organization of the city it is the smallest local unit. [pp. 579-80]

This description captures many of the dimensions one finds in subsequent descriptions and definitions of neighborhoods. In particular, it includes the two core elements of most contemporary definitions—geography and social interaction. Still, this description, like many that have come since, suffers from ambiguities that pose challenges to neighborhood theory and research, challenges that we believe should be particularly salient to neighborhood researchers interested in wellness.

Neighborhood researchers have long recognized the definitional ambiguities inherent in the neighborhood construct. The rigid boundaries that must be used by neighborhood researchers and social agents to define neighborhoods are normally somewhat arbitrary. This is partly because all neighborhoods have, to some extent, the organic nature that Park [1915] described, growing from and reflecting the interests of citizens, and partly because neighborhoods are open systems whose boundaries fluctuate over time and are often unspecified. Many neighborhoods simply do not have precise, widely recognized boundaries. Moreover, research consistently has shown that neighbors, when asked to describe or define their neighborhood, are likely to give different responses [Aber et al. 1998; Coleman 1978;

Haeberle 1988; Lee & Campbell 1997]. In addition to variability in where they draw the boundaries of the neighborhood, their descriptions often differ in the relative emphases placed on factors used to define the neighborhood, including the nature and meaning of social relations in the locale, the role and importance of social institutions, and the extent to which residents personally identify with the neighborhood. Residents' descriptions are also likely to differ from the formal neighborhood designations employed by the school district, church parish, municipal government, and park district to which they belong. Each of these, in turn, is likely to differ from one another and from the proxy measures most neighborhood research has relied on to represent neighborhoods—census tracts. Clearly, there are many ways to define and measure neighborhoods, and no consensus as to which is best.

While definitional difficulties abound, a neighborhood literature has developed based on the belief and common experience that neighborhoods are recognized and recognizable. In Chaskin's [1997] words, "Neighborhood is known, if not understood, and in any given case, there is likely to be wide agreement on its existence, if not its parameters" [p. 523]. Indeed, belief that neighborhoods provide a viable unit of analysis in understanding the ecology of human development and social interaction underlies the recent resurgence of scientific interest in neighborhoods. That neighborhoods have meaning and significance to residents has long been a core belief of neighborhood organizers and today fuels policies that target police, municipal, and human services to the neighborhood level. With the exception of neighborhood influences on crime, however, empirical support for these beliefs is scant. A pluralistic neighborhood theory must explicitly recognize and confront the ambiguity and complexity inherent in the neighborhood construct.

Reflecting on this state of affairs, we agree with Chaskin [1997] who concluded:

> [N]eighborhoods must be identified and defined heuristically, guided by specific programmatic aims, informed by a theoretical understanding of neighborhood and a recognition of its complications on the ground, and based on a particular understanding of the meaning and use of neigh-

borhood (as defined by residents, local organizations, government officials, and actors in the private sector) in the particular context in which a program or intervention is to be based. [p. 541]

Indeed, perusal of the neighborhood literature reveals that some definitions reflect particular disciplinary concerns (e.g., the planning perspective of Glass [1948]), and some the particular interests of individual scholars [e.g., Park & Burgess 1925]. Other definitions consider only a few of the many forms neighborhoods take, while still others emphasize some select set of the many functions neighborhoods may serve for their residents (e.g., Kotler's [1969] emphasis on the political functions of neighborhoods). One implication of this view is that what constitutes a useful definition or operationalization of neighborhood for the purposes of studying wellness will differ from that designed to study problem outcomes. The MacArthur Network on Psychopathology and Development has recently come to a similar conclusion with respect to understanding the effects of social contexts more generally on psychopathology, arguing that "contexts should be selected for assessment in light of specific questions or outcomes [Boyce et al. 1998]. We will consider this issue in more detail below when we examine the implications of social disorganization theory for the study of wellness. For now it suffices to say that pluralistic neighborhood theory emphasizes residents' perceptions of and definitions of their own neighborhoods. In particular, residents' perceptions of neighborhood history, boundaries, strengths, and resources are all viewed as very important to our understanding of psychological wellness.

## Community or Neighborhood?

Even if this volume was not dedicated to Emory Cowen, by all counts a leading figure in community psychology, we would be remiss not to mention the relation between the terms "neighborhood" and "community," because much of the theory upon which current neighborhood studies rely has been developed in terms of community, not neighborhood. The situation is complicated further by the fact that much neighborhood and community theory has failed to articulate the parameters of the geographical and/or social unit to which it applies, often not distinguishing neighborhoods from communities. Still, a meaningful distinction can be made.

The term "community" most generally is used to refer to a collection of people who have a common bond, usually based in some combination of shared circumstances, interests, beliefs, or concerns. The source of the bond that joins together members of a community may (as in the case of local communities referred to in many community social organization theories), but need not, derive from place. Communities of faith, professional communities, ethnic communities and others, typically transcend geographic areas. Even in local communities, the defining characteristics of the community are the common bonds that contribute to some shared identity for its members.

By contrast, nearly all definitions of "neighborhood" include reference to a circumscribed place or geographical area. Typically such areas are recognized as subunits of larger areas [Chaskin 1997]. Most definitions do not specify much about these physical areas other than that they are, to some extent, residential and in some way distinct from surrounding areas. Thus, it is generally agreed neighborhoods are quite diverse, varying widely in size, from several residences on a single city block to square miles. Some neighborhoods have well-recognized names and/or boundaries, while others do not [Keller 1968]. Some are recognized by external factors, while few nonresidents would recognize others.

In addition to the spatial dimension, most neighborhood definitions implicitly or explicitly assume neighborhood residents have some level of social interaction with and/or connection to one another, though the nature and extent of these relations are often left unspecified, again accommodating a wide range of social interaction across neighborhoods [Chaskin 1997]. In some areas, social interaction may be limited to acknowledging familiar neighbors or exchanging greetings. Residents of such neighborhoods may share little more than the common conditions that attend their physical proximity. In other neighborhoods, extensive and intimate social relations exist, sometimes based on shared historical, ethnic, cultural, or religious background, and sometimes based on common circumstantial, social, economic, or political concerns. Each of these dimensions, among others, can serve to give a particular neighborhood its distinctive quality.

To the extent that residents of a particular geographical area share common circumstances, interests, and concerns that derive from the neighborhood, the neighborhood serves as a source of community. In this sense, if for no other reason than that residents of neighborhoods share a common geographic area, all neighborhoods are to a limited extent communities, if by community we mean a group of people who share a common bond. A good number of references to community in urban sociological theory, however, appear to refer to local geographic areas that are larger in size and often more diverse than is true of either the modal neighborhood referent in the literature, or the "smallest local unit" of social and political life that Park [1915] had in mind when he described neighborhood [see e.g., Bursik 1984]. It remains for empirical research to illuminate the extent to which specific community theories apply to neighborhoods more narrowly construed. To our knowledge, no systematic analysis of the conceptual and operational match between these constructs has been attempted. We believe such analysis would benefit the field. Meanwhile, as we venture to extract the relevance of past work for understanding neighborhood effects on psychological wellness, we must be careful to distinguish the various meanings of neighborhood and community. Failure to do so will slow theory testing and development, and impair the comparison and integration of research results. Moreover, in future work we must strive both to articulate more clearly the definitions of these constructs and to minimize the difference between each definition and how we operationalize it in research. Otherwise, overreliance on artificially bounded, purely geographic designations of neighborhoods (e.g., census block groups and tracts) will continue. This, in turn, will constrain and obscure our understanding of neighborhood social processes that extend beyond artificially defined neighborhood boundaries.

Of course, progress clarifying and validating these constructs, by itself, will not completely solve our problems. For most researchers, collection of neighborhood level data is prohibitively expensive, forcing reliance on archival data sources that are usually not organized by neighborhood (such as census tracts, planning districts, catchment areas, precincts, wards, etc.). Consequently, most neighborhood research will not focus, and, strictly speaking, has not focused on neighborhoods *per se*. As a guide to ethnographic research, social action, and interpretation of large N neighborhood studies using such proxy measures, however, such progress remains sorely needed. Moreover, research should examine the implications of using census designations of various sizes (like tracts and block groups) to represent neighborhoods. In particular, we should work to identify those neighborhood processes and individual outcomes that are most sensitive to variations in the geographical unit used to define neighborhood [Gephart 1989].

Finally, explicit and clear definitions are necessary to ease the development of theory attuned to historical change in the nature of neighborhoods and their meaning to residents and external actors. As mentioned above, much of the original theory that laid the foundation for and has guided recent and ongoing neighborhood research was developed with urban community areas circa 1920–1940 in mind [e.g., Park & Burgess 1925; Shaw & McKay 1942]. Arguably, much about neighborhoods has changed since then. Contemporary theoretical accounts must capture the dynamics and realities of contemporary neighborhoods and can only benefit from explicit and clear definition(s). We turn to one such theory now.

## Implications of Social Disorganization Theory for Wellness

### Overview

Shaw and McKay's [1942, 1969] social disorganization theory, probably the most influential neighborhood theory among psychologists today, was developed to explain differential rates of crime and delinquency across Chicago neighborhoods. The theory grew from two observations. First, crime rates were higher in neighborhoods closest to the business centers of the city and generally decreased as one moved away from them. Second, these crime patterns tended to remain stable over decades, even though the population in the areas changed. Shaw and McKay took these facts to indicate that something about the social structure of the areas, not their residents, produced the differences in crime. In comparison to the structural features of low-crime areas, high-crime areas were found to have lower socioeconomic status, higher residential mobility, and greater ethnic heterogeneity.

Shaw and McKay proposed the construct of social disorganization to link neighborhood structure to crime and delinquency. A neighborhood or community's social organization refers to its ability to realize its common interests and values and solve its common problems. Local social networks and collective attachment are the fundamental vehicles for the development of social organization. The relation between the social organization of a community and the rules and social expectations for its members is seen as interactive and dynamic. Social organization both serves as a source of rules and expectations and reflects what the community views as important. Social institutions such as schools, churches, social clubs, and block associations constitute a primary source of formal organization in the community. They establish, promote, and enforce the community's rules and expectations. There also exists an array of informal structures including local friendship and acquaintanceship networks that provide social organization, actively shaping attitudes and behavior and being shaped by them. Anything that implicitly or explicitly diminishes the ability of social institutions, formal and informal, to perform their designated functions is expected to reduce community social organization.

In general terms, Shaw and McKay hypothesized that community social organization mediates the effects of poverty, residential mobility, and ethnic heterogeneity on juvenile crime patterns. Poverty, mobility, and ethnic heterogeneity exert negative influences on the development of social interaction, communication, and social ties. Neighborhoods with these characteristics have difficulties establishing and maintaining the social organization necessary for adults in the neighborhood to exert social control over youth crime.

Research following in the tradition of Shaw and McKay has expanded the ways social organization has been conceptualized and measured [Coleman 1986; Buckner 1988; Kasarda & Janowitz 1974;

Sampson 1988]. Moreover, broader sets of population characteristics, community structures, and individual developmental outcomes have been incorporated into this general framework [Brook-Gunn et al. 1997; Sampson 1992; Shaw & McKay 1969]. Despite these advances, the dominance of the general community social organization perspective has limited the scope of neighborhood research. Most research on neighborhood effects still takes a problem orientation, attempting either to identify neighborhood characteristics that indicate or lead to weakened social organization, or to demonstrate deleterious influences of these factors on child and adolescent behavior and development. This work has directed attention to the presumed weaknesses of poor neighborhoods, particularly to weaknesses in their abilities to control deviant behavior, and away from neighborhood strengths and indications of psychological wellness. Thus, we have studied in some detail the influence of neighborhood structure on crime and delinquency, but we have not systematically asked what aspects of neighborhoods influence the prosocial development of adolescents. Nor have we examined influences on the health or wellness of residents more generally, nor characteristics reflecting the health and wellness of the neighborhood itself.

Building on Cowen's [1994] suggestions for studying influential social environments, a wellness-oriented neighborhood research agenda might seek to address the following kinds of questions: What neighborhood characteristics promote psychological wellness outcomes? "What are the different ways, structurally in which ... [neighborhoods] ... can pursue their mandates? What relationships exist between these ways and wellness outcomes for ... [neighborhood] inhabitants?" [p. 157].

Community social organization theories provide a potentially useful starting point from which to address these questions insofar as they articulate dimensions of social structure such as poverty and employment rates, ethnic composition, and residential mobility that, at least theoretically, are relevant to individual level behavior. Equally important, they highlight the role that community-level social processes such as social organization might play in mediating the relation between social structure and individual behavior. Thus, this general framework might be applied usefully to the study of individual level psychological wellness. We must proceed cautiously, however. These theories make a number of questionable claims and rest on several problematic assumptions that must be interrogated before the theories will be of much use to the wellness research agenda. Below, we examine several assumptions related to ideal neighborhoods and the measurement of social disorganization. We also briefly examine claims about the effects of social organization and explore the concept of neighborhood-level protective factors. By challenging erroneous assumptions and claims, we hope not only to minimize the damage they wreak on future research, but also to illuminate related issues relevant to the examination of neighborhood effects on wellness from the perspective of pluralistic neighborhood theory.

## Social Disorganization's Implicit Ideal Neighborhood

Perhaps the most important assumptions implicit in community social organization theories concern what constitutes normal, healthy, and ideal neighborhoods. In the same way that psychopathology is often characterized in terms of deviations from normal development and healthy psychological functioning [Cicchetti 1989], social disorganizational accounts of neighborhood problems are built on implicit notions of what constitutes normal and ideal neighborhoods. These notions, though rarely articulated explicitly, are likely to play a prominent role in our thinking about how neighborhoods influence psychological wellness and therefore deserve careful scrutiny.

Because community social organization theories were developed to explain community problems, these theories rarely include direct or explicit consideration of positive neighborhood characteristics. Instead, to the extent that they can be found at all, positive references are usually imbedded in descriptions of the failures of low-income neighborhoods. Few of the characteristics of neighborhoods that are presumed to be healthy have been empirically evaluated. Rather, most have been inferred from work that treats them as implicit standards against which troubled neighborhoods are compared. Thus, much of what neighborhood researchers believe constitutes "healthy" neighborhoods derives from inferences from studies of what makes "unhealthy" neighborhoods. From studies showing that neighborhoods with high poverty rates tend to have low levels of social organization and high crime rates, it is inferred that healthy neighborhoods are wealthy, should have high levels of social organization and, thereby, low crime rates. As we will see, many of these assumptions may not be tenable.

The ideal community conjured up by Park [1915] harked back to earlier times when, he argued, "simpler and more primitive forms of society" prevailed [p. 582]. Park's ideal reflected the prototypic small, rural American town of the late 1800s; its residents were demographically homogeneous, residentially stable, knew each other well, and shared common interests. Perhaps most importantly, from Park's perspective, residents had a common and clear understanding of the values and social expectations governing individual and community life. In such a community, Park argued, conformity to an agreed set of values and social expectations was rewarded. Deviance could not flourish there because the entire community reacted against deviant attitudes and behaviors.

Park argued that some urban neighborhoods of the 1920s came closer to approximating this ideal than others. For example, he described neighborhoods that were so completely segregated by vocational class that they made it "possible within the limits of the city to live in an isolation almost as complete as that of some remote rural community" [p. 595]. Similarly, first-generation immigrant neighborhoods—where European languages dominated daily commerce, social interaction, and newspapers—tended to have independent social and political organization and to preserve "the social ritual and the moral order which these immigrants brought with them from their native countries" [p. 596].

Park also argued that as communities grew and members became exposed to a diversity of views and social practices, local attachments were weakened, as were the social restraints and inhibitions born of such attachments. Under these circumstances, community institutions in charge of promoting a particular set of values and behaviors became less influential in shaping the attitudes and daily activities of their members, and vice and crime were given room to grow. For these reasons, Park believed, social control based on traditional mores broke down in immigrant communities in the second generation. Park [1915] noted that "Under the complex influences of ... city life, what

may be called the normal neighborhood sentiment has undergone
many curious and interesting changes, and produced many unusual
types of local communities ... anything and everything that tends to
render the population unstable, to divide and concentrate attentions
upon widely separated objects of interest [threatens and weakens
neighborhoods]" [p. 580-581]. Thus, the modernization of communication and transportation that accompanied industrialization in the
early 1900s was thought "to destroy the permanency and intimacy of
the neighborhood" [p. 582]. He noted in this regard:

> In a great city, where the population is unstable, where
> parents and children are employed out of the house and
> often in distant parts of the city, where thousands of people
> live side by side for years without so much as a bowing
> acquaintance ... intimate relationships of the primary group
> are weakened and the moral order which rested upon them
> is gradually dissolved [p. 594].

These views of normal and ideal neighborhoods have shaped how
neighborhoods have been studied. First, they have promoted the idea
that ethnically homogeneous neighborhoods are healthier than heterogeneous ones. Second, and related to the first idea, they have
artificially restricted how neighborhoods have been defined and
measured. We briefly examine both of these issues and attempt to
draw out their implications for the study of psychological wellness.

### The Ethnic Homogeneity Assumption

The assumption that ethnic homogeneity represents a healthy ideal
for neighborhoods is widespread. This idea most probably derives in
part from the fact that most neighborhoods exhibit moderate to high
degrees of homogeneity. People are not and never have been distrib-
uted randomly throughout the city. In fact, in many metropolitan
areas like Chicago, residential segregation by ethnicity/race is more
common than not [see e.g., Brown et al. 1997]. Thus, the ethnic
homogeneity assumption partly reflects the unfounded but common
tendency to equate what is statistically normative with what is
healthy. It is also likely that this assumption derives part of its allure
from the well documented fact that most people prefer to live in

communities mainly populated by people like themselves [Massey 1990; Massey & Eggers 1990; Massey et al. 1992]. Clearly, the desire for homogeneity shapes the composition and functioning of most communities. Yet, neither the fact that homogeneity is normative nor the fact it is desired by residents constitutes evidence that it promotes well-being generally or psychological wellness in particular. Whether it does is an empirical question, the answer to which is still very much open to debate.

In contrast to social disorganization theory, which posits that the beneficial effects of ethnic homogeneity are ubiquitous, pluralistic neighborhood theory suggests that homogeneity has positive effects only for some people and some purposes at particular times and places. In order to understand the effects of homogeneity, it will be important to take into account how and why homogeneity has come to be. It may be useful, for example, to consider whether and why residents want it, to differentiate voluntary segregation from involuntary redlining, and to consider the historical power dynamics that give rise to, are reflected in, and are re-created by the maintenance of segregated neighborhoods. Indeed, there are a variety of social, economic, and political dynamics that lead demographically similar people to settle in close proximity. Some of these—immigrant settlement patterns, housing costs, proximity to or availability of certain types of employment and services—might exert a positive influence on psychological wellness. Others, like redlining, might have the opposite effect.

Wilson's [1996] recent work documents the damaging effects of "white flight" on the increasingly homogenous African American and Latino populations left behind in inner cities, and thus, directly challenges the homogeneity assumption. In doing so, it also exposes a related problem: the difficulty of studying the unique effects of either ethnicity or socioeconomic status in contemporary American cities where these variables are strongly correlated with one another. A neighborhood wellness research agenda conducted from the perspective of pluralistic neighborhood theory must promote more sophisticated work to replace past and current research that employs ethnicity as a proxy for poverty and thereby fuels racial stereotypes [Figueira-McDonough 1991]. Moreover, traditional methods of statistically partialing the effects of highly correlated predictors are seriously limited. At best, valid application of such methods depends on a sound theoretical model. Too often, however, efforts to "control for" the effects of either race or SES while examining the effects of the other are pursued without sufficient theory to guide the analysis and result in misleading or meaningless results. The problem is particularly thorny when cross-sectional data are used and the underlying processes that given rise to the relations between race, SES, and some outcome of interest are multidirectional or transactional. The sources of these interpretive and data analytic difficulties are numerous and space precludes discussing them here [see Cohen and Cohen 1983; McDonald 1985; and Pedazur 1982 for more thorough discussions]. Suffice it to say that these difficulties point to the need for future quantitative and qualitative research to more clearly articulate and analyze those processes through which neighborhood race, ethnicity, and socioeconomic status combine to influence individual well-being.

Even when desired by residents, ethnic homogeneity at the neighborhood level has some troubling implications for a society as diverse as ours. Arguably, under certain conditions, individuals' desires to live in segregated communities conflict with society's need to combat and reduce ethnic and racial misunderstanding, prejudice, discrimination, and animosity [Blau 1977]. Data documenting the extent of the general unwillingness of white Americans to live alongside people of color are telling. The fact is that white Americans typically consider moving out of a neighborhood when the proportion of minority residents approaches 20% [Massey & Denton 1993]. What is more, white Americans tend to grossly overestimate the proportion of minority residents in their communities [Chiricos et al. 1997] and in the country as a whole [Nedau et al. 1993].

These findings point to the need to understand the motivations people have in seeking ethnic homogeneity in their neighborhoods. In order to understand the implications of neighborhood ethnic homogeneity for wellness, research will need to examine the extent to which segregation is motivated by fear, ignorance, and animosity. It will also need to examine how these dynamics contribute to the development of neighborhood stereotypes, and how these in turn effect the wellness of residents, both those propagating the stereotypes and those who are targets of them. From our perspective, these types of research questions are not well served by theories that view neighborhood homogeneity as an ideal.

Cowen [1994] has suggested that wellness might be usefully thought of in terms like gratification in living [Rappaport 1981], life satisfaction [Rappaport 1987], sense of efficacy [Bandura 1977] and sense of coherence [Antonovsky 1979]. These dimensions of wellness might frame our inquiry into peoples' motivations to live in segregated neighborhoods. We should ask ourselves and our neighbors what it is about neighborhood ethnic composition that contributes to our sense of well-being; what makes living in a relatively segregated or integrated neighborhood gratifying, satisfying, efficacy enhancing, and/ or productive of coherence and sense of community? When we ask these questions, we may find that the residents of low-income, minority neighborhoods are interested in a different amount of homogeneity, and for different reasons, than those in high-income, white neighborhoods. The answer to these questions promise to have wide-ranging policy implications. At a practical level such information may be useful to communities (geographic, ethnic, and racial among them) that are struggling to predict the probable effect of policies that promote segregation or integration across class, race, ethnic, and other demographic lines.

*Implications for Neighborhood Definition and Measurement*

The assumption that a normal neighborhood should have the characteristics of a small, demographically homogeneous rural town is reflected in how neighborhoods have been defined and measured. When the U.S. Census Bureau initially created census tracts and block groups, for instance, it chose boundaries for these units, insofar as it was feasible, in a manner that both honored the integrity of identifiable neighborhoods *and* maximized the demographic homogeneity of the residents. Periodic redrawing of census tract boundaries also has sought to promote neighborhood homogeneity. Researchers have tended to adopt the same strategy, combining block groups and/or census tracts that have similar demographic characteristics when they have sought to form larger units such as social areas [Shaw & McKay 1942] or neighborhood clusters [Sampson et. al. 1997].

This approach to neighborhood definition has both advantages and disadvantages. On a practical level, city planners and community developers find homogeneous neighborhoods useful when applying to federal and state agencies that make receipt of aid contingent on the identification of target neighborhoods and communities that are defined in terms of concentrated disadvantage. From a research perspective, one advantage of this approach is that it provides a cost-effective way to use census information to identify reasonable proxies for true neighborhoods without having to survey residents or engage in direct observation. Another advantage is that neighborhoods defined this way facilitate comparisons across neighborhoods based on the demographic characteristics of their populations.

However, this definitional approach has disadvantages that, from the perspective of pluralistic neighborhood theory, outweigh its advantages. From this perspective, two disadvantages stand out, both of which are related to the fact that the tendency on the part of planners and researchers to define all neighborhoods as if they are homogeneous decreases the likelihood that neighborhoods that are, in fact, heterogeneous will be identified and targeted for inclusion in research or intervention. The first of these problems follows from how people define their own neighborhoods. There is some evidence that people define their neighborhoods in ways that enhance their perceived positive qualities. Thus, people tend to exclude undesirable areas from their neighborhoods [Aber et al. 1998] and to include adjoining areas they deem more desirable (safer, higher property values, etc.) [Coleman 1978]. This dynamic drives both affluent and less affluent residents to identify with the relatively wealthy in their community and, thus, to differentiate their own neighborhoods from adjoining areas where property values are lower and/or populated by people perceived as undesirable. The result is that the wealthy tend to define their neighborhoods in ways that produce racial and class segregation, while the poor tend to define their neighborhoods in ways that produce heterogeneity. Thus the homogeneity ideal assumed by planners and researchers matches the self-definitions of the affluent considerably better than those of the poor. To the extent that neighborhood self-definitions serve as resources to their residents, the homogeneity ideal serves the interests of the affluent better than it does the poor. Neighborhood researchers who aim to understand how neighborhoods and the resources they provide are related to the psychological wellness of residents will do well to attend to these dynamics.

The second significant disadvantage of this definitional approach is that it inhibits examination of certain types of questions. For example, defining neighborhoods in ways that encourage between neighborhood comparisons (across socioeconomic level, cultural group, level of residential mobility, historical tradition, etc.) has the simultaneous effect of directing attention away from examination of variation within neighborhood group. Thus, research based on definitions that privilege homogeneity is more likely to generate findings that might inadvertently reify unfair and damaging stereotypes (e.g., that poor neighborhoods are weak, that the social relationships in them are inadequate or inferior to those in wealthy neighborhoods).

Pluralistic neighborhood theory posits that examination of within-neighborhood group variation is essential for a valid understanding of neighborhood effects. Thus, definitions that facilitate such inquiry are critical to the neighborhood wellness research agenda. Such definitions can provide the starting place for investigations that eschew the view that there is a single standard for healthy neighborhoods, or suggests that the statistical norm is healthiest and that deviations are problematic. Good clinical and community psychologists are familiar with the limitations and weaknesses of many of these approaches to defining health and their limiting implications for understanding wellness. Examination of within-group variation promises to expose additional sources of influence on the social processes of neighborhoods, over and above social organization. This type of work is less likely to lead to intervention suggestions that essentially call for poor neighborhoods (and the individuals who reside in them) to become more like those that are wealthy. Of course, we are not advocating that poor neighborhoods should not pursue economic wealth, or access to jobs or other resources that they deem desirable and/or that research shows to be of value [to the contrary, see Aber 1998]. Rather, we are interested in decreasing the likelihood that social interventions will call for the residents of poor neighborhoods to behave in ways that residents of wealthy neighborhoods are presumed to do, but actually do not, or to do so without needed resources.

## Measuring Social Organization

Most empirical examinations of social disorganization theory have proceeded as if social organization can be measured in the same way across different types of neighborhoods [e.g., Sampson et al. 1997; Shaw & McKay 1969; Simcha-Fagan & Schwartz 1986]. From the perspective of pluralistic neighborhood theory, this is a serious mistake. By contrast, this theory posits that the meaning of participation in informal social interaction or formal organizations can vary depending on the socioeconomic status of the neighborhood.

Take, for example, the case of resident councils, which are often organized in public housing neighborhoods with the goal of building social organization. Often, such councils maintain close relations with paid housing staff. Moreover, many public housing authorities have policies that punish residents with eviction for allowing friends or relatives who are not on the lease to live in their apartments, or punish residents financially for earning unreported income. Given this context, failure on the part of residents to participate in the resident council, where they will come into regular contact with housing authority staff, may reflect more about the nature of the relationship between residents and housing staff than about social organization among the residents themselves. Residents may choose not to participate because they believe their participation will not be taken seriously by housing authority staff, or staff will not have their best interests at heart. Similarly, failure to establish, or low rates of participation in, neighborhood watch groups and park district programs located in low-income minority neighborhoods often reflects more about the antagonistic and/or distrustful relations between residents and the police and city and park district officials than it does about the social relationships or organization among residents. These examples challenge the assumption that participation in formal social organizations and groups are always good measures of social organization or the ability of residents in low-income neighborhoods to realize their common interests. Similarly, they raise questions about the willingness of residents to reveal the true nature of their social relations to researchers who are identified with distrusted social institutions.

This perspective is bolstered by research that has documented other forms of supportive and meaningful social organization in poor neighborhoods [see e.g., Borchert 1980; Dash 1989; MacLeod 1987; Stack 1974]. When researchers have looked for social organization in such neighborhoods we often have found it, even if not always in the same places or forms that we find it in middle- or upper-class neighborhoods. When we know where to look and what to look for, we find things that we did not see before. We are not suggesting that there are not unhealthy aspects of economically poor neighborhoods. The organization that we find may not be purely positive or healthy. But this should not surprise us. Even a cursory observation of participation in social organizations in relatively affluent communities reveals the same complexity—families and individuals hurt by hostile exclusion from social clubs and organizations, and families and individuals hurt *by participating in* social organizations whose members for one reason or another target them for ostracism. We do want to emphasize, however, that our efforts to study social organization in low-income neighborhoods must take into account the fact that the forms social organization will take will reflect people's experience with formal systems that typically are inhospitable to their needs and ways of understanding the world. Participation in many public organizations—schools, municipal government advisory bodies, community service organizations, and so forth—is often discouraged by the stigmatizing and blaming attitudes these organizations have of low-income and minority people. Such persons are often treated in such settings as outsiders and/or as recipients of experts' charity, services, and knowledge. Their voices are usually ignored, there is little meaningful change that results from participation, the process is infantilizing, and the style of communication is condescending. We must remember this when we study neighborhoods, especially when we aim to understand strengths and wellness. Participation in public settings that appears to be simple, straightforward indications of health and well-being in some neighborhoods may not have the same meaning in other neighborhoods, particularly when the setting is controlled by persons who have different life experiences, life goals, values, and cultural views. In much the same way that Giroux [1983] has characterized marginalized students' lack of attachment to school, lack of participation by low-income adults may not reflect personal, cultural, or social dysfunction, but may be a form of resistance to domination and oppression born of moral and political indignation.

Even when participation by residents from different status neighborhoods can reasonably be thought to reflect a common form of social organization, there may be sufficient differences in the nature of the organizations/institutions themselves (how they are structured, who controls them, their social climate, etc.) and in how their members experience them, that participation has different types of effects. We know for example that the ways that schools socialize students differ across neighborhoods, depending on social and economic status [Bowles & Gintis 1976]. Schools serving working class and poorer neighborhoods provide a different type of socialization experience to their students than do schools serving upper-class children. Schools serving students from working-class neighborhoods tend to be more regimented and place a higher value on rules and behavioral control, while suburban schools tend to have more open classrooms that "favor greater student participation, less direct supervision, more student electives, and, in general, a value system stressing internalized standards of control" [Bowles & Gintis 1976; p. 132]. Oftentimes, this differential treatment of children is evident within a single school through tracking [Oakes 1985; Oakes et al. 1990]. Parallel differences, though not as well documented, exist in the nature of the social experiences of parents in their children's schools. Thus, pluralistic neighborhood theory posits that in order to understand the effects of neighborhood social organization on wellness, neighborhoods must be viewed in the context of social dynamics like classism and racism, which correlate with, but cannot be reduced to, the "social composition effects" of class and race.

## The Effects of Social Organization

Implicit in community organization theories is the idea that social organization is a ubiquitous good. Research by Rieder [1985] in the Canarsie community of New York City suggests otherwise. Rieder's work shows that when neighborhood residents are threatened from population turnover and increasing heterogeneity, high levels of social organization can lead to violence. He found that the more tightly organized Italian neighborhoods used substantially more violence to resist an influx of blacks than did the less organized Jewish neighborhoods in the area. The violence was initially restricted to fighting among young boys; when condoned by highly organized adults, it eventually escalated to include bombing of homes and a race riot at the high school. In this case, while social disorganization may have served to promote the perceived interests of the neighborhood, it failed not only to mitigate against criminal behavior, but arguably diminished the psychological wellness of the Italian youth. Thus, from a pluralistic neighborhood theory perspective, understanding the implications of social organization for the development of psychological wellness requires articulation of how other factors at various levels of analysis may condition the effects of social organization.

### Neighborhood-Level Protective Factors

An additional step toward incorporating a wellness focus into neighborhood research could build rather directly on existing findings which demonstrate the negative effects of toxic neighborhood conditions on human behavior. Without minimizing the importance of these findings, pluralistic neighborhood theory argues it is critical to the wellness agenda that we not over-interpret them. Even research demonstrating moderately strong relations between neighborhood structures and neighborhood rates of problem outcomes suggests that many youth living in "risky" neighborhoods do not become delinquent, or drop out of school, or bear children (in fact, typically *most* do not), while many youth living in "good" neighborhoods do. This points to the opportunity to examine resilience in the neighborhood context, or the capacity of many youth at risk for problem outcomes to "beat the odds" by adapting and developing successfully, an idea that is central to the wellness agenda [Cowen 1994].

Already, considerable work on resilience has been pursued at the individual level [Cicchetti & Garmezy 1993; Cowen et al. 1990; Garmezy et al. 1984; Werner & Smith 1982, 1992; Luthar, Cicchetti, & Becker, in press]. Much of this work starts by asking what it is about the resilient person that enables her to withstand or overcome difficult circumstances. This approach has led to exciting and important findings concerning the strengths of successful copers. A calm and sociable temperament, good social skills, and problem solving abilities, among others, have each been implicated as characteristics of resilient children. But, as Cowen et al. [1990; 1997] have noted, the processes underlying resilience are not fully understood. Consideration of neighborhood context should help to elucidate at least some of these processes.

Conceptually, resilience may represent an interaction between the individual and her conditions, an interaction that moderates the impact of some risk condition. Pluralistic neighborhood theory focuses on the cross-level effects of neighborhoods on individual adjustment and asks whether there is anything about the neighborhood context, rather than the individual, that might account for such positive outcomes. Put another way, might the reason why some neighborhood conditions impact some persons negatively, and others not at all, be found in the nature of the conditions themselves rather than in individual differences among those exposed to the conditions? One might ask why some neighborhoods that have high rates of poverty, mobility, and/or ethnic heterogeneity still have relatively high rates of social organization, or low rates of crime.

Consider the case of neighborhood-level poverty. Residents of neighborhoods with high poverty rates might experience and view the meaning of their neighborhoods' economic conditions differently, depending on whether those conditions are declining or improving. If, as has been documented before [e.g., Korbin et al. 1998; Seidman et al. 1998], experiences and perceptions mediate the impact of neighborhood conditions on adjustment, we would expect resident adjustment to vary across neighborhoods that are on different trajectories. Note that this is not a hypothesis about the direct impact of neighborhood change on residents, but rather a hypothesis that the impact of difficult neighborhood conditions might depend on the trajectory of those conditions. It is a hypothesis about an interaction among neighborhood level factors, or if the analogy is appropriate, the operation of a neighborhood-level protective factor.

While this case is similar to research that identifies individual differences as the source of resilience, in the sense that residents in this example differ in their experiences and perceptions of neighborhood, we emphasize that the focus is different from most resilience research to date because the reason for the individual differences in perception is sought and located in the external conditions of the neighborhood, rather than in the person, and this has important implications for how we think about intervention. Suppose that residents develop a sense of (personal and/or collective) optimism or efficacy about neighborhood life when they see their neighborhood is on the way up. If one looked for individual but not neighborhood level protective factors, one might mistakenly conclude that optimism moderates the impact of neighborhood poverty on adjustment. Thus, neighborhood research stands to advance the wellness agenda not only by focusing our attention on important contexts within which to examine resilience, but also by directing our attention to potential alternative explanations for positive individual outcomes under high-risk conditions. What might appear as individual level resilience processes, in fact, can sometimes be accounted for by factors operating at the neighborhood level.

A word of caution is in order with respect to interpreting the operation of neighborhood risk factors in cross-level research on resilience (where the interest is to understand the impact of neighborhood level variables on individual level ones). For certain neighborhood level risk factors or stressors, it may be unwise to assume that all residents of the neighborhood are equally exposed, or even exposed at all. Take, for example, the case of risk from neighborhood violence. We know that all youth living in the same neighborhood are not equally exposed to such risk. Some youth simply live in a safe corner of what is an otherwise dangerous neighborhood and avoid danger without any deliberate effort. We would not want to confuse these youth with those who successfully cope with potential exposure to violent situations by actively avoiding dangerous street corners or houses where drug trafficking is known to take place. Failure to distinguish these two groups of youth who appear unaffected by neighborhood violence would substantially reduce our power to identify the latter group of active copers. Of course, depending on the method, the same validity threat may exist in the assessment of risk located at other levels of analysis (classroom, family, individual). However, the process of aggregation by which many neighborhood variables are constructed and the mere size of neighborhoods relative to other social settings, we believe makes this problem a more likely threat at the neighborhood level.

## Conclusions and Future Directions

The wellness orientation poses a challenge to neighborhood research to develop a conceptual framework that allows for the examination of how neighborhoods function in relation to the interests of both their residents and the larger social context. By focusing attention on the social functions that neighborhoods serve for their residents and the social interaction among them, a wellness-oriented neighborhood research agenda can help to provide an antidote to the problems of individualism in psychology. Pluralistic neighborhood theory posits that we enhance our chances of discovering the places and ways that neighborhoods promote wellness if we focus on what actually happens in neighborhoods, rather than if we come to them with preconceived ideas about what is problematic about them. Thus, the wellness orientation leads us to challenge the adequacy of current problem-focused frameworks, an important first step toward modifying them and developing alternatives. While social organization has proven useful for describing some neighborhood social processes, problems stemming from the implicit ideal inherent in this conceptualization and the dominant strategies used to measure both neighborhoods and social organization expose the limitations of this framework. Our review points to several issues that will be important to advancing a wellness-oriented neighborhood research agenda.

Pluralistic neighborhood theory abandons the deterministic conceptualization of community organization theories. The simple unidirectional model of relations inherent to these theories is replaced by a model that accounts for the transactional relations between social structure, social processes, and individuals. Not only do neighborhood social structures and processes shape residents' experiences and understandings of their neighborhoods, but residents' responses actively shape those processes and structures.

Additionally, pluralistic neighborhood theory and the wellness research it generates, like all attempts to delineate environmental features that promote healthy development, considers how and why individuals differ in their adjustment to the same environmental conditions. Neighborhood characteristics and processes that promote healthy development in one child (or group of children) may be detrimental to others. These issues will be particularly important if we seek to promote neighborhoods that are heterogeneous with respect to race, culture, ethnicity, and social class. Success addressing this challenge will require that we reconsider our notions of what constitutes an ideal neighborhood, search for neighborhood-level protective factors, and relinquish the idea that there are single standards for neighborhood health and psychological wellness in favor of a more pluralistic view. These demands, in turn, call on us to go beyond social organization to explore a broader range of neighborhood mediating structures and mechanisms.

Our review also suggests that the identification of neighborhood level constructs that promote wellness will demand attention to the ethnocentric bias in traditional community organization and human development frameworks. As we have described, current conceptions and measures of social organization do not generalize well across socioeconomic class. Toward this end, it will be important to view neighborhoods in their broader ecological, social, political, and historical contexts in order to understand the meaning of neighborhoods to their residents, and the impact of neighborhood characteristics on individual, family, and group development. We should not be surprised, for example, to discover that the implications of living in an ethnically heterogeneous neighborhood in the year 2000 differ from those in the 1920s through the 1940s when the Chicago School sociologists developed their theories. Similarly, it will not do to create housing policies for a particular neighborhood without taking into account the overall demographic and economic trends for the city and region.

The size of the broader community in which neighborhoods are located will also be an important contextual consideration from the perspective of pluralistic neighborhood theory. Past neighborhood and community theory has paid scant attention to differences between large metropolitan areas and smaller sized cities and towns situated in otherwise rural areas. Most such theory has been developed with urban neighborhoods in mind. Pluralistic neighborhood theory posits that, for many purposes, it is unwise to assume that neighborhoods in large urban areas like New York City and Chicago function in the same way as those in the suburbs, rural areas, or smaller cities and towns. Wilson's [1996] work showing that the effects of neighborhood poverty differ across areas, depending on how heavily concentrated poverty is in surrounding neighborhoods, offers just one example of how community size might matter.

Finally, Cowen [1994] points out that defining and operationalizing positive developmental outcomes necessarily involve issues of values. Indeed, many of the concerns that are central to a wellness-oriented research agenda and that pluralistic neighborhood theory aims to address are inexorably infused with questions of values. How to define neighborhoods? Who gets to define them? What is desirable, healthy, and ideal about neighborhoods? How do we understand the relevance of race and class in analyses of neighborhood social structure and processes? These questions will not and cannot be resolved by resorting to even the most sound theory and research. They challenge us to confront head on our hopes and dreams for the kinds of neighborhoods and communities that we want to live in, indeed, how we want to live with our neighbors. Pluralistic neighborhood theory, by exposing some of the value-laden assumptions of community organization theories, highlights this challenge. By seeking to complement attention to wellness at the individual level with concern for defining and understanding wellness at the neighborhood level, it acknowledges that sometimes what is good for the neighborhood, may not be good for all, or even most, of the individuals who live there. Should affordable housing in the neighborhood be razed to support the expansion of a commercial strip mall? Future answers to such questions call for us to think about how to balance the interests of the neighborhood and the individuals who live in them, and to create public processes to define and pursue the proper balance.

# References

Aber, J. L., Gephart, M., Brooks-Gunn, J., & Connell, J. P. (1997). Development in context: Implications of studying neighborhood effects. In J.

Brooks-Gunn, G. J. Duncan, & J. L. Aber (Eds.), *Neighborhood poverty: Context and consequences for children* (pp. 44–61). New York: Russell Sage Foundation.

Aber, M. S. (1998). *Building self sufficiency and improving social welfare: Linking community and economic development*. Grant proposal funded by University of Illinois's Partnership Illinois Initiative. Champaign-Urbana.

Aber, M. S., Nieto, M., & Langhout, R. (1998). *Resident views of neighborhood: Implications for community involvement in neighborhood schools*. Manuscript in preparation. Champaign: University of Illinois.

Antonovsky, A. (1979). *Health, stress and coping*. San Francisco: Jossey-Bass.

Bandura, A. (1977). Self-efficacy: Toward a unifying theory of behavior change. *Psychological Review, 84*, 191–215.

Blau, P. (1977). *Inequality and heterogeneity*. New York: Free Press.

Borchert, J. (1980). *Alley life in Washington: Family, community, religion and folklike in the city, 1850–1970*. Urbana: University of Illinois Press.

Bowles, S. & Gintis, H. (1976). *Schooling in capitalist America*. New York: Basic Books.

Boyce, W. T., Frank, E., Jensen, P. S., Kessler, R. C., Nelson, C. A., Steinberg, L., & the MacArthur Foundation Research Network on Psychopathology and Development. (1998). Social context in developmental psychopathology: Recommendations for future research from the MacArthur Network on Psychopathology and Development. *Development and Psychopathology, 10*, 143–164.

Brooks-Gunn, G. J., Duncan, & Aber, J. L. (Eds.) (1997). *Neighborhood poverty: Context and consequences for children* (pp. 44–61). New York: Russell Sage Foundation.

Brooks-Gunn, J., Duncan, G. J., Klebanov, K., & Sealand, N. (1993). Do neighborhoods influence child and adolescent development? *American Journal of Sociology, 99*, 353–394.

Brown, K., Heumann, L., Winter-Nelson, K., Lukehart, J., & Bird, J. (1997). *An analysis of fair housing impediments in the State of Illinois*. Final report prepared by the University of Illinois at Urbana-Champaign Building Research Council and the Leadership Council for Metropolitan Open Communities for the State of Illinois and the Illinois Housing Department Authority.

Buckner, J. (1988). The development of an instrument to measure neighborhood cohesion. *American Journal of Community Psychology, 16*, 771–791.

Burgess, E. W. (1925). The growth of the city. In G. A. Theodorson (Ed.), *Urban patterns: Studies in human ecology* (pp. 35–41). University Park: Pennsylvania State University.

Bursik, R. J. (1984). Urban dynamics and ecological studies of delinquency. *Social Forces, 63*(2), 393–413.

Chaskin, R. J. (1997, December). Perspectives on neighborhood and community: A review of the literature. *Social Service Review,* 521–547.

Chiricos, T., Hogan, M., & Gertz, M. (1997). Racial composition of neighborhood and fear of crime. *Criminology, 35,* 107–131.

Cicchetti, D. (1989). Developmental psychopathology: Past, present, and future. In D. Cicchetti (Ed.), *Rochester Symposium on Developmental Psychopathology* (Vol. 1) (pp. 1–12). Hillsdale, NJ: Erlbaum.

Cicchetti, D. & Aber, J. L. (Eds.). (1998). Contextualism and developmental psychopathology [Special Issue]. *Development and Psychopathology, 10*(2).

Cicchetti, D. & Garmezy, N. (Eds.). (1993). Milestones in the development of resilience. *Development and Psychopatholoqy, 4,* 497–783.

Cohen, J. & Cohen, P. (1983). *Applied multiple regression/correlation analysis for the behavioral sciences* (2nd ed.). Hillsdale, NJ: Erlbaum Associates.

Coleman, R. P. (1978). *Attitudes toward neighborhoods: How Americans choose to live* (Working Paper No. 49). Joint Center for Urban Studies of MIT and Harvard University.

Coleman, J. (1986). Social theory, social research, and a theory of action. *American Journal of Sociology, 91,* 1309–1335.

Cowen, E. L. (1994). The enhancement of psychological wellness: Challenges and opportunities. *American Journal of Community Psychology, 22*(2), 149–179.

Cowen, E. L., Work, W. C., & Wyman, P. A. (1997). In S. S. Luthar, J. A. Burack, D. Cicchetti, & J. R. Weisz (Eds.), *Developmental psychopathology: Perspectives on adjustment, risk and disorder* (pp. 527–547). New York: Cambridge.

Cowen, E. L., Wyman, P. A., Work, W. C., & Parker, G. R. (1990). The Rochester Child Resilience Project (RCRP): Overview and summary of first year findings. *Development and Psychopathology, 2,* 193–212.

Crane, J. (1991). The epidemic theory of ghettos and neighborhood effects on dropping out and teenage childbearing. *American Journal of Sociology, 96,* 1226–1259.

Dash, L. (1989). *When children want children: An inside look at the crisis of teenage parenthood*. New York: Penguin Books.

Dornbusch, S. M., Ritter, L. P., & Steinberg, L. (1991). Community influences on the relation of family statuses to adolescent school performance: Differences between African Americans and Non-Hispanic Whites. *American Journal of Education, 38*(4), 543–567.

Duncan, G. J. (1994). Families and neighbors as sources of disadvantage in the schooling decisions of white and black adolescents. *American Journal of Education, 41*, 20–53.

Duncan, G. & Aber, J. L. (1997). Neighborhood models and measures. In J. Brooks-Gunn, G. Duncan, & J. L. Aber (Eds.), *Neighborhood poverty: Context and consequences for children: Vol. 1. Six studies of children in families in neighborhoods* (pp. 62–78). New York: Russell Sage.

Elliot, D. S. & Huizinga, D. (1990). The mediating effects of the social structure in high risk neighborhoods. Paper presented at the Annual Meeting of the American Sociological Association, Washington, D.C.

Feagin, J. R. (1973). Community disorganization: Some critical notes. *The Community*, 123–146.

Figueira-McDonough, J. (1991, March). Community structure and delinquency: A typology. *Social science review*, 68–91.

Garmezy, N., Masten, A. S., & Tellegen, A. (1984). Studies of stress resistant children: A building block for developmental psychopathology. *Child Development, 55*, 97–111.

Garner, C. L. & Raudenbush, S. W. (1991). Neighborhood effects on educational attainment: A multilevel analysis. *Sociology of Education, 64*, 251–262.

Gephart, M. A. (1989). Neighborhoods and communities in concentrated poverty. *Items, 43*, 84–92.

Giroux, H. (1983). Theories of reproduction and resistance in the new sociology of education: A critical analysis. *Harvard Educational Review, 53*, 289.

Glass, R. (1948). (Ed.) *The social background of a plan*. London: Routledge and Kegan Paul.

Haeberle, S. H. (1988). People or place—variations in community leaders' subjective definitions of neighborhood. *Urban Affairs Quarterly, 23*, 616–634.

Hojnacki, W. P. (1979, Sept./Oct.). What is a neighborhood? *Social Policy,* 47–52.

Hoyt, H. (1939). The pattern of movement of residential rental neighborhoods. In G. A. Theodorson (Ed.), *Urban patterns: Studies in human ecology* (pp. 42–49). University Park: Pennsylvania State University, 1982.

Kasarda, J. & Janowitz, M. (1974). Community attachment in mass society. *American Sociological Review, 39,* 328–339.

Korbin, J. E., Coulton, C. J., Chard, S., Platt-Houston, C., & Su, M. (1998). Impoverishment and child maltreatment in African American and European American neighborhoods. *Development and Psychopathology, 10*(2), 215–233.

Kotler, M. (1969). *Neighborhood government: The local foundations of political life.* New York: The Bobbs-Merrill Company, Inc.

Keller, S. (1968). *The urban neighborhood: A sociological perspective.* New York: Random House.

Lee, B. A. & Campbell, K. E. (1997). Common ground? Urban neighborhoods as survey respondents see them. *Social Science Quarterly, 78,* 922–936.

Luthar, S., Cicchetti, D., & Becker, B. (In press). The construct of resilience: A critical evaluation and guidelines for future work. *Child Development.*

MacLeod, J. (1987). *Ain't no makin' it.* Boulder, CO: Westview Press.

Massey, D. S. (1990). American apartheid: Segregation and the making of the underclass. *American Journal of Sociology, 96*(5), 329–358.

Massey, D. S. & Denton, N. A. (1993). *American apartheid: Segregation and the making of the underclass.* Cambridge, MA: Harvard University Press.

Massey, D. S. & Eggers, M. L. (1990). The ecology of inequality: Minorities and the concentration of poverty, 1970–1980. *American Journal of Sociology, 96,* 1153–1188.

Massey, D. S., Gross, A. B., & Eggers, M. L. (1992). Segregation, the concentration of poverty, and the life chances of individuals. *Social Science Research, 20*(4), 397–420.

McDonald, R. P. (1985). *Factor analysis and related methods.* Hillsdale, NJ: Erlbaum Associates.

Miller, Z. L. (1981). The role and concept of neighborhood in American cities. In R. Fisher & P. Romanosfsky (Eds.), *Community organization for urban social change: A historical perspective* (pp. 3–32). Westport, CT: Greenwood.

Nadeau, R., Niemi, R. G., & Levine, J. (1993, Fall). Innumeracy about minority populations. *Public Opinion Quarterly, 57,* 332–347.

Oakes, J. (1985). *Keeping track: How schools structure inequality.* New Haven, CT: Yale Press.

Oakes, J., Ormseth, T., Bell, R., & Camp, P. (1990). *Multiplying inequalities: The effects of race, social class, and tracking on opportunities to learn mathematics and science (R-3928-NSF).* Santa Monica, CA: Rand Corporation.

Park, R. E. (1915). The city: Suggestions for the investigation of human behavior in the city environment. *American Journal of Sociology, 20*(5), 577–612.

Park, R. E. (1936). Human ecology. In G. A. Theodorson (Ed.), *Urban patterns: Studies in human ecology* (pp. 50–54). University Park: Pennsylvania State University.

Park, R. E. & Burgess, E. W. (1925). *The city.* Chicago: University of Chicago Press.

Pedazur, E. J. (1982). *Multiple regression in behavioral research: Explanation and prediction* (2nd ed.). Chicago: Holt, Rinehart and Winston.

Rappaport, J. (1981). In praise of paradox: A social policy of empowerment over prevention. *American Journal of Community Psychology, 9,* 1–25.

Rappaport, J. (1987). Terms of empowerment/exemplars of prevention: Toward a theory of community psychology. *American Journal of Community Psychology, 15,* 121–148.

Rieder, J. (1985). *Canarsie: The Jews and Italians of Brooklyn against liberalism.* Cambridge, MA: Harvard University Press.

Sampson, R. J. (1988). Local friendship ties and community attachment in mass society: A multilevel systemic model. *American Sociological Review, 53,* 766–779.

Sampson, R. J. & Groves, W. B. (1989). Community structure and crime: Testing social disorganization theory. *American Journal of Sociology, 94,* 774–802.

Sampson, R. J. (1992). Family management and child development: Insights from social disorganization theory. In J. McCord (Ed.), *Advances in criminology theory: Vol. 3. Facts, frameworks and forecasts* (pp. 63–93). New Brunswick, NJ: Transaction Press.

Sampson, R. J., Raudenbush, S. W., & Earls, F. (1997). Neighborhoods and violent crime: A multilevel study of collective efficacy. *Science, 277,* 918–924.

Seidman, E., Yoshikawa, H., Roberts, A., Chesir-Teran, D., Allen, L., Friedman, J. L., & Aber, J. L. (1998). Structural and experiential neighborhood contexts, developmental stage, and antisocial behavior among urban adolescents in poverty. *Development and psychopathology, 10*(2), 259–281.

Shaw, C. & McKay, H. (1942). *Juvenile delinquency in urban areas.* Chicago: University of Chicago Press.

Shaw, C. & McKay, H. (1969). *Juvenile delinquency and urban areas* (Rev. ed.). Chicago: University of Chicago Press.

Simcha-Fagan, O. & Schwartz, J. (1986). Neighborhood and delinquency: An assessment of contextual effects. *Criminology, 24*(4), 667–704.

Stack, C. (1974). *All our kin.* New York: Basic Books.

Taylor, R., Gottfredson, S., & Brower, S. (1984). Block crime and fear: Defensible space, local social ties, and territorial functioning. *Journal of Research in Crime and Delinquency, 21,* 303–31.

Werner, E. E. & Smith, R. S. (1982). *Vulnerable but invincible: A study of resilient children.* New York: McGraw-Hill.

Werner, E. E. & Smith, R. S. (1992). *Overcoming the odds: High risk children from birth to adulthood.* Ithaca, NY: Cornell University Press.

Willis, P. E. (1977). *Learning to labor.* Aldershot: Gower.

Wilson, W. J. (1987). *The truly disadvantaged: The inner city, the underclass, and public policy.* Chicago: Chicago University Press.

Wilson, W. J. (1996). *When work disappears: The world of the new urban poor.* New York: Alfred A. Knopf.

# 7

# Health Promotion as a Strategy in Primary Prevention

*Joseph A. Durlak*

In the early 1990s, the Institute of Medicine convened a committee of experts for a 24-month study of the field of prevention. The publication emanating from this project [Institute of Medicine 1994] is an impressive volume that clarifies terminology regarding prevention, evaluates representative outcome studies, and offers recommendations for future research and practice. While there is much to praise in this report, ultimately, the committee chose NOT to include health promotion as a major form of prevention because of the interpretation that health promotion was not primarily designed "to prevent psychological or social problems, or mental disorders" [p. 27]. This chapter offers an alternative view.

Not all health promotion programs have a prevention goal, but those that do should be seen as viable approaches in primary prevention. While part of the support for health promotion as a preventive strategy can be made on conceptual grounds, the major evidence is present in outcome studies. Many contemporary health promotion programs have been successful as preventive interventions, and have obtained results comparable to those achieved by other approaches to prevention. In other words, empirical data suggest that promoting health is one way to prevent later problems.

This chapter is divided into two major sections. In the first, a model of adjustment is presented that incorporates healthy functioning and serves as a context for understanding prevention through health promotion. The second section summarizes outcome data on the success of health promotion prevention programs. The emphasis throughout this chapter is on programs for children and adolescents, which constitute the bulk of prevention intervention research.

## A Model of Adjustment

Figure 1 offers a heuristic, multidimensional model of adjustment for children and adolescents modified from another source [Durlak 1997]. The model does not depict adjustment solely in terms of pathology (i.e., problems), but as a combination of competencies (i.e., healthy aspects of functioning) and problems. Just because someone does not have problems does not necessarily mean they are well-adjusted. Therefore, adjustment refers to the presence of decidedly positive characteristics or competencies. For instance, in the psychological domain these characteristics might refer to high levels of self-esteem and self-efficacy; in the social domain, they might include effective social skills and positive attachments to others, and so on.

In the model there are four main domains of functioning: physical, psychological, social, and academic. Within each domain, there are two major dimensions, one representing different types of competencies and the other different types of problems. Only a few representative competencies and problems are listed in each area. This model conceives of competencies and problems in continuous rather than dichotomous terms. That is, the degree or level of each competency and problem can be assessed along a continuum (e.g., from very low to very high).

Furthermore, competencies and problems within each domain are listed separately rather than as end points of the same continuum. Data suggest that although competencies and problems are related, they tend to fall on separate factors or dimensions of adjustment. For example, subjective mental health is a combination of positive factors such as happiness and life satisfaction, and negative factors such as depression and anxiety [Bryant & Veroff 1984]. In studying children's peer relationships, it is important to consider peer rejection and peer acceptance separately because they are not merely the opposite of each other [Asher & Coie 1990].

All children have some problems, or at the least, limitations (no one is perfect). All have some competencies or capacities for growth (no one should be viewed only from a pathological perspective). Therefore, children's adjustment is determined by how the interplay among their competencies and problems affects their functioning in each of the four major adjustment domains depicted in figure 1.

**Figure 1. A Heuristic Model of Adjustment Illustrating Representative Competencies and Problems in Four Major Domains. Modified from Durlak [1997]**

## A MODEL OF ADJUSTMENT

### PHYSICAL DOMAIN

| *Competencies* | *Problems* |
|---|---|
| Physical Indices: muscle tone, cholesterol level, blood pressure<br>Behaviors: eating habits, exercise levels | Various medical problems<br>Physical injuries and disabilities<br>Sexually transmitted diseases |

### PSYCHOLOGICAL DOMAIN

| *Competencies* | *Problems* |
|---|---|
| Psychological well-being<br>Self-efficacy<br>Self-esteem<br>Adaptive skills: coping, emotional regulation, behavioral self-control | Clinical disorders<br>Subclinical-level problems<br>Drug misuse<br>Risky behaviors: drinking and driving, unprotected intercourse |

### SOCIAL DOMAIN

| *Competencies* | *Problems* |
|---|---|
| Peer acceptance<br>Altruism<br>Attachments/bonds with others<br>Social skills: communication, assertiveness, conflict-resolution | Peer rejection<br>Social isolation<br>Social anxiety<br>Violence, delinquency |

### ACADEMIC DOMAIN

| *Competencies* | *Problems* |
|---|---|
| Full development of cognitive talents and abilities<br>Metalearning (learning how to learn)<br>Higher order thinking skills | Underachievement<br>Test anxiety<br>School dropouts |

Several determinations are relative to adjustment. How competent is a child in each of the four domains (physical, psychological, social, and academic) and what levels of problems exist within each domain? Judgments about adjustment can be made for each domain separately and for overall functioning. Children can be relatively healthy or have problems in one domain of functioning (e.g., at school), but not necessarily in other areas of adjustment (e.g., at home or with peers).

Finally, the four dimensions of adjustment have bidirectional influences on each other as suggested by figure 2. This is important to keep in mind because good functioning in one domain might help a child compensate for limitations in another domain. The exact relationships among different aspects of adjustment at different developmental time periods and for different competencies and problems are just now being uncovered. For instance, children with physical health problems are at risk for problems in other areas; those with serious behavior problems are at risk for school problems and vice versa, and problems in peer and family relationship can influence psychological or academic health [Durlak 1997]. The relationships between competencies across domains has been less frequently studied, although some research has suggested that improving competencies in one domain (e.g., academics or social skills) can lead to positive changes in other domains [Caplan et al. 1992; see also Durlak & Wells 1997a; Yoshikawa 1995].

In summary, the model suggested by figures 1 and 2 emphasizes that adjustment is best viewed holistically by not only identifying multiple competencies and problems in different domains of functioning, but also by considering how these competencies and problems influence each other within and across domains and over time.

### Rationale Behind Health Promotion as Prevention

What is health promotion? Different terminology has been used in reference to health promotion interventions such as wellness, competency, well-being, and empowerment [e.g., Cowen 1994; Elias 1995; Rappaport 1987; Weissberg et al. 1997]. Others have discussed how theory and research on empowerment is emerging as a new paradigm

## Figure 2. An Illustration of Bidirectional Influences Among the Four Domains of Adjustment

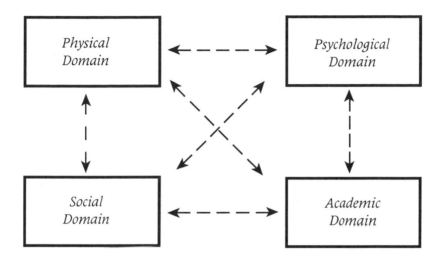

for prevention [Chinman & Linney 1998; Kim et al. 1998]. This chapter summarizes research on preventive-oriented health promotion programs that emphasize skill building—interventions that have a major emphasis on promoting specific competencies or skills in target populations in order to prevent future problems. Multicomponent programs containing a mixture of strategies are considered relevant as long as their major elements focus on health promotion.

It is important to stress that the philosophy behind health promotion does not rest on a deficit model that asserts that youths need competencies to compensate for their deficiencies. Rather, health promotion believes that individuals have high capacities for growth and development if their physical and social environments provide them sufficient opportunities, guidance, and support.

The basic rationale behind health promotion when it is used in prevention is that enhancing competencies in children should reduce later problems. Investigators target different competencies, but the general notion is that, if characteristics such as self-efficacy or social skills can be increased, then children should be better able to master future developmental challenges and tasks and deal more effectively with stress and negative events. As a result, future problems should be less likely. For example, in more concrete terms, if you enhance children's social skills, then they will be less likely to develop later behavior problems. If you increase interpersonal problem-solving skills, children will not be as aggressive or as rejected by peers. If you develop adolescents' refusal skills, they will be capable of resisting peer pressures to take drugs, and so on.

There is, of course, the question of which competencies should be targeted in prevention programs. Some studies focus on single competencies to test their value in prevention. However, because of the growing realization that most, if not all, outcomes are multiply determined, many effective preventive programs are multicomponent interventions. Such programs might improve children's social skills, help teachers in classroom management, and promote more effective parental child-rearing practices in the belief that targeting multiple competencies is more likely to produce positive results than targeting only one.

Multicomponent prevention programs also illustrate how attempts to change individuals directly (so-called person-centered approaches) can be combined with attempts to modify the social environment such as the home and school (sometimes called environment-centered approaches). Therefore, health promotion can be directed at changing individuals, changing environments, or doing both of these things simultaneously.

In summary, Figure 1 offers one way to view health promotion prevention programs. Investigators adopting this approach concentrate on the positive side of adjustment; they seek to enhance one or more competencies in one or more of the four domains of functioning in order to reduce future problems. Figure 2, which illustrates the interconnectedness of the four domains, suggests that improvement of key competencies in one domain may also eventually generalize to other aspects of functioning. Therefore, it should be possible to prevent multiple problems across domains through a single intervention, which has been found in some outcome research [Durlak & Wells 1997a].

## Program Outcomes

By the end of 1997, over 1200 outcome studies targeting children and adolescents had appeared [Durlak 1997]. No one has counted how many of these interventions can be classified as health promotion programs, and it is impossible to do justice to all outcome research in this chapter. Therefore, the following sections highlight representative health promotion programs in several preventive areas.

### Mental Health

Durlak and Wells [1997b] reviewed 177 preventive mental health programs that were intended to prevent various behavioral and social programs such as aggression, school disruption, and internalizing problems. Durlak and Wells [1997b] presented outcome data for studies grouped into several conceptually distinct categories, but the studies have been regrouped here to focus on health promotion.

The 66 programs qualifying as health promotion programs fell into two main categories (affective education and interpersonal problem solving), and a third miscellaneous category combining interventions focusing on different types of competencies such as specific social skills. Affective education seeks to increase children's awareness and expression of feelings and their social-cognitive skills relative to understanding the possible reasons behind their own as well as their peers' behaviors. Spivack and Shure [1984] have been the foremost proponent of interpersonal problem-solving training programs and have suggested that the ability to solve interpersonal problems is an important mediator of adjustment.

Mean effect sizes for preventive mental health programs are presented in Table 1 separately for outcomes measuring competencies and problems. Competencies reflect a composite of such variables as assertiveness, interpersonal problem-solving skills, self-esteem and self-efficacy, and measures of prosocial behavior. Problems included a combination of internalizing and externalizing symptoms, peer rejection, and academic underachievement.

With the exception of problem outcomes for interpersonal problem solving programs, all of the means in Table 1 differ significantly from zero, and none of the means differ significantly from each other.

## Table 1. Mean Effect for Different Categories of Preventive Mental Health Program

| | | Outcomes | |
|---|---|---|---|
| *Program Category* | *N* | *Problems* | *Competen-cies* |
| All Programs | 177 | 0.29 | 0.38 |
| All Health Promotion | 76 | 0.30 | 0.41 |
| Affective Education | 46 | 0.34 | 0.32 |
| Interpersonal Problem Solving | 18 | 0.15[1] | 0.61 |
| Miscellaneous Health Promotion | 12 | 0.35 | 0.47 |
| All Other Programs | 101 | 0.28 | 0.36 |

[1] Only mean effect not significantly different from zero.

*Note: Data are drawn from Durlak and Wells [1997b]*

In other words, most types of preventive mental health programs emphasizing health promotion were successful in significantly reducing problems and significantly increasing competencies in target populations.

Analyses of follow-up data suggested that program effects held over time. There were no significant differences between the mean effects obtained at post and follow-up for all outcomes combined, or when results were divided into more specific categories such as internalizing or externalizing problems, or measures of academic achievement. Once again, health promotion and non-health promotion programs showed a similar pattern of findings. Unfortunately, only 25% of the studies collected any follow-up data, and few studies followed participants for longer than six months.

Durlak and Wells' [1997b] meta-analysis included studies that had appeared by the end of 1991. Subsequent publications have continued to confirm the preventive value of health promotion. For example, skill training interventions for children, teachers, and parents have been effective in a variety of contexts [LaFreneiere & Capuano 1997; Miller-Heyl et al. 1998; O'Donnell et al. 1995; Sandler et al. 1992; Caplan et al. 1992; Wolchik et al. 1993]. There have also been positive outcomes in areas not reviewed by Durlak and Wells [1997b] such as delinquency prevention [see Gottfredson 1990; Lipsey 1992] and infancy programs [van Ijzendoorn et al. 1995]

For instance, in a meta-analysis of interventions designed to promote secure infant attachment, distinctions were made between preventive and therapeutic interventions [van Ijzendoorn et al. 1995]. The therapeutic interventions involved mothers with adjustment problems, whereas the preventive interventions did not. Both types of programs attempted to increase maternal sensitivity to infant signals and to help mothers become more responsive to these signals. Although each of the therapeutic programs produced negative effects, none of the preventive interventions did, and the latter's mean effect with secure attachment as an outcome was a moderately high 0.42. There is no straightforward relationship between attachment and later functioning, but the absence of a secure infant attachment is one risk factor for later psychopathology [Cicchetti et al. 1995].

There are some notable successes among preventively-oriented attachment interventions. For instance, van den Boom [1994, 1995] reported that a home visiting intervention was successful in enhancing maternal sensitivity to their infants. Compared to controls, intervention mothers were more responsive, stimulating, visually attentive, and appropriately controlling of their 9-month-old infant's behavior. This program had positive long-term effects. At 18 months of age, almost three times more intervention than control children were securely attached (72% versus 26% respectively). At a 33-month follow-up, when the children averaged 3-1/2 years of age, intervention children demonstrated more positive and less negative behaviors than controls.

In summary, outcome data indicate that mental health programs emphasizing health promotion reduce later problems. These findings argue for considering health promotion programs as legitimate preventive interventions.

## Drug Use

Health promotion is popular in drug abuse prevention. Nearly all of the 418 projects funded by the Center for Substance Abuse Prevention since 1987 have emphasized skill training as a core program component [Sambrano et al. 1997], although the outcomes of every one of these projects has not been carefully evaluated.

One of the most extensively evaluated and effective drug prevention programs, however, is Life Skills Training (LST), which was developed by Botvin and his colleagues [Dusenbury et al. 1990]. LST trains school children in multiple skills applicable to drugs and other personal and social situations. These skills include communication and assertiveness skills, decision making and goal setting, self-directed behavior change strategies, and methods of coping with anxiety and social pressure. Replications have confirmed the efficacy of LST in reducing future drug use, and the core program has been modified successfully for different cultural groups and for community settings other than schools [Botvin et al. 1994; St. Pierre et al. 1992]. Research on the implementation of LST is also consistent with other findings in prevention. That is, better effects are obtained when the program is faithfully and consistently conducted [Durlak 1998a].

## Learning Problems

Most academically-oriented prevention programs promote learning-related competencies. Interventions conducted during the preschool period often focus on school readiness as an important intermediate goal. School readiness refers generally to the effective maturation of physical, cognitive and social skills so that children can complete a formal academic curriculum successfully. Up to one-third of children are not fully ready for school entry, and those who are least prepared are at greater risk to do more poorly in school [Lewit & Baker 1995].

To develop school readiness, successful preschool interventions often combine early childhood education with services to families that are designed to help parents create and sustain a positive learning environment at home. Barnett [1995] described how several well-done preschool interventions were able to prevent later learning problems over an average eight-year follow-up period.

There have also been several successful academic interventions conducted at the elementary school level, which usually concentrate on developing children's competencies in basic subjects such as reading through intensive academic training and tutoring. Slavin, Karweit, and Wasik [1994] provide an excellent synthesis of this research.

## Physical Health Programs

Physical health programs are another area of prevention where many interventions have a health promotion focus [Perry et al. 1997]. The general intent is to develop positive health-related practices that will prevent later problems. For example, interventions may seek to improve the medical health of pregnant women and teach new mothers effective infant care behaviors and the importance of well-baby checkups and immunizations for their children. Interventions for school-age populations focus on eating and exercise patterns to improve nutritional intake and levels of physical fitness. Some programs have also involved parents so that both the school and home support children's new health behaviors. Programs to prevent smoking, adolescent pregnancy, and AIDS are also relevant as they often employ skill-training components related to assertiveness, peer resistance skills, and the development of safe sexual behaviors [for reviews, see Durlak 1997; Sagrestano & Paikoff 1997].

Similar to other areas of prevention, there have been several notable successes among physical health programs indicating practical, as well as statistically significant impact on future problems. For instance, studies indicate it is possible to reduce the percentage of low birthweight infants by 42% [Ershoff et al. 1990]; rates of youthful smoking by 39% [Perry et al. 1992]; adolescent pregnancies by 41% [Allen et al. 1994]; medical problems and rates of child abuse by up to 50% [Olds et al. 1986] and the intake of nonnutrious foods by up to 47% [Simons-Morton et al. 1991]. Although the short-term effects of the above programs have been dramatic, more data are needed on the long-term impact of physical health promotion.

There have also been some carefully done, large-scale, multisite studies of physical health programs focusing not only on outcomes, but also on program dissemination and implementation [Connell et al. 1985; Resnicow et al. 1996]. These investigations are important in suggesting that health promotion can be effectively introduced into many different settings and are appropriate for diverse populations.

## Critical Questions for Health Promotion

If health promotion is to assume a prominent place in prevention, then research must answer four important questions:

1. Can competencies be significantly improved through inter-vention?

2. Do health promotion interventions significantly reduce problems?

3. Are the results of intervention relatively enduring?

4. Does prevention occur through the mediating role of health promotion?

These above questions are listed in order of the challenge or difficulty they pose for researchers. Accordingly, there is less available information for each successive question, but there are some positive data relevant to each one.

### Question # 1: Are Competencies Improved?

The answer to this question is clearly "yes." Hundreds of studies exist indicating that it is possible to significantly improve different compe-tencies in children [see Durlak 1997; Weissberg et al. 1997]. It is also clear that systematic training is necessary for children to acquire and maintain new competencies. Merely telling children what to do does not have much effect. Many successful interventions have used social learning principles to promote new competencies. In this approach, each competency is first carefully defined and its effective use is then modeled. If necessary, complicated skills are broken down into their components, and training takes a step-by-step approach. Youth re-ceive immediate feedback and support for practicing the modeled competencies until mastery is achieved. Booster sessions and environmental supports may be added to maintain the performance of newly-learned skills. Many different types of personal and social competencies have been significantly increased using social-learning training principles such as assertiveness, communication, and interpersonal problem solving; levels of self-efficacy; habits related to nutrition, exercise, and safe sexual practices; and mastery of basic academic tasks and other learning demands [see Durlak 1997].

The consistent success of systematic skill training stands in stark contrast to the general ineffectiveness of didactically-oriented programs that assume that increasing knowledge will make a difference. "We know what does not work in prevention. Programs that rely on informational strategies to change behavior have not been effective in any area of prevention in which they have been tried. In fact, the evidence is overwhelming that such programs do not significantly change behavior. The use of information-only programs in prevention should be abandoned" [Durlak 1997, pp. 192-193].

Efforts to promote health and prevent problems by modifying the social environment have also been successful. For example, there is growing evidence that changing the organization and structure of school environments can result in higher levels of academic achievement, fewer behavioral and social problems, and more positive peer relationships [Baker et al. 1998; Durlak 1997; Good & Brophy 1986].

## Question # 2: Are Problems Also Reduced?

This chapter has reviewed representative programs in mental health, drug use, education, and physical health to show that preventively-oriented health promotion programs significantly reduce future problems. Not every program has been able to simultaneously improve health and reduce problems, but the convergent evidence across multiple areas of prevention suggests that health promotion has preventive impact. These findings offer a strong justification for the value of preventively-oriented health promotion programs.

## Question #3: Do Effects Last?

There is relatively less positive evidence in answer to this question than for the previous two questions. However, this is not because data suggest that intervention impact has dissipated over time, but due to the relative absence of many sustained follow-up studies. Follow-up studies are in the minority in all areas of prevention, and when investigators do track participants over time, most follow-up periods are less than a year. Nevertheless, available follow-up data indicate that the effects of health promotion persist, at least over the shorter term. The most impressive long-term follow-up data of program effects are in the early childhood education literature [Barnett 1995]. More data are needed in other areas on the enduring impact of health promotion.

## Question # 4: Does Health Promotion Mediate Outcomes?

Is it the promotion of one or more competencies that is responsible for preventive effects when they are obtained? Unfortunately, there is the least amount of information for this question. At the same time, however, the active or causal elements of all types of preventive interventions, health promotion or otherwise, are unknown. Actually, this is not surprising. Prevention is a relatively young science, and the first stages of intervention research usually involve demonstrating that programs are effective and can be replicated, before investigators try to determine what it is about a program that produces its results.

Regardless of whether an intervention produces positive, negative, or mixed effects, it is worthwhile to document if targeted competencies were modified as planned. If they were not, this might be the reason why the full impact of an intervention was not obtained [e.g., Hostetler & Fisher 1997].

There are several ways to explore how a program works. Structural equation modeling (SEM) is one technique well-suited to examining the longitudinal effects of large-sample preventive interventions. SEM can be used first to evaluate how well relevant constructs have been measured, and then to test a program's intended outcomes. Moreover, SEM encourages theory-building and theory-testing because it requires that researchers propose an a priori model that specifies a program's direct and indirect effects on measured variables.

Preventionists are beginning to use SEM. For instance, Wolchik et al. [1993] examined which of five possible mediators explained the results of their skill training program for divorced mothers. They found that an improvement in the mother-child relationship was a significant mediator in the reduction of child problems. At the same time, they found that not all of the possible mediators were significantly modified by the intervention (e.g., discipline practices and contact with noncustodial fathers). This is important because it suggests the need to strengthen future interventions in order to put these possible mediators to an adequate test.

As another example, Spoth and his colleagues [Spoth et al. 1998] have reported several analyses of skill-building, family-focused interventions targeting children's future drug use. To examine if the program worked as theorized, they tested a model whereby specific parenting practices targeted in the intervention (e.g., communication skills and greater involvement in child activities) had increased as predicted, and then whether changes in these practices were associated with positive changes in broader constructs such as the parent-child relationship and parents' general management style. Analyses supported the existence of these hypothesized direct and indirect effects [Spoth et al. 1998].

Even negative findings are helpful in improving programs. For example, the fact that interpersonal problem-solving programs significantly increased competencies (primarily problem-solving skills) but did not, as a group, significantly reduce mental health problems [Durlak & Wells 1997b] would seem to suggest that problem-solving skills did not mediate adjustment. This finding is consistent with the results of individual studies in which adjustment gains have occurred in target groups, but there was no significant relationship between improvement in problem-solving skills and improvement in adjustment [e.g., Weissberg et al. 1981; Work & Olsen 1990]. Therefore, negative findings can still be helpful by directing investigators to more profitable areas of inquiry.

In summary, as we move through the four evaluative questions regarding health promotion programs, there is less information to answer each successive question. Different competencies in children can definitely be enhanced, and many programs promoting competencies also reduce problems. Because follow-ups are in the minority and usually involve brief periods of time, the durability of program effects needs more documentation. Finally, the exact processes responsible for change in successful programs are only now beginning to be explored.

Nevertheless, there are sufficient data on hand to encourage further research and practice on health promotion programs as preventive interventions.

## Future Directions

Health promotion can have a bright future in prevention *if* adequate funding and administrative support are forthcoming. Current outcome data offer justification for recognizing the potential of appropriately crafted health promotion efforts as legitimate preventive interventions. It may take persistent advocacy to convince funding agencies of this fact, but empirical evidence can be marshaled to support a strong argument. Health promotion is actually a flexible strategy that can be integrated with other prominent approaches such as biopsychological models, principles of developmental psychopathology, and community-based empowerment and collaboration. Purists might grimace at this blending of approaches, but with mounting evidence suggesting that most positive and negative outcomes are multiply determined, there is a need for integrative paradigms.

There is also a need for more multidisciplinary collaboration. Investigators trying to prevent different types of negative outcomes (e.g., learning difficulties, drug use, behavioral or health problems), often target a common set of risk and protective factors [Durlak 1998b]. Collaboration among preventionists should eventually reduce any reluctance to embrace health promotion as a preventive strategy as investigators come to recognize the many commonalities that exist across disciplines and research areas. Furthermore, cross-disciplinary collaborations are likely to emerge as the most cost-effective way to achieve multiple positive outcomes from interventions and thus can more efficiently use the relatively few resources that funding and service agencies usually devote to prevention.

Over the long term, another good way to increase support for both prevention in general and health promotion in particular is to include these elements in professional training programs. Few disciplines currently give prevention and health promotion a very prominent place in training curricula. Because professionals are most likely to support approaches consistent with their training and experience, professional programs need to be modified so that all students become familiar with preventive health promotion strategies.

# References

Allen, J. P., Kuperminc, G., Philliber, S., & Herre, K. (1994). Programmatic prevention of adolescent problem behaviors: The role of autonomy, relatedness, and volunteer service in the Teen Outreach Program. *American Journal of Community Psychology, 22*, 617–638.

Asher, S. R. & Coie, J. D. (Eds.). (1990). *Peer rejection in childhood*. New York: Cambridge University Press.

Baker, J. A., Terry, T., Bridger, R., & Winsor, A. (1998). Schools as caring communities: A relational approach to school reform. *School Psychology Review, 26*, 586–602.

Barnett, W. S. (1995). Long-term effects of early childhood programs on cognitive and school outcomes. *The Future of Children, 5*, 25–50.

Botvin, G. J., Schinke, S. P., Epstein, J. A., & Diaz, T. (1994). Effectiveness of culturally focused and generic skills training approaches to alcohol and drug abuse prevention among minority youth. *Psychology of Addictive Behaviors, 8*, 116–127.

Bryant, F. B. & Veroff, J. (1984). Dimensions of subjective mental health in American men and women. *Journal of Health and Social Behavior, 25*, 116–135.

Caplan, M., Weissberg, R. P., Grober, J. S., Sivo, P. J., Grady, K., & Jacoby, C. (1992). Social competence promotion with inner-city and suburban young adolescents: Effects on social adjustment and alcohol use. *Journal of Consulting and Clinical Psychology, 60*, 56–63.

Chinman, M. J. & Linney, J. A. (1998). Toward a model of adolescent empowerment: Theoretical and empirical evidence. *Journal of Primary Prevention, 18*, 393–413.

Cicchetti, D., Toth, S. L., & Lynch, M. (1995). Bowlby's dream comes full circle. In T. H. Ollendick & R. J. Prinz (Eds.), *Advances in clinical child psychology* (Vol. 17) (pp. 1–75). New York: Plenum.

Connell, D. B., Turner, R. R., & Mason, E. F. (1985). Summary of findings of the school health education evaluation: Health promotion effectiveness, implementation, and costs. *Journal of School Health, 55*, 316–321.

Cowen, E. L. (1994). The enhancement of psychological wellness: Challenges and opportunities. *American Journal of Community Psychology, 22,* 149–180.

Durlak, J. A. (1997). *Successful prevention programs for children and adolescents.* New York: Plenum.

Durlak, J. A. (1998a). Why program implementation is important. *Journal of Prevention and Intervention in the Community, 17,* 5–19.

Durlak, J. A. (1998b). Common risk and protective factors in successful prevention programs. *American Journal of Orthopsychiatry, 68,* 512–520.

Durlak, J. A. & Wells, A. M. (1997a). Primary prevention mental health programs: The future is exciting. *American Journal of Community Psychology, 25,* 233–243.

Durlak, J. A. & Wells, A. M. (1997b). Primary prevention mental health programs for children and adolescents: A meta-analytic review. *American Journal of Community Psychology 25,* 115–152.

Dusenbury, L., Botvin, G. J., & James-Ortiz, S. (1990). The primary prevention of adolescent substance abuse through the promotion of personal and social competence. In R. P. Lorion (Ed.), *Protecting the children: Strategies for optimizing emotional and behavioral development* (pp. 201–224). Binghamton, NY: Haworth.

Elias, M. J. (1995). Primary prevention as health and social competence promotion. *Journal of Primary Prevention, 16,* 5–24.

Ershoff, D. H., Quinn, V. P., Mullen, P. D., & Lairson, D. R. (1990). Pregnancy and medical cost outcomes of a self-help prenatal smoking cessation program in a HMO. *Public Health Reports, 105,* 340–347.

Good, T. L. & Brophy, J. E. (1986). School effects. In M. C. Wittrock (Ed.), *Handbook of research on teaching* (3rd ed.) (pp. 570–602). New York: Macmillan.

Gottfredson, D. C. (1990). Changing school structures to benefit high-risk youths. In. P. E. Leone (Ed.), *Understanding troubled and troubling youth* (pp. 246–271). Newbury Park, CA: Sage.

Hostetler, M. & Fisher, K. (1997). Project C.A.R.E. substance abuse prevention program for high-risk youth: A longitudinal evaluation of program effectiveness. *Journal of Community Psychology, 25,* 397–419.

Institute of Medicine. (1994). *Reducing risks for mental disorders: Frontiers for preventive intervention research.* Washington, DC: National Academy Press.

Kim, S., Crutchfield, C., Williams, C., & Hepler, N. (1998). Toward a paradigm in substance abuse and other problem behavior prevention for youth:

Youth development and empowerment approach. *Journal of Drug Education, 28,* 1–17.

LaFreniere, P. J. & Capuano, F. (1997). Preventive intervention as means of clarifying direction of effects in socialization: Anxious-withdrawn preschoolers case. *Development and psychopathology, 9,* 551–564.

Lewit, E. M. & Baker, L. S. (1995). School readiness. *The Future of Children, 5,* 128–139.

Lipsey, M. W. (1992). Juvenile delinquency treatment: A meta-analytic inquiry into the variability of effects. In T. D. Cook, H. Cooper, D. S. Cordray, H. Hartman, L. V. Hedges, R. J. Light, T. A. Louis, & F. Mosteller (Eds.), *Meta-analysis for explanation: A casebook* (pp. 83–127). New York: Russell Sage Foundation.

Miller-Heyl, J., MacPhee, D., & Fritz J. J. (1998). DARE to be you: A family-support, early prevention program. *Journal of Primary Prevention, 18,* 257–285.

O'Donnell, J., Hawkins, J. D., Catalano, R. F., Abbott, R. D., & Day, L. E. (1995). Preventing school failure, drug use, and delinquency among low-income children: Effects of a long-term prevention project in elementary schools. *American Journal of Orthopsychiatry, 65,* 87–100.

Olds, D. L., Henderson, Jr. C. R., Chamberlin, R., & Tatelbaum, R. (1986). Preventing child abuse and neglect: A randomized trial of nurse home visitation. *Pediatrics, 78,* 65–78.

Perry, C. L., Kelder, S. H., Murray, D. M., & Klepp, K. I. (1992). Community-wide smoking prevention: Long-term outcomes of the Minnesota Heart Health Program. *American Journal of Public Health, 82,* 1210–1216.

Perry, C. L., Story, M., & Lytle, L. A. (1997). Promoting healthy dietary behaviors. In R. P. Weissberg, T. P. Gullotta, R. L. Hampton, B. A, Ryan, & G. R. Adams (Eds.), *Healthy children 2010: Enhancing children's wellness* (pp. 214–249). Thousand Oaks, CA: Sage Publications.

Rappaport, J. (1987). Terms of empowerment/exemplars of prevention: Toward a theory of community psychology. *American Journal of Community Psychology, 15,* 121–148.

Resnicow, K., Robinson, T. N., & Frank, E. (Eds.). (1996). The multicenter Child and Adolescent Trial for Cardiovascular Health (CATCH): Promoting cardiovascular health through schools. [Special Issue]. *Preventive Medicine, 25*(4).

Sagrestano, L. M. & Paikoff, R. L. (1997). Preventing high-risk sexual behavior, sexually transmitted diseases, and pregnancy among adolescents. In R. P. Weissberg, T. P. Gullotta, R. L. Hampton, B. A. Ryan, & G. R. Adams (Eds.), *Healthy Children 2010: Enhancing children's wellness* (pp. 76–104). Thousand Oaks, CA: Sage.

Sambrano, S., Springer, J. F., & Hermann, J. (1997). Informing the next generation of prevention programs: CSAP's cross-site evaluation of the 1994–95 high-risk youth grantees. *Journal of Community Psychology, 25,* 375–395.

Sandler, I. N., West, S. G., Baca, L., Pillow, D. R., Gersten, J. C., Rogosch, F., Virdin, J., Beals, J., Reynolds, K. D., Kallgren, C., Tein, J., Kriege, G., Cole, E., & Ramirez, R. (1992). Linking empirically based theory and evaluation: The Family Bereavement Program. *American Journal of Community Psychology, 20,* 491–521.

Simons-Morton, B. G., Parcel, G. S., Baranowski, T., Forthofer, R., & O'Mara, N. M. (1991). Promoting physical activity and a healthful diet among children: Results of a school-based intervention study. *American Journal of Public Health, 81,* 986–991.

Slavin, R. E., Karweit, N. L., & Wasik, B. A. (1994). *Preventing early school failure.* Needham Heights, MA: Allyn & Bacon.

Spivack, G. & Shure, M. (1974). *Social adjustment of young children: A cognitive approach to solving real-life problems.* San Francisco: Jossey Bass.

Spoth, R., Redmond, C., & Shin, C. (1998). Direct and indirect latent-variable parenting outcomes of two universal family-focused preventive interventions: Extending a public health-oriented research base. *Journal of Consulting and Clinical Psychology, 66,* 385–399.

St. Pierre, T. L., Kaltreider, L., Mark, M. N., & Aiken, K. J. (1992). Drug prevention in a community setting: A longitudinal study of the relative effectiveness of a three-year primary prevention program in Boys and Girls Clubs across the nation. *American Journal of Community Psychology, 20,* 673–706.

van den Boom, D. C. (1994). The influence of temperament and mothering on attachment and exploration: An experimental manipulation of sensitive responsiveness among lower-class mothers with irritable infants. *Child Development, 65,* 1457–1477.

van den Boom, D. C. (1995). Do first-year intervention effects endure? Follow-up during toddlerhood of a sample of Dutch irritable infants. *Child Development, 66,* 1798–1816.

van Ijzendoorn, M. H., Juffer, F., & Duyvesteyn, M. G. C. (1995). Breaking the intergenerational cycle of insecure attachment: A review of the effects of attachment-based interventions on maternal sensitivity and infant security. *Journal of Child Psychology and Psychiatry, 36,* 225–248.

Weissberg, R. P., Gesten, E. L., Rapkin, B. D., Cowen, E. L., Davidson, E., de Apodaca, R. F., & McKim, B. (1981). The evaluation of a social problem-solving training program for suburban and inner-city grade children. *Journal of Consulting and Clinical Psychology, 49,* 251–261.

Weissberg, R. P., Gullotta, T. P., Hampton, R. L., Ryan, B. A., & Adams, G. R. (Eds.). (1997). *Healthy Children 2010: Enhancing children's wellness.* Thousand Oaks, CA: Sage.

Wolchik, S. A., West, S. G., Westover, S., Sandler, I. N., Martin, A., Lustig, J., Tein, J., & Fisher, J. (1993). The Children of Divorce Parenting Intervention: Outcome evaluation of an empirically based program. *American Journal of Community Psychology, 21,* 293–331.

Work, W. C. & Olsen, K. H. (1990). Evaluation of a revised fourth grade social problem solving curriculum: Empathy as a moderator of adjustive gain. *Journal of Primary Prevention, 11,* 143–157.

Yoshikawa, H. (1995). Long-term effects of early childhood programs on social outcomes and delinquency. *The Future of Children, 5,* 51–75.

## Acknowledgments

Early in my career, Emory Cowen treated me as though I were a long-lost prodigal son. He invited me to come to Rochester to "present" a paper at one of his week-long school workshops, analyzed the outcome data for me from my first prevention study (several times, in fact, until it was correct), and could not refrain from revising some, I should say most, well, actually, it was all of my initial manuscript before I submitted it for publication. I will always be grateful for his support and kindness, which continue to this day. It was Emory who suggested to the editors that I be asked to contribute this chapter. I am complimented to be part of this volume honoring Emory Cowen.

# 8

## Wellness in the Schools: The Grandfather of Primary Prevention Tells a Story

*Maurice J. Elias and Roger P. Weissberg*

This chapter is written in the format of a dialogue between Emory Cowen and one of his young grandchildren. We wrote it in this way for a few reasons. First, we have seen Grandfather Cowen in action with young children. He is warm, caring, and engaging with them. Second, Professor Cowen is a master teacher and mentor of school-based prevention and wellness. He has educated hundreds of scholars and practitioners who have devoted their careers both to prevention research and practice (including the authors of this chapter), as well as to training a new generation of preventionists and wellness-enhancers. Third, Scholar Cowen has been obsessed for many decades with clarifying the definitions of terms like primary prevention [Cowen 1977, 1983] and wellness [Cowen 1994, 1997a, 1997b]. We believe he would appreciate our efforts to describe "wellness in schools" so that even a child could understand it!

During his career Emory has excelled in making kid-helping contributions that translated research and theory into practical applications that have benefitted literally thousands of children. His committed approach to work is symbolized less by academic high tea than by morning bagel. We aspired to reflect that aspect of his "mensch-like" working style and his scholarly contributions in the form of our chapter, not only in content.

The format also reflects Emory's interest in wellness and in resilience in children—one strong empirical finding is how competence is enhanced through dialogues in caring relationships, such as the one depicted in this chapter. We also took a cue from Cowen's [1995, p. 11] writing:

A prime task is to enhance wellness in the many using diverse approaches (e.g., strengthening early caregiver attachments; promoting competence acquisition in children; engineering settings and environments that favor positive adaptation; empowerment; teaching stress-coping), as adapted to 'fit' the needs and life situations of different age and sociocultural groups.

We opted to use a divergent format to engage readers in ways complementary to the more conventional style used by other authors in this volume [see Consortium on the School-based Promotion of Social Competence [1994] or Weissberg and Greenberg [1998] for two recent comprehensive, traditional reviews of school-based prevention and wellness-enhancement programs].

Finally, we know that while Emory wants to make the world a better place for all children, and especially children whose life circumstances place them at great risk for harm, his foremost commitment is to making the world a better place for his own grandchildren. We want to salute that and ensure that Emory, his readers, and, when they are old enough, his grandchildren, know how this man of great scholarship is driven by the love of children. We honor this along with his contributions to the field.

## The Story Begins: The Prevention Parable and PMHP

**Child:** Grandpa, will you tell me a story?

**Grandfather Cowen:** Of course I will! Would you like the Three Bears, or would you like me to read you a Dr. Seuss book?

**C:** No, Grandpa, tell me the story about the river and the children.

**G:** Are you sure?

**C:** Yes. Please!

**G:** Well, one day, I was walking by the river and I saw a lot of children in the river. They looked like they were having trouble swimming. I saw someone, a man I didn't know, trying to help the children come out of the river. He had a long stick with a net on it, and would scoop up as many children as he could. But there were a lot of children and he couldn't help them all. I started to help him, but even with me there, we couldn't help everyone.

**C:** So what did you do, Grandpa? Is that when you took the walk?

**G:** Yes, that's what I did. I took a walk up to the place in the river where the children were falling in. There was a problem with a bridge and when they walked over it, a lot of them fell in.

**C:** Did you do the Pim Hip?

**G:** Yes, we started our Primary Mental Health Project (PMHP), or Pim Hip, and fewer kids were falling into the river. This also made it a lot easier for the man to help the ones that did fall in.

**C:** What is PMHP?

**G:** PMHP is special program that helps kindergarten through third-grade children succeed in school [Cowen et al. 1996]. It began in one Rochester, New York, school more than 40 years ago, and now it is in about 1,000 schools around the world!

**C:** Wow!

**G:** Sometimes children have problems getting along in school. Some get into fights, others are sad or have trouble making friends, and some have trouble following class rules or getting their work done.

**C:** I have a few friends like that.

**G:** Actually there are lots of kids who have problems like these. PMHP works with teachers and parents to find out which children need help. Then really nice counselors work and play with the children once or twice a week and help them to feel better about themselves and school.

**C:** Grandpa, you're great!

**G:** I think we need a snack.

## Key Integrated Social Services and the Development of Wellness

**C:** Grandpa, while we are having a snack, will you tell me the story about being well?

**G:** Are you sure? It's long and it gets a little complicated.

**C:** I like the way you tell stories, Grandpa.

**G:** Okay, Okay, I'll tell you. You know how much I love you, don't you?

**C:** Yes, Grandpa.

**G:** And you know that you are healthy. You almost never get sick, you are happy most of the time, you have a lot of friends, you have a lot of confidence,...

**C:** What's that?

**G:** It means that when you need to get something done, you feel like you can do it. Remember when you couldn't open your desk drawer? You didn't cry, you didn't run to mommy or daddy or ask for help, you tried to open it yourself. Do you remember how you did it?

**C:** Uh, I pushed it in and shook it from side to side a couple of times and then when I tried it again, it opened.

**G:** That's right. There are a lot of things that have to happen so that you and your friends are healthy. My old friend Eli Bower said that a lot depends on whether or not you get a good kiss when you are very young.

Eli loved children very much and he believed that the more adults take care of what he called the "Key Integrated Social Services" (KISS), the healthier children would be [Bower 1972]. When your mommy was pregnant with you, she had very good doctors. She visited them all the time. When you were born, a pediatrician came to look at you right away. She and the nurses showed your mommy and daddy how to take care of you, you know, like changing your diaper and giving you a bath and feeding you. She kept going to the doctor all the time until you were a year old, and then she went every six months for a while.

You got off to a healthy start, but it made a big difference that your family was ready for you. They couldn't wait to teach you things, to read to you, to hold you, and just do what they could to take care of you. I think they—with some help from me—got you off to a good start. Don't you think so?

**C:** Yeah!

**G:** When you started school, you began the third part of Eli's KISS. Do you remember your preschool?

**C:** Sure. It was fun. We had two great teachers, and we had blocks and dress-up and the kitchen area and we had a snack every day.

**G:** Some children whose parents don't have the money to go to a preschool like you did go instead to Head Start. There, they learned a lot of the same things that you did. But they also met doctors who checked their eyes, hearing, teeth, and their health, and their parents met people who helped them with housing, giving them ideas about how to take care of kids, getting around town, even help in finding a job if they needed it. It's still strange to me that once these kids start kindergarten, they and their parents usually don't get this extra help anymore unless they pay for it, even though they really still need it.

Anyhow, the next KISS system is your friends, kids your age. I have watched you play with your friends, learn from them, copy them sometimes, ask them questions, like how to play that new computer game you got for your birthday, and argue with them and make up and be friends again. You are pretty good at this! When you get to be a teenager, your friends will be even more important to you than they are now.

**C:** Why, Grandpa?

**G:** Well, you will be at an age where you will want to find out more things for yourself, without always asking mom or dad. You can always come to me, of course! Your friends and you will talk about jobs, colleges, even religion.

**C:** But I want to ask mommy and daddy.

**G:** And you still will. Speaking of mommy and daddy, there are some things that influence what they do as parents—things like how much time they have to spend with you, how tired they are when they are with you, and what kind of mood they are in. Jay Belsky [1984] called these things by the fancy name of micro and exosystems, and he has written about how they affect not only parents, but other caregivers.

**C:** Sometimes when Daddy comes home from work, he says he is tired or upset.

**G:** True, and I have seen him also come home excited, like the time he took us all out to dinner because things went so well on his project. Remember?

**C:** Yeah, that was good!

**G:** Another thing that makes a difference to your parents is what they do for leisure or recreation, like neighborhood clubs; country clubs; bowling teams; golfing partners; Sunday morning softball teams; season tickets to sporting events; health clubs; morning walks, Tai Chi groups, meditation, poker games, horse racing, legal betting, college basketball, sewing and quilting groups, cooking clubs; attending concerts of any and all kinds; reading and use of libraries; having a porch to sit on; coffee klatches, whether at one's home, at school, or in a coffee place or big bookstore; community organizations, which include parents' groups affiliated with schools; Neighborhood Watch; shelters for homeless or victims of domestic violence; groups such as Kiwanis, Scouting, Rotary, Lions, Moose, Elk, B'nai B'rith, CYO, or Mothers Against Drunk Driving; local Chambers of Commerce and other business associations; associations of realtors and manufacturers; and advocates for beautification/preservation of one's town.

**C:** Sometimes you say a lot of stuff I don't all understand, Grandpa. What's legal burping?

**G:** That's betting, not burping, and, well, if you have questions like that, later you can ask your mom or dad. There is one more thing that also influences how well parents and caregivers do their jobs, and that is the range of human service organizations, which include United Way agencies; supervised housing; halfway houses; formal service agencies such as Child Protective Services, Juvenile Justice, and Family Courts; the range of inpatient, partial hospitalization, and outpatient or community based services for those with difficulties related to mental health and mental retardation; local counseling centers; Safe Homes; pastoral counseling and other religiously-affiliated individual and family service agencies; and managed care and HMO services and systems.

**C:** Wow! No wonder they get tired so early sometimes!

**G:** Did I notice a new computer in your room?

**C:** Yup! It has a WXYZ-997 Wizbang Gizmo with a Nonfat Seminuclear Nonchocolate Chip, and it's superfast!

**G:** Well, things like media, the Internet, and cyberspace are things that Eli Bower never thought much about, but these now should be thought of as part of his KISS. People worry about what children watch on TV and see on the Internet, not to mention what you listen to through those headphones of yours. I wonder if all this is the best way for you to spend your time. How much time is being taken from things like playing with your friends? How do families deal with all of the channels and magazines and e-mails and things that are pouring into our homes? To what should children be exposed? At what ages? For that matter, to what should adults be exposed? At the same time, how fair is it that you and your sister and your friends have all these electronic things, but other kids in your school don't? They can't do their homework easily on the Internet.

**C:** I don't know. If it's not so good for me, maybe they are better off.

**G:** That's a good thought. But it would be fair if they had the same choices, don't you think? Well, Eli Bower always liked to say that when the KISS systems work as they are supposed to, they provide health care, schooling, parenting, friendships, and spiritual supports they were intended to, and individuals passing through them would find themselves possessing considerable strengths and being very supported. But, as we know, not too many things work perfectly. Some schools, families, and hospitals are a lot better places to be than others. Training and supervision that help professionals work at their very best are not always provided or available. And the extent to which all the KISS systems work together can be quite different in different places. Rochester is a pretty good place that tries hard to keep things working together. But I have been to other places where this doesn't happen too well at all.

**C:** Why not, Grandpa? Can't it hurt kids if adults don't work together or do a good job?

**G:** Yes, it can. Since you are a grown-up kind of kid, I will tell you a sad example. In some hospitals, in some communities, moms come in to give birth to their kids and it almost always goes very well, just like it did for you. But there are other places where things don't always go so well, where the babies are more likely to be sick, or even die.

**C:** Die?

**G:** Yes. And the even sadder thing is that people sometimes know about these places, and not too much is done about it—I think because they are in poorer neighborhoods.

**C:** That's not fair!

**G:** No, it's not. When things don't go so well in the KISS systems, Eli Bower said that it is important for people to find good help fast so that they can feel better and get back to whatever it was they were doing. So, when you get sick, you go to a doctor, and pretty soon, you are back in school. Other kinds of special help are guidance counselors and special services staff in schools, mental health clinics of different kinds, police, a crisis center, an emergency room at a hospital, and people in workplaces that help when employees are upset or having a lot of stress or other troubles.

C: Grandpa, I remember last time you told me something about being cold.

G: What a good memory you have! Eli did say that sometimes life can be very cold for people. They cannot get the help they need, and so they have to go to special places where it sometimes takes a long time to get better. He called this ICE—llness Correctional Endeavors. ICE is provided by psychiatric hospitals, prisons, and long-term health care facilities. These may appear like places where those in need of a lot of help can go so they can return to KISS, but it often can be easier to enter ICE institutions than it is to leave them to return to KISS systems. It's kind of complicated and gets into matters of money and politics that I would rather not talk to you about on such a beautiful day.

## Maintaining and Enhancing Children's Wellness

C: Okay, Grandpa, that's a good idea. Is now when you tell me about the things that make people stay well?

G: You know, when I was going to school, to graduate school, we spent a lot of time talking about all the things that made people sick or unhappy. I remember my teachers would take a card with an ink blot—you know, something like this, where you put some ink on a page and then fold the page over and, just like this, it makes a funny shape that's pretty much the same on both sides of the page. You see?

C: Yeah, Grandpa, that one looks like a tree and a farm.

G: Well, we would ask people to tell stories about a lot of these things and then we would write reports and go in meetings and talk about all the problems we thought the person had.

C: You mean, like there would be bugs on the trees or the cows got sick and they had no milk?

G: Something like that. After a while of doing that, I started to ask myself, what did I really know about these people, about their interests, their hopes, the things that made them happy, the ways in which they tried to take good care of themselves? Not very much. So, I spent more and more of my time trying to understand what helped people get or stay healthy. And some other people started doing the same thing [Cowen 1997b; Elias 1994; Garmezy 1991; Haggerty et al. 1994; Rutter 1987; Weissberg & Greenberg 1998; Weissberg, Gullotta, et al. 1997; Werner & Smith 1992]. And do you know what?

    **C:** What?

    **G:** We started learning a lot about what makes people...

    **C:** Well!

    **G:** Right! There are so many ways of thinking about this. Let me tell you about three things that I think make a big difference.

## 1. How Much Does Your Environment Support You?

During the day, at school or work or home or with your friends or even just around the neighborhood, how much do people let you know you are doing a good job, reward you when you accomplish things, and generally give you a lot more smiles than frowns? And when things don't go so well, like when you have a problem or important people in your life are sick or in trouble and need help, how much support do you get? Does the support kind of find you, or do you have to go and look a lot for it? It's like that cartoon we saw, where the two fish were having problems and every place one fish turned for help closed their doors, said he was the wrong kind of fish, told him they were not open now, and the other fish not only got help everywhere, but you remember what happened when he was floating along thinking about what to do next?

    **C:** That's when that squid thing came over and said, "You look like you need a tentacle" and gave him three or four to hold on to!

    **G:** And he grabbed on and the squid...

    **C:** Pulled him along on a kind of fun ride, and pretty soon the fish started to smile, and right after that he got a great idea about how to solve his problem.

    **G:** That fish was in what I call a wellness-enhancing environment. And people just feel better and do better when they are in that kind of situation [Cowen 1994; 1997a].

## 2. How Supportive Is Your Family Environment?

We spend a lot of time with our families, and the more supportive they are, the more wellness gets spread around to everyone. What really matters is that we feel connected, close, to at least one person in our family.

**C:** I feel close to you, Grandpa.

**G:** And I feel very close to you, too. Just thinking about our time together helps keep me feeling well. It makes me want to take care of myself, stay healthy, and learn about new things so I can share them with you. And I even watch some cable TV things and try some computer games that I otherwise might not, because I know that you like them.

**C:** And I even listen to some of that music, that Artie Krupa and Elephant Geraldine and that clarinet guy—I just remember Beany Babies.

**G:** You are thinking of Benny Goodman, aren't you?

**C:** Yeah! You like that stuff more than I do, but the guy who plays the xylophone is pretty cool. And those sisters who sing about beer.

**G:** Actually, it's Bei Mir Bis Du Shayne. It also helps when family members feel that they are supported by other members of the family, and there is not a lot of conflict in the house. It is not fun coming home to a place where there is a lot of anger and fighting.

**C:** You might not even want to come home! Timmy once came to our house after school because he said he was afraid his Dad would yell at him when he got home.

**G:** When that happens, Timmy is at least lucky that he could come to your house, instead of just hanging out on the street or something. There is one more thing that is important to people's wellness:

## 3. What Is the Person Like?

It's true that people can learn and change, but sometimes you start out in a better place than others. Some people can have a lot of upsetting things happen to them and they still handle it, they still feel hopeful that things will work out, and they work hard and actively to solve their problems, to make things better, to figure out what is going on around them and how to make the best of things. They have learned how to ask for help from others, to look ahead and think about the consequences of their ideas for themselves and for others, and they just have an overall sense that, "I can do it and it will work out okay in the end."

**C:** Is that what you called, let me remember, Slovakian Epiphany?

**G:** Wow! What a memory! That's pretty close—it's self-efficacy. There are people who don't feel these ways and don't have these skills, and it is harder for them to feel well.

**C:** That's like Mrs. Gristle in school. She is always telling us we will never learn this and we will never learn that, and we will never finish what we are doing on time. She is always taking aspirin for her headaches. The good thing is that she is absent a lot. Oops, I didn't mean that.

**G:** But what you are saying is important—a lot of times, people get what they think is physical sickness as a result of too much stress and not enough support or skills to deal with stress.

**C:** And that's why you started working with kids like me, in schools, right Grandpa?

**G:** Right again! Some of my friends [Masten, Best, & Garmezy 1990] point out that there are three kinds of situations relating to children that we need to worry most about: good outcomes in high-risk children, sustained competence in children under stress, and recovery from trauma. The way to help kids in all these situations is similar. They need positive relationships with competent adults, good learning and problem-solving skills, good social-approach and social-engagement skills, and they need to know that they have some things they are good at—"areas of perceived competence" in fancy language—and that they feel they are important to themselves, to other people, and even to their neighborhoods and society.

As I looked around, I saw lots of things that made it hard for a lot of kids to get well or stay well. And a lot of things have gotten a little better, but not fast enough. And some things have gotten worse.

**C:** What kinds of things, Grandpa? Do you mean not enough to eat?

**G:** Yes. Child poverty; deepening social intolerance of differences in a time of greater and greater diversity; and growing difficulty in making ends meet, so that both parents are working, making it harder and harder for adults and children to have positive relationships. When these things happen, not all kids have the same access to the best instruction in school, to models and chances to learn interpersonal skills, thoughtful problem solving, and positive, patient social approach and engagement skills. It's hard for kids to look around and around and say to themselves, "I'm as important as anyone else, I matter a lot, my future is important." Poverty also leads kids to be less healthy, which also takes away their strengths and makes kids less able to show resilience, especially under sustained or acute adversity.

**C:** I remember a couple of kids in school who kept coming in hungry and they never brought lunch. It was a problem, and then one day a kid in the class asked us all to take some of our lunches and give it to these kids at lunchtime. They got so happy! The rest of the afternoon went better in school, too, because they didn't get in trouble. The teacher called their house and I don't know what happened after that, but they weren't hungry anymore, except when they had that yucky soup in school—everyone was hungry after that.

**G:** That's some story! It shows me that you really understand what we are talking about.

## Promoting Wellness in Schools

**C:** Grandpa, can you tell me now some stories about making things better? You showed me that book with the big 14 on it—14 oxes, or something?

**C:** Close! *14 Ounces of Prevention* [Price et al. 1988], actually. But it might have been called 14 oxen, because each of the 14 programs in that book had to be strong as an ox to keep going and help the people involved.

**G:** Can you tell me about some of them?

**C:** Okay, I will. But then, I want to tell you also about some things that have been happening lately that I think make for a happier story than the one I might have told five years ago.

In 1988, the American Psychological Association published a set of articles describing 14 programs that had been selected from over 500 as the "best" examples of prevention across the life span. To get picked, the programs have to have data to show that what they said they were doing really worked, and they had to have been in "real" operation for at least a period of several years.

Myrna Shure and George Spivack [1988] looked at children's preschool teachers, and how they could learn to carry out a curriculum to children that would increase their interpersonal cognitive problem solving (ICPS, now known as "I Can Problem Solve") skills.

**C:** What's a curriculum?

**G:** You know, that's a wonderful question. A lot of people think it's a book with lessons you give to a teacher and then the teachers just carries it out in the classroom. But that's not true. A curriculum is a way of thinking about things, a way of organizing a classroom and even a school for an entire year. The curriculum has lessons in it but it also gives the teachers an idea of how to handle situations that come up with students all the time.

For ICPS, what was most important was that a set of caregivers were being helped to deliver not only certain content to children, but to give children opportunities to practice the skills being taught and then to apply the skills at other times during the school day. The centerpiece of ICPS is teaching caregivers to "dialogue" with children. In essence, "dialoguing" involves asking open-ended questions first, to promote children's own thinking and problem solving, reverting to more a "telling" mode only as needed. That is what ICPS, and an entire group of problem-solving and decision-making approaches to wellness that has evolved from this pioneering work, tries to do for children of preschool through high school age [Elias & Clabby 1992; Weissberg et al. 1991].

**C:** There were other stories in there also, right Grandpa? Like some about teenagers, and adults who lost their jobs.

**G:** Yes, but I don't want to tell you all the same stories all the time! How about a new one? This has a big sounding name: Report of the Committee on Prevention of Mental Disorders of the Institute of Medicine (IOM) [Mrazek & Haggerty 1994]. It is over 600 pages of both prevention research and prevention programs. What really surprised me is that they put wellness-type programs in their own chapter, calling them programs designed to promote competence.

**C:** Isn't that better, Grandpa? Then people can see that you don't always have to worry about keeping somebody from catching something, it's okay to just help them be healthy.

**G:** I think you should join the IOM! Anyhow, the report talks a lot about the Social Development Model [Hawkins et al. 1992] as a universal prevention approach focused on elementary schools. It addresses the need to teach skills to children, but also to change the norms of the setting around things like smoking and violence and drugs and healthy eating, and make sure that there are lots of opportunities to try out the new skills. Teachers were trained in classroom management, cooperative learning, and the use of the ICPS curriculum; there also was a part for parents, to help create norms in homes for self-control on the part of children and for academic work as important. Following first graders into fifth grade, the authors found that children from the intervention group were less likely than what is called a control group to start alcohol use, and data on family communication and involvement and attachment to school and school rewards and norms were all better.

Elias, Gara, Schuyler, Branden-Muller, and Sayette [1991] looked at the impact of an elementary school version of ICPS, the Social Decision Making and Problem Solving Program [Elias & Tobias 1996], on problem behaviors. One difference from the ICPS program is that the SDM/PS program spends a lot of time and energy on a set of "Readiness" skills designed to build students self-control and group participation and to foster norms in classrooms that support these skills, and an "Application Phase" in which the skills of the program are systematically used in all parts of the school routine, including the discipline system, academic areas such as language arts and social studies, and community service. They found that students followed up six years after receiving a two-year program in their elementary schools showed significantly less likelihood than controls of being involved in alcohol and smoking.

The most successful programs directed toward adolescents have combined an informational part, a curriculum part most often targeted to substance abuse prevention with a social influence resistance approach that teaches students how to identify and combat peer and media pressure to engage in substance use, and a part designed to change students' norms about the prevalence and acceptability of peer drug use [Weissberg, Barton, et al. 1997]. Positive post-program results in the area of alcohol use have been found for such approaches as Adolescent Prevention Trial [Hansen & Graham 1991] and ALERT Drug Prevention [Ellickson & Bell 1990], but enduring effects have been rare.

It also helps if the legal age for drinking alcohol goes up, and if taxes on alcohol purchases also go up [Cook & Tauchen 1982; O'Malley & Wagenaar 1991]. When we look at the data, it seems as if doing these kinds of policy-level things lead to less alcohol use, alcohol-related illness, and alcohol-related fatal car crashes.

**C:** I know a kid in my school who buys cigarettes from the store and smokes them in back of the field house.

**G:** Well, we also know that if the laws are not enforced, children do not benefit as much. Many more communities are checking up on their stores, though, to make sure they don't sell tobacco or alcohol to children.

Speaking of smoking by the field house, the IOM Report also included programs designed to change school environments. In the School Transitional Environmental Project (STEP) [Felner & Adan 1988], ninth graders remained with kids their age for more of their classes and had fewer different teachers. Homeroom teachers also were taught to handle more of the students' guidance needs. Results of a matched control study showed that students in the STEP program had better school grades and fewer absences, and they also had a more positive view of the school environment The IOM Report said that gains like these make the school less violent by reducing the risk of conduct disorder.

Another friend of mine, Dan Olweus [1991], works in Norway. He believed that if schools were focused and motivated, they could be "bully proof." His intervention involved sending an educational book-let on bullying to all students and parents, showing them a video depicting the lives of victims of bullying, and having strong school rules that labeled even nasty verbal comments as bullying. When any bullying takes place, the bully would be removed from the playground or classroom or wherever it takes place. Repeated bullying leads parents to have to come into the school.

**C:** I wish they did this in my school. The playground scares me sometimes.

**G:** Well, I will have to look into this. You won't be surprised to know that where this program has been put in, kids feel improvements in satisfaction with school life, feelings of comfort and safety, and, most importantly, there is less bullying of others; replications in the United States also have been effective.

**C:** Grandpa, you are starting to sound like a college professor instead of a grandpa!

**G:** Sorry! What I really like about these stories is that they are not just about what individual people can do to get or stay well. These stories tell us that the kind of school you go to, how it is set up, and even the habits and rules in the neighborhood you live in can make a difference in lots of people's wellness [Cowen et al. 1992].

**C:** Like, if I don't keep my room clean, I start to sneeze from all the dust and dirt. If Mom and Dad didn't keep the whole house clean, I would feel sick a lot of the time, even if my own room was neat.

**G:** *Mazal tov*! You understand this very well! Speaking of your mom and dad, how is your friend Gary, who was in the group for children whose parents have been divorced?

**C:** He's good! At first, he was so mad. He wasn't fun to play with, and he was making all his friends angry at him. But then he went to that thing you got started, and since then, he's been, well, he's like Gary again.

**G:** You mean CODIP—the Children of Divorce Intervention Program [Pedro-Carroll 1997]. That program is something we are very proud of. It takes some of the ideas of social problem solving and of PMHP and puts them together. It gives children going through hard times around the divorce of their parents some ways to solve the problems that result, and it gives them a place to feel supported and cared about, and understood.

**C:** Understood?

**G:** Yes. The other children there are going through many of the same things, and have many similar feelings. Also, the group leader uses curriculum materials developed by Joanne Pedro-Carroll and her colleagues, and the materials have lots of things that kids are going through, like wondering if their parents will get back together, how will it be to spend time in two houses, and how to deal with some of the confusing feelings that happen when you want to get along with both of your parents, but they don't get along with each other. They evaluated their program and have a lot of data showing how well it works. When children don't go through a program like CODIP, they are more likely to stay angry, which makes it harder for them to learn in school and more likely that they will get into fights and other troubles.

**C:** Grandpa, is this how come we keep hearing in the news about people with guns, kids shooting other kids, and bad things like that? If there are so many good programs and things, why does all this bad stuff still happen?

**G:** Those are very hard questions. When children live in households that are unhappy or where parents are not doing a good job, it certainly contributes to violence. But there are many reasons. And you know a lot about programs and things in part because I am your Grandpa. But other kids in other places, whose Grandpas do different things, don't know about wellness. In fact, too few places seem to know even as much as you do! But we are making progress. Having said that, it's also true that too many people are reading old stuff that talks about individual people, instead of the things we were just talking about that make whole schools and neighborhoods places where wellness is encouraged and people look out for each other more [Cowen 1997b]. We talked before about those risk factors, but it's one thing to talk about them and another for people to do something about them. I am trying with the PMHP, and we are reaching more and more people all the time. But we have a long way to go.

**C:** I get scared, Grandpa, that someone is going to come in my school with a gun and start shooting.

**G:** Well, we know a lot of things that can make such a thing even less likely to happen than it is now. Of course, the number one thing is for parents to watch what kids are doing and to make sure they never handle guns. I think it would be great if there were a lot fewer guns around, even for adults. But still, it's people that have to load and shoot the guns. We know that when certain things happen in schools, violence and vandalism are less likely. Here they are [Hawkins & Lam 1987; Hunter & Elias 1998]:

1. Students perceive their courses to be relevant.

2. Students perceive that they have some control over what happens to them at school.

3. Students perceive school discipline policies as firm, fair, clear, and consistently enforced.

4. Students see that there is a rational reward structure in the school that recognizes students for their achievement.

5. There is a strong and effective school governance, with a consistent structure of order and strong principal leadership.

6. Ways are found to decrease the impersonality of the school and increase the amount of continuing contact between students and teachers.

How a school handles discipline also is important. When the focus is on punishment rather than correction and skill building, and when consequences don't clearly follow infractions, schools can get out of control. Wager [1992/3] provides a good case example of what happens when schools keep careful track of incidents of violence and come together as an entire faculty to design appropriate discipline procedures. Working in the context of what she describes as a "shared ethical culture," Wager calls for each school to develop "ten commandments of behavior," a process for handling violations, a system of rewards for positive behaviors, and an elimination, or severe restriction, of suspension of students. That's a lot like the kind of thing that Dan Olweus does, except it covers things beyond bullying and also includes good ways people should treat each other.

In Wager's school, disciplinary incidents were reduced to only one significant incident per week, few suspensions each year, and significant increases in time spent by staff on academic reform and renewal, resulting in dramatic increases in quality of teaching and academic performance. The crowning achievement was being named a "Blue Ribbon School." These changes provide a clear example of the radiating effect of change beginning with one key facet of the school environment.

People are realizing that to make schools safer, it is important to raise the levels of interpersonal skills and prosocial behaviors in students overall [Pepler & Slaby 1994]. We know what areas need the most focus: self-control, group participation and social awareness skills, and skills for reacting to and thinking through everyday problems and decisions and making difficult choices when under stress. Children who have these skills are able to be effective learners and citizens in the many communities of which they are a part. School violence is prevented when children find they have the social and life skills to be real parts of competent communities [Cottrell 1976].

**C:** It sounds like a lot of things have to happen for me to be safe in school.

**G:** That's true, but if you don't feel safe, I don't know how you can concentrate on your learning.

## New Ways in School-Based Wellness Enhancement: The Collaborative to Advance Social and Emotional Learning

**G:** And, to help bring this long story to an end, I want to tell you something I am so proud of, involving Uncle Roger, Uncle Maurice, and some of his friends [Elias et al. 1997; Weissberg et al. 1997].

**C:** I like Uncle Roger and Uncle Maurice. They're funny.

**G:** I like them, too. And they do pretty good work. They and some of their friends are working with teachers and principals all over the United States and even in places like Israel and Brazil and Norway and Koreaand Japan and Canada to help them see that well children learn better, behave better, and become better citizens when they get older. They realized that using the word "wellness" might get some school folks nervous, or else they would get sent to talk to the health or gym teachers only. So, they tried something a little different. They call it *Promoting Social and Emotional Learning: Guidelines for Educators* [Elias, et al. 1997].

Uncle Maurice and his friends who wrote the book all together, and a lot of other people, made a kind of a group or a club in 1995. It has a big name, The Collaborative to Advance Social and Emotional Learning, but a short abbreviation—CASEL. They did this to increase awareness of educators, trainers of school-based personnel, the scientific community, policymakers, and the public about the need for, and the effects of, systematic efforts to promote the social and emotional competencies of children and adolescents, and to facilitate the implementation, ongoing evaluation, and refinement of comprehensive programs in social and emotional learning throughout all grade levels.

**C:** Grandpa, do you mean that they wanted to do things kind of like PMHP and Social Problem Solving and CODIP and the other stuff you and Uncle Dirk [Hightower 1997] and all the other people you have been working with have been doing?

**G:** Well, I guess that's one way of saying it. You know, a lot of times an idea has to keep coming back, stated in different ways, until it is understood. Remember how many times and ways you tried to convince your mom and dad to let you stay up later on school nights?

**C:** Yeah, that was hard. But when I talked to you, I got a good idea and it worked. And whenever I get up without a hassle in the morning, I can stay up later at night!

**G:** It's the same idea. CASEL was able to talk about social and emotional learning because Dan Goleman wrote a book called *Emotional Intelligence* [1995] and it helped people realize that our minds, our feelings, and our bodies are all connected. We can't learn well when we are too unhappy or unhealthy. That's why poverty is such a big risk factor for kids.

**C:** Do they talk about PMHP, Grandpa?

**G:** Of course they do! But only because it met what they called their "criteria." Like other sound programs, PMHP is supported by the best available research evidence; it has been operating in practice in the schools for multiple years as part of the normal service system of the school, not as a grant-funded or demonstration project; and it has received recognition by practitioners as a theoretically sound and practically effective approach.

The book talks about programs and, more importantly, guidelines for making them work, which cover a variety of ecological contexts: classrooms, school buildings, and school districts. Some of the programs featured in the book include ones we have talked about (e.g., I Can Problem Solve; Social Decision Making and Problem Solving; Primary Mental Health Project, of course) and others that we haven't mentioned (PATHS—Mark Greenberg; School Development Program—James Comer; Responsive Classroom—Chip Wood; Second Step—Committee for Children/Karin Frey; Resolving Conflict Creatively—Linda Lantieri; Raising Healthy Children—Kevin Haggerty; Success for Life—Raymond Pasi).

They mention 39 Guidelines, but for now, I just want to share the number one guideline:

*Number 1* : Educators at all levels—elementary, middle, and high school—need explicit plans to help students become knowledgeable, responsible, and caring. Efforts are needed to build and reinforce skills in four major domains of social and emotional learning:

A. Life skills and social competencies;

B. Health promotion and problem behavior prevention skills;

C. Coping skills, conflict resolution, and social support for transitions and crises;

D. Positive, contributory service.

This forces schools to realize that if they really want students like you to be safe and to learn and to grow up to be caring, responsible, and involved members of the school and community, they have to be sure to give you the social and emotional and academic nourishment you need!

**C:** Wow! That sounds great! I just hope they can get it past Mr. DiPilliamo. He says we just have to read and write and add and subtract all the time and we will be good people.

**G:** Well, Guideline 31 has some good advice for us concerning this:

*Number 31:* Long-lasting social and emotional learning programs are highly visible and recognized. These programs "act proud" and not "snuck in" or carried out on unofficially "borrowed time." They do not act in opposition to school or district goals, but rather are integral to these goals.

We don't have to sneak around, and I am proud of Roger, Maurice, and their friends for being willing to stand up and say the truth, like it is.

**C:** Grandpa, is this just a story or can it be real?

**G:** Not only can it be real, but, if CASEL keeps going the way it is going, it WILL be real in a lot of places. Sometime soon, we should look at CASEL's web site (www.casel.org) to see all they are doing and sharing with people around the world! What CASEL wants to encourage is the presence of actively engaged educators, parents, and community leaders who create activities and opportunities before, during, and after the regular school day that teach and reinforce the attitudes, values, and behaviors of positive family and school life and, ultimately, of responsible, productive citizenship.

We can't let this turn into a fad, like those upside-down reading books you had last year. The work of Howard Gardner [1983], Dan Goleman [1998], James Comer [1988], and Carol Gilligan [1987], among others, tell us why. Social and emotional development and the recognition of the relational nature of learning and change are the fundamentals of human learning, work, and accomplishment. Until this is given proper emphasis, we cannot expect to see progress in making your school or any schools safer, drug free, with fewer students who don't care and want to drop out, or with better tolerance of people who are different.

To me, wellness is less important than the ideas it represents. What Uncle Roger, Uncle Maurice, and their friends are doing is taking good science and turning it into real helping. I taught Uncle Roger and some of his friends a little of the science and a few things about making a difference in the real world. Even before you grow up, I hope that we will see that the real challenge in our schools is not whether to attend to the social and emotional life of students, but how. We need to blow the *shofar* and wake everyone up and get some action. Enough writing, enough talking! Let's get moving!

**C:** Do you want to play a game with me instead of telling me any more about this story? How about "Operation"?

**G:** Sounds like a lot of fun—and wellness—to me!

**C:** Grandpa, thanks for being such a great grandpa. All the kids in school tell me they feel like you are their grandpa, too.

**G:** You're welcome. *Zei gezundt*, someday, it should happen to you!

## Notes

Correspondence about this chapter may be sent to: Maurice J. Elias, Department of Psychology, Rutgers University, Livingston Campus, New Brunswick, NJ 08903 (e-mail: hpusyme@aol.com); or Roger P. Weissberg, Department of Psychology (M/C 285), University of Illinois at Chicago, 1007 West Harrison Street, Chicago, IL 60607-7137 (e-mail: rpw@uic.edu).

## Acknowledgments

Both authors gratefully acknowledge the support of several funders of the Collaborative to Advance Social and Emotional Learning (CASEL) including the Fetzer Institute, the Joseph P. Kennedy Foundation, the Irving B. Harris Foundation, the Surdna Foundation, the United States Department of Education, and the University of Illinois at Chicago (UIC). Roger Weissberg also acknowledges the NIMH's Prevention Research Branch and Office on AIDS for their support of UIC's Prevention Research Training Program in Urban Children's Mental Health and AIDS Prevention (1-T32-MH19933). He also appreciates the support of the Office of Educational Research and Improvement of the U.S. Department of Education through a grant to the Mid-Atlantic Laboratory for Student Success at the Temple University Center for Research in Human Development and Education.

## References

Belsky, J. (1984). The determinants of parenting: A process model. *Child Development, 55*(1), 83–96.

Bower, E. (1972). Education as a humanizing process and its relationship to other humanizing processes. In S. Golann & C. Eisdorfer (Eds.), *Handbook of community mental health* (pp. 37–49). New York: Appleton-Century-Crofts.

Comer, J. P. (1988). Educating poor minority children. *Scientific American, 259*(5), 42–48.

Consortium on the School-based Promotion of Social Competence. (1994). The school-based promotion of social competence: Theory, research, practice, and policy. In R. J. Haggerty, N. Garmezy, M. Rutter, & L. R. Sherrod (Eds.), *Stress, risk, and resilience in children and adolescents: Processes, mechanisms, and interventions* (pp. 268–316). New York: Cambridge University Press.

Cook, P. & Tauchen, G. (1982). The effect of liquor taxes on heavy drinking. *Bell Journal of Economics, 13*, 379–390.

Cottrell, L. S. (1976). The competent community. In B. H. Kaplan, R. N. Wilson, & A. H. Leighton (Eds.), *Further explorations in social psychiatry* (pp. 195–209). New York: Basic Books.

Cowen, E. L. (1977). Baby-steps toward primary prevention. *American Journal of Community Psychology, 5*, 1–22.

Cowen, E. L. (1983). Primary prevention in mental health: Past, present, and future. In R. D. Felner, L. A. Jason, J. N. Moritsugu, & S. S. Farber (Eds.), *Preventive psychology: Theory, research, and practice* (pp. 11–25). New York: Pergamon.

Cowen, E. L. (1994). The enhancement of psychological wellness: Challenges and opportunities. *American Journal of Community Psychology, 22*(3), 149–179.

Cowen, E. L. (1995). Forty years of community psychology: Time goes by fast when you're having fun. *The Community Psychologist, 22*(3), 10–13.

Cowen, E. L. (1997a). On the semantics and operations of primary prevention and wellness enhancement (or will the real primary prevention please stand up?). *American Journal of Community Psychology, 25*(3), 245–256.

Cowen, E. L. (1997b). Schools and the enhancement of children's wellness: Some opportunities and some limiting factors. In R. P. Weissberg, T. P. Gullotta, R. Hampton, B. Ryan, & G. Adams (Eds.), *Healthy children 2010: Establishing preventive services* (pp. 97–123). Thousand Oaks, CA: Sage.

Cowen, E. L., Hightower, A. D., Pedro-Carroll, J. L., Work, W. C., Wyman, P. A., & Haffey, W. G. (1996). *School-based prevention of children at risk: The Primary Mental Health Project.* Washington, DC: American Psychological Association.

Cowen, E. L., Wyman, P., Work, W., & Iker, M. (1992). A preventive intervention for enhancing resilience among highly stressed urban children. *Journal of Primary Prevention, 15*(2), 247–260.

Elias, M. J. (1994). Capturing excellence in applied settings: A participant conceptualizer and praxis explicator role for community psychologists. *American Journal of Community Psychology, 22*(3), 293–318.

Elias, M. J. & Clabby, J. (1992). *Building social problem solving skills: Guidelines from a school-based program.* San Francisco: Jossey-Bass.

Elias, M. J., Gara, M. A., Schuyler, T. F., Branden-Muller, L. R., & Sayette, M. A. (1991). The promotion of social competence: Longitudinal study of a preventive school-based program. *American Journal of Orthopsychiatry, 61*(4), 409–417.

Elias, M. J. & Tobias, S. E. (1996). *Social problem solving interventions in the schools.* New York: Guilford.

Elias, M. J., Zins, J., Weissberg, R., Frey, K., Greenberg, M., Haynes, N., Kessler, R., Schwab-Stone, M., & Shriver, T. (1997). *Promoting social and emotional learning: Guidelines for educators.* Alexandria, VA: Association for Supervision and Curriculum Development.

Ellickson, P. & Bell, R. M. (1990). Drug prevention in junior high: A multi-site longitudinal test. *Science, 247,* 1299–1305.

Felner, R. D. & Adan, A. (1988). The school transition environment project: An ecological intervention and evaluation. In R. Price, E. L. Cowen, R. Lorion, & J. Ramos-McKay (Eds.), *14 ounces of prevention: A casebook for practitioners* (pp. 111–122). Washington, DC: American Psychological Association.

Garmezy, N. (1991). Resilience in children's adaptation to negative life events and stressed environments. *Pediatric Annals, 20,* 459–466.

Gardner, H. (1983). *Frames of mind.* New York: Basic Books.

Gilligan, C. (1987). Adolescent development reconsidered. In C. E. Irwin, Jr. (Ed.), *Adolescent social behavior and health: New directions for child development* (No. 37) (pp. 63–92). San Francisco: Jossey-Bass.

Goleman, D. (1995). *Emotional intelligence.* New York: Bantam.

Goleman, D. (1998). *Working with emotional intelligence.* New York: Bantam.

Haggerty, R., Sherrod, L., Garmezy, N., & Rutter, M. (Eds.). (1994). *Stress, risk, and resilience in children and adolescents.* New York: Cambridge University Press.

Hansen, W. & Graham, J. W. (1991). Preventing alcohol, marijuana, and cigarette use among adolescents: Peer resistance training versus establishing conservative norms. *Preventive Medicine, 20,* 414–430.

Hawkins, J. D., Catalano, R. F., Morrison, D., O'Donnell, J., Abbot, R., & Day, L. (1992). The Seattle Social Development Project: Effects of the first four years on protective factors and problem behaviors. In J. McCord &

R. E. Tremblay (Eds.), *Preventing antisocial behavior: Interventions from birth through adolescence* (pp. 139–161). New York: Guilford.

Hawkins, J. D. & Lam. T. (1987). Teacher practices, social development, and delinquency. In J. D. Burchard & S. N. Burchard (Ed.), *Prevention of delinquent behavior* (pp. 241–274). Newbury Park, CA: Sage Publications.

Hightower, A. D. (1997). Primary Mental Health Project. In G. W. Albee & T. P. Gullotta (Eds.), *Primary prevention works* (pp. 191–212). Thousand Oaks, CA: Sage.

Hunter, L. & Elias, M. J. (1998). Violence in the high schools: Issues, controversies, policies, and prevention programs. In A. Roberts (Ed.), *Juvenile justice: Policies, programs, and services* (2nd ed.) (pp. 71–94). Chicago: Nelson-Hall.

Masten, A. S., Best, K., & Garmezy, N. (1990). Resilience and development: Contributions from the study of children who overcome adversity. *Development and Psychopathology, 2(*4), 425–444.

Mrazek, P. & Haggerty, R. J. (Eds.). (1994). *Reducing risks for mental disorders: Frontiers for preventive intervention research. A Report of the Institute of Medicine.* Washington, DC: National Academy Press.

Olweus, D. (1991). Bully/victim problems among school children: Basic facts and effects of an intervention program. In D. J. Pepler & K. H. Rubin (Eds.), *The development and treatment of childhood aggression* (pp. 411–448). Hillsdale, NJ: Erlbaum.

O'Malley, P. & Wagenaar, A. (1991). Effects of minimum drinking age laws on alcohol use, related behaviors and traffic crash involvement among American youth: 1976–1987. *Journal of Studies on Alcohol, 52,* 478–491.

Pedro-Carroll, J. (1997). The Children of Divorce Intervention Program: Fostering resilient outcomes for school-aged children. In G. W. Albee & T. P. Gullotta (Eds.), *Primary prevention works* (pp. 213–238). Thousand Oaks, CA: Sage.

Pepler, D. J. & Slaby, R. (1994). Theoretical and developmental perspectives on youth and violence. In L. Eron, J. Gentry, & P. Schlegel (Eds.), *Reason to hope: A psychosocial perspective on violence & youth* (pp. 27–58). Washington, DC: American Psychological Association.

Price, R., Cowen, E., Lorion, R., & Ramos-McKay, J. (Eds.). (1988). *14 ounces of prevention: A casebook for practitioners.* Washington, DC: American Psychological Association

Rutter, M. (1987). Psychosocial resilience and protective mechanisms. *American Journal of Orthopsychiatry, 57(*3), 316–331.

Shure, M. B. & Spivack, G. (1988). Interpersonal cognitive problem solving. In R. Price, E. L. Cowen, R. Lorion, & J. Ramos-McKay (Eds.), *14 ounces of prevention: A casebook for practitioners* (pp. 69–82). Washington, DC: American Psychological Association.

Wager, C. (1992/3). Toward a shared ethical culture. *Educational Leadership, 49*(5), 19–23.

Weissberg, R. P., Barton, H., & Shriver, T. P. (1997). The social competence promotion program for young adolescents. In G. W. Albee & T. P. Gullotta (Eds.), *Primary prevention works* (pp. 268–290). Thousand Oaks, CA: Sage.

Weissberg, R. P., Caplan, M., & Harwood, R. L. (1991). Promoting competent young people in competence-enhancing environments: A systems-based perspective on primary prevention. *Journal of Consulting and Clinical Psychology, 59*, 830–841.

Weissberg, R. P. & Greenberg, M. T. (1998). Social and community competence-enhancement and prevention programs. In W. Damon (Series Ed.) & I. E. Sigel & K.A. Renninger (Vol. Eds.), *Handbook of child psychology: Vol. 4. Child psychology in practice* (5th ed.) (pp. 877–954). New York: John Wiley & Sons.

Weissberg, R. P., Gullotta, T. P., Hampton, R. L., Ryan, B. A., & Adams, G. R. (Eds.). (1997). *Healthy children 2010: Enhancing children's wellness.* Thousand Oaks, CA: Sage.

Werner, E. E. & Smith, R. (1992). *Overcoming the odds: High risk children from birth to adulthood.* New York: Cornell University Press.

# 9

# Educational Reform as Ecologically-Based Prevention and Promotion: The Project on High Performance Learning Communities

*Robert D. Felner*

The current paper provides a discussion of the evolution, theoretical basis, and representative emerging findings of the Project on High Performance Learning Communities [Felner, Kasak, et al. 1997]. The Project seeks to employ an ecological perspective to guide the systematic restructuring of educational settings in ways that enhance the well-being, adaptation, and overall "wellness" [Cowen 1991, 1994] of students, teachers, and parents. The past half-century has seen profound changes in societal approaches taken to address the social, emotional, behavioral, physiological needs, and well-being of Americans. At the midpoint of the century, interventions were primarily aimed at those with serious difficulties and only undertaken by highly trained professionals in tertiary care settings. Ground-breaking efforts, such as those of the Primary Mental Health Project in Rochester New York [Cowen et al. 1975], shifted the focus toward efforts to identify early signs of disorder and reverse emerging difficulties before they could lead to more serious disorder and negative life consequences. These efforts also brought with them dramatic shifts in the settings in which these interventions now took place—schools and community settings rather than mental hospitals and physicians' offices—and brought to the efforts a whole new range of nontraditional interventionists, including teachers and trained nonprofessionals. In other ways, however, these initiatives often looked remarkably like "clinical" work in that they were "person-focused" in both their choice of targets and the locus of the changes sought [Cowen 1985].

Over the past three decades, new, often dramatic changes have occurred, so that approaches that were once controversial are now routine (e.g., widespread preventive efforts). The focus has now shifted to next generation issues that were only brought clearly into focus as a result of the "baby-steps" [Cowen 1977] forward of the past 50 years of social intervention, prevention, and policy efforts. Now, the powerful association between positive social and emotional adaptation and risk for physical heath problems or health-risk behaviors is widely recognized. Formal efforts to improve the adaptive functioning and well-being of the population have continued to evolve. Cowen [1985] noted that what we [Felner & Felner 1989] have termed "second generation" prevention and promotion efforts emerged, which typically sought to enhance specific competencies through direct training or by providing experiences that promote the acquisition of the skills [Cowen 1985]. New "competence" enhancement program efforts were based on a "three-step conceptual paradigm." The primary elements of this are: (1) Identification, through empirical investigation of skills or competencies that are associated with the presence or absence of adequate adaptation; (2) The development of age-appropriate programs to impart these skills; and (3) Demonstration of the outcomes of the intervention efforts.

A basic assumption of these efforts is that, "Acquiring such skills and/or having such experiences is presumed to radiate positively to adjustment" [Cowen 1985]. Adjustment here is used in the general sense, independent of particular setting or situational circumstances. Such programs are based on the view that individuals who have deficiencies in the competencies that are emphasized in the training program are at greater risk for maladjustment, either in a broad range of areas or in some subgroups of these programs, specific disorders or types of disorders. Clearly, these programs are far more proactive than those that focus on the remediation of early behavioral dysfunction. Still, it must also be clear that, at their heart, they are again deficit-reduction models that largely ignore, except in a very general sense, the contribution of factors external to the individual in the trajectory to disorder.

Recently, Cowen [1991, 1994] has argued that although great strides have been seen in these efforts to forestall human misery and enhance well-being, it is still the case that most programmatic and policy efforts typically have, as their primary focus, only one element of the two core strategies of primary prevention. The two core elements are: (1) preventing dysfunction, including conditions of known risk; and (2) promoting psychological well-being. Although in definitions of prevention both sides of the prevention equation are given equal weight, in reality Cowen [1994] notes that "there has been a strong trend in influential quarters to define primary prevention, de facto, as disease prevention and for such a program to guide the allocation of program and research monies." [p. 153]. In the face of this imbalance, efforts that focus on "wellness" and the promotion of settings and competencies that support and sustain wellness and positive life adaptation have received scant attention. Here, interventions and ecological alterations that are concerned with wellness are seen to address, systematically and intentionally, life outcomes and patterns of daily functioning such as positive work and family life and adjustment, the mastery of age- and ability-appropriate tasks, having a sense of connectedness to others, engagement in key social settings, and a sense of efficacy in these interactions.

Emerging "third generation" efforts at primary prevention sought to be more truly focused on the developmental transactions and ecology in which people grew and functioned [Felner & Felner 1989]. Although the reduction of disorder is still a goal, there are critical differences in these approaches from those of the past, which make them a sharp break from "person-focused" settings and are far more consistent with wellness promotion efforts. First, it must be understood that for ecologically-focused intervention and policy efforts, the locus of risk and important sources of protective factors are seen to be almost entirely outside the child or adult. An ecological frame also enables us to see that those developmental processes that produce healthy outcomes also produce what may appear to be deviance but are, in fact, appropriate and highly positive attempts to adapt to contexts and conditions that are incompatible with those required in other contexts or in the larger society [Felner & Felner 1989]. Finally, it is also the case that efforts seeking to enhance the developmental contexts and resource of individuals or to remove developmentally hazardous circumstance will, with few exceptions, produce positive adaptive consequences in a broad array of domains, further strengthening the overall wellness of the person.

Viewed in this fashion, it should be clear that an ecological approach to school improvement and reform will, in fact, shift the focus from the strategies of traditional programs focused primarily on struggling students, to an approach that naturally embraces and encompasses the five main pathways to wellness articulated by Cowen [1994]. Like Cowen's five wellness pathways, these ecological school reform and improvement strategies: (1) seek to build on understandings of developmental ecology to create and otherwise modify primary developmental settings, such as schools, in ways that favor and *actively foster* the acquisition of wellness outcomes, such as key developmental competencies and skills and feelings of belonging, connectedness, and efficacy in those settings; and (2) actively pay attention to the connections between the strengths and competencies they require and foster, and those that are required both concurrently and in the future in the persons life for them to have a sense of efficacy and control as well as to be able to cope adequately with the demands they confront. If the first two aspects are successfully accomplished, when targeted at children and youth, these ecological strategies result in their becoming empowered adults, who have a full-range of life choices and possibilities for finding stable and satisfying work and life situations. That is, ecological interventions seek to create contexts in which students, as part of the day-to-day transactions within that setting, acquire both age-appropriate competencies and those they need to continue to successfully acquire new competencies in future settings, such as those required to be effective lifelong learners in all of their primary developmental contexts and systems.

Ecologically-focused efforts may have as their target a number of particular elements of the person's environment, either singly or in combination. The family system, peer groups, and the school's social, organizational and physical characteristics are among those to which educational efforts are most often targeted.

In this paper we describe the evolution of the Project on High Performance Learning Communities (Project HiPlaces). This Project was developed in response to the needs of policy makers and practitioners for a more fully developed and practical knowledge base about "what works" in educational reform—both at the school and in the surrounding conditions and policies that shape the potential for creating and sustaining effective reforms in the teaching and learning context.

Of particular concern in the development of the Project was the ways in which an ecological framework for guiding the ongoing improvement of schooling could serve to systematically inform these efforts. Although this seems an obvious step in America's efforts to improve its schools, the use of an ecological perspective has, in fact, been obvious neither to policymakers nor educators and other social scientists. They have not started with such basic questions as:

"What would schools look like... if they were to attend to the goals embodied in the big idea that guides this work ... such as seeking school readiness and connectedness, effective learning, and high achievement and performance for all students—i.e., like that fostered wellness outcomes and the acquisition of key age-appropriate competencies." Instead, educational policymakers have more often begun with discussions of who should fund schools, who should run them, [Sarason 1998] or what should students know, but in both cases with little attention to what would be required to create an effective teaching and learning environment that promoted these outcomes and the acquisition of the intermediate processes and outcomes required to attain the focal goals. As noted by Cowen [1994], the tropism of those attempting to work with schools to improve student outcomes has been to try to "fix the problem kids" rather than start with a intentional, systematic focus on modifying the educational context to foster wellness in the students, and, critically, the teachers, on whom the success of the former efforts so strongly rests [Sarason 1990]. Illustrative of this issue and the degree to which there is a pervasive failure to embrace the "promotion/wellness" side of the primary prevention definition even in the thinking of the field, we have often run into the situation where, as we present or submit discussions of this project to policymakers, researchers, and practitioners, we hear the statement, "It is school improvement, but what does it have to do with prevention?" Only when those concerned with wellness understand that school reform based on the premises of "wellness" *is true prevention—and even more so wellness promotion*—will they start to move from the blinders of professional socialization that constrain such perspective [Sarason 1983].

## Understanding the Changing Competencies That Must Be Provided for in American Public Schools.

Before we can adequately design school settings that foster the competencies required by children and adolescents for age-appropriate functioning and future success, it is important to understand the changing contexts in which these students must be able to cope and function throughout life. As never before, these conditions have brought profound changes to the tasks of public education. Now, more than at any time in American history, the environment and curriculums in schools and educational outcomes are critically linked to empowerment and positive work and life adjustment, both while in school and in later life. This understanding helps to make sense out of what is otherwise one of the most perplexing problems in American public policy discussions. That is the apparent disconnection between the current performance of public schools and the way they are viewed by the American public. American pubic schools are, at least from a historical perspective, "doing better" than ever. Dropout rates are at all-time lows. More students than ever are in public schools. The absolute levels of literacy and numeracy of the population and our youth are at all-time highs. Why, then, isn't the public singing the praises of public schools? Simply put, the standards and expectations that the public holds for schools have increased far faster than has the rate of improvement of public education. The reasons for this state of affairs are, at least in part, the result of the wide gulf between the goals and tasks that American public schools were designed to address, and the demands the 21st century world have thrust upon them.

Dramatic changes in American society and the world economy have changed the definition of a successful school. When widespread public education emerged, the types and levels of proficiency to be mastered by the masses were quite different from anything envisioned in the standards that are recommended today. At the dawn of the 20th century, for most students there were no learning targets beyond basic ciphering, literacy, and the development of the citizenship base to function in the ideal of the "melting pot" society. In 1900, only 25% of American youth entered 9th grade and as few as 12% completed high school. By the middle of the century, it was still the case that nearly half of the students in the United States failed to complete high school but there was little concern about the dropout rate as these students posed no problems in the economy of post-World War II America. The country's need for unskilled labor, and the limited resources and funding base for public schools, not only made it acceptable for public schools to be designed to tolerate such educational "casualties" [Felner, et. al. 1997a] but, in fact, made it important that some level of casualties were built into the assumptions that guided the design of public schools. If there were no casualties, there would both be no workers to fill these important jobs and there would be insufficient resources to educate all of the students who remained. When prior generations arrived or began their ascent out of poverty, America's need for non-skilled labor allowed them to elevate their economic status [Wilson 1987]. Their children could then complete k-12 public school, and many could go on to college. Hence, when public education was designed, the surrounding context made clear that school failure and early leaving neither meant becoming or remaining a "casualty" in the broader society. Instead, it often provided the first step on the ladder out of poverty for a family.

The subsequent 50 years have, however, seen significant changes in the consequence of schooling and school failure. The reality now is that failure in school will relegate students to an almost inescapable impoverished state, leaving them at far greater risk for a host of social, emotional, and health difficulties [American Psychological Association 1997]. Educational casualties are now at significant risk to become casualties in all others all areas of life. A high school degree has gone from being the "entry ticket" to economic self-sufficiency to being merely one necessary but insufficient step toward obtaining that ticket.

In defending the difficulty of the challenge to educate all students, we often hear, *"But we have different kids today."* But what is the real nature of the *"differences"* between today's disadvantaged students and their counterparts earlier in the century? In both cases we find children of poor immigrants, many of whom did not or do not speak English as their first language. Others came, and still come, from groups where pervasive poverty has been the result of generations of oppression and unequal access to quality schools and economic opportunity.

What is different is that public education *must now retain and succeed with these students.* For those seeking to adequately frame the task that modern public education faces, it is far more important to understand that the critical *"difference"* lies in the societal and economic circumstances that faced past generations of immigrants and other impoverished Americans and their children versus those of today and tomorrow. These circumstances require that today educators be charged with helping all students learn and achieve at levels far beyond those of previous generations—independent of the resources of their families or their prior preparation and early experience. No longer can public education operate on the assumption that there is some level of "acceptable casualties." Instead, operating principles must start with the assumption that public education will be judged against a standard of preparing 100% of its students to learn and succeed in school and life. The goal now must be sustainable high performance and achievement, and the acquisition of the skills and motivation for learning required for 100% of students to be effective lifelong learners. This goal brings with it the recognition that neither high achievement nor wellness in one area of functioning will result without the other, requiring schools to focus on the wellness of the whole child, in all areas of development.

Hence, although students are not "different" from those of the past in the degree to which they are somehow more difficult to educate, the challenge facing educators is that they must now educate and retain a more *complete set of students.* This set now includes those students who in previous generations left school because they were not well suited to the design of public education, who had family needs that required them to leave early, or who lacked the support or school readiness necessary to succeed in those school settings. Many of these students do not learn best in the "traditional" models of schooling or do not come to school with the requisite nutrition and health to benefit fully from schooling. They may need more support or different instructional strategies or school regularities to succeed than those who come in with backgrounds, preparation, and support systems that enable them to be successful in traditional instructional settings.

Exacerbating the difficulties of the new demands on public education is that, although in the past students confronted a life in which the "one life/one career imperative" [Sarason 1977] was the norm, American workers can now anticipate that they will change jobs or careers several times across their lifetimes, with the skills and knowledge to fill those roles increasing at astonishing rates. Public education must not only educate all of its students—including that 40% who were previously acceptable casualties—but they must do so at far higher levels and equip them with skills to continue to learn, problem solve, and function in environments and in tasks that often may not yet even exist.

The "bar" that American public schools must jump is further raised by yet another significant change in the context around them. Public school systems are, at last, moving away from norm-referenced assessment approaches that compare students on some population distribution. On these tests it is quite possible for a student to have significant gaps in proficiency but still score "average" or above. But states and districts are now moving to assessments of school and student performance on which all students must reach some absolute levels of performance proficiency. Further, the domains of proficiency assessed and against which schools are judged have been broadened from the basic skills that most norm-referenced assessments have traditionally focused on, to include assessments of problem solving and concept learning, as well as "authentic performance" in which students are actually called upon to write, explain their computation, and otherwise show more than the receptive/recognition skills required in responding to multiple choice questions. Assessments such as these have led to schools and districts receiving what has often been shocking news—schools that had scores showing their students to be "average" or above on norm-referenced tests were also ones in which 50% of more of *all* students were lacking key proficiencies in core subject areas [c.f., Rhode Island Department of Education 1998].

All of these changes have underscored the interdependence of the future success of public education and the social, emotional, and physical well-being of the students that come to them. The changes in societal context bring significant changes in the consequences of school failure. So, too, do they require that we have a student population with levels of social, emotional, and physical well-being that do not impede the degree to which they can benefit from educational innovation and improvement. Students with social and emotional difficulties or a lack of adequate health care and nutrition enter school "not ready to learn." Students who do not learn and perform at levels that meet increasingly high standards in core subject and competency areas are ever less likely to be able to effectively participate in society and attain wellness. Those who fail in school and/or do not acquire the necessary skills while there are at far higher levels of risk for all forms of social, emotional, and health difficulties, ranging from a life of crime, to mental heath problems, to severe physical disorder and shortened life span. Illustratively, the National Institutes of Health have, for the first time, identified a failure to learn in school—i.e., a failure to achieve adequate levels of *literacy*—as a major public health issue. They note the strong linkages between a lack of adequate levels of literacy to function in today's society and a wide array of social, behavioral, and physical ills. They recognize the ever-changing and increasing demands of the new economy for students with high levels of competencies in both literacy and numeracy. Now, students need not only to have performed well in school, but must also be prepared *to be effective lifelong learners* [Lyon 1999]. To accomplish this goal, students must obtain age-appropriate social and academic competencies at each point in their journey through schooling.

To summarize, a significant source of the criticism of American public education stems not from their being somehow less effective than in the past but, rather, that they face a vastly different societal ecology than did public schools in the past. These societal changes have brought a far more daunting set of tasks and expectations than public schools were ever designed to meet. The new societal contexts in which schools operate has led educators and other policymakers to move away from a stance that expects and even condones some prevailing rate of failure and dropouts for students and subgroups of students, to a stance that reflects an "all kids" agenda based on the goal that all students can learn and will succeed. These professionals and policymakers recognize that many of the original assumptions of public education are no longer viable. Public education can no longer have as its operating premise the idea that there are "acceptable casualties" [Felner et al. 1997]. Now, public elementary, middle, and secondary schools must educate a far greater percentage of students—100%—to far higher levels of skill and performance, *typically in the same numbers of days and hours* as was true of schooling 50 years ago or more. More than ever before, as reflected in our guiding big idea, schools must attend to the positive growth and wellness of the whole child to prepare them to be fully participating and effective members of a democratic society. Certainly, addressing the far greater demands in the same amount of time requires significant reconsideration of the means and methods we have built upon in the past and the redesign and transformations of schools and schooling in order to allow them to serve our children well.

At a recent conference of the American Psychological Association on "Bringing to Scale Educational Innovation and School Reform: Partnerships in Urban Education" [American Psychological Association 1997], conference participants noted that, "psychology departments too often view education as a fringe interest not equal to other specialties, such as child development or cognitive psychology [and] that attitude has taken its toll on the nation's schools." Participants further suggested that, "Today, American education is minimally informed and rarely takes seriously what psychologists have learned about learning." The Project on High Performance Learning Communities seeks to help bridge this divide by helping educators and policymakers meet the new challenges raised by the societal ecology in which they must function, by adding to a more fully developed and practical, empirically-grounded and-theory-based knowledge base about "what works" in educational reform.

# The Project on High Performance Learning Communities

## *Theoretical Model*

The initial stages of the Project on High Performing Learning Communities (*Project HiPlaces*) began more than two decades ago. It is grounded in theoretical models of human ecology [Bronfenbrenner 1979] and the transactional-ecological perspective on intervention that has derived from it [Felner & Felner 1989; Felner et al. 2000]. This approach is also ideally suited to an approach to educational reform and improvement that seeks to build student strengths, competencies, and achievements while removing hazards and barriers to those developmental outcomes. It is also one that, because of its focus on broad-based transcategorical areas of student outcomes, enables schools to use their resources efficiently and change efforts to be respectful of the full range of agendas and demands to which schools must respond. It meets the standard of the vision articulated in the recent report of the Institute of Medicine that "the principles of prevention [should be built] into the ordinary activities of everyday life and into community structures to enhance development over the entire life span" [Mrazek & Haggerty 1996, p. 298-299]. Finally, it meets the standard of creating developmental settings that actively foster wellness [Cowen 1994]. In school settings, reform efforts or approaches to prevention and promotion that fail to meet these standards, no matter how well conceived otherwise, may predictably fail to be mounted with fidelity, requisite intensity, or to be sustainable, since they are typically not syntonic or ecologically congruent with the other demands and needs of the setting or those of the lives of the students [Felner, et al. 2000].

That such psychological theory may provide an important building block for efforts to aid educational settings in meeting their new tasks is made clear by Lee and Smith [1994]. They note the need for theory-driven evaluation research on school reform and state, "Despite its growing popularity among school people and educational policy specialists, the reform movement, embodied in the term 'restructuring' rests on thin and inconsistent theory" [p. 1]. Sarason [1992] adds to the case for the importance of a coherent theoretical base to guide reform by noting that there is a critical need for a vision and "big idea" around which school reform efforts is organized, to have any hope for success. Reform efforts that are derived from a central "big idea" have, as a primary hallmark, coherence of the elements and strategies that comprise them. Coherence of the elements and strategies that comprise comprehensive reform frameworks lead to the development of school improvement strategies that make sense to participants, whose steps follow logically, and whose elements form more than a loose knitting together of discrete components.

As noted, for the development of the HiPlaces model, the "big idea" that best summarizes the questions with which the Project is concerned and the developmental ecological approach in which it is grounded is, "*How do we create educational contexts in which all children and youth are nurtured and challenged in ways that lead them to be highly effective learners, achieve and perform at high levels, and be healthy, responsible, and productive citizens in our democracy.*" The theoretical framework offered by the developmental ecology big idea also provides for a systematic approach to understanding the ways in which the elements of schools and other developmental settings and systems (e.g., schools, families, communities, districts, and state education agencies) fit together—within and across contexts—and for considering the ways in which such interactions shape the developmental pathways and outcomes of the children and adults in those settings and contexts or impacted by them. A comprehensive theoretical framework also guides all actions and provides for a lens through which all potential reform elements could be judged and evaluated for their potential utility.. That is, it provided for the coherence and comprehensiveness we sought. If the goal is continuous refinement and improvement of educational reform, rather than a "thumbs up, thumbs down" test, the "model" we employ needed to be one whose assumptions are clearly testable against the outcomes sought and that provided both guidance and flexibility concerning the incorporation of lessons learned. The ecological perspective both in its general form, and the specific application of it that we have evolved from it to guide educational reform, described below, do all of this.

## Goal of Project HiPlaces

A primary goal of the Project continues to be to respond to the needs of practitioners and policymakers for a knowledge base that guides *systematic* and *increasingly effective* reforms in public education for all students. We seek to help provide a model for "what works" in educational reform for adolescents, both at the school level and in the conditions and policies that surround schools, and shape the potential for creating and sustaining changes in the teaching and learning contexts that promote the highest levels of performance, achievement, and positive developmental outcomes for students. In organizing our programmatic, research, and school change support efforts to address these issues, we have identified four fundamental questions that, in one form or another, are repeatedly asked by policymakers and practitioners, and that must be addressed for any reform effort to be successful:

- If you did "it," would it "work"?

- What does "it" look like, and what elements, practices, and processes are necessary and sufficient ingredients of "it"?

- What are the necessary conditions, both inside the school and in the broader educational system, to get "it" to happen?

- How do you sustain and continuously improve "it"?

Core goals of this paper are to provide an overview of our emerging understanding of the answers to these questions and strategies for getting change to happen in ways that reflect the lessons learned.

## The School Transitional Environment Project.

The Project began in the mid-1970s with focus students who were at "high risk" because of the transition to high school. This work sought to transform the organizational norms of large high schools in order to prevent the dramatic declines in academic adjustment and sharp increases in behavioral and socioemotional difficulties that have been found to frequently follow the transition from elementary or middle grade schools to secondary settings. During this early phase, we developed the School Transitional Environment Project (Project STEP), the precursor of HiPlaces. STEP sought to reduce the levels of developmentally hazardous conditions that characterize large high school environments, while at the same time modifying the social climate and the support available to students from faculty. The primary elements of this initiative were ones that would now be viewed as central to the creation of "small communities for learning," "small schools," "schools within schools," and what would now be labeled as "teaming" and "teacher-based advisory." High school staff and students were organized into small (120-student or less) teams for all of their academic subjects, kept in the same area of the building for these classes, and were introduced to teacher-based advisory programming. Although increasingly used in middle schools since the mid-1980s, in the late 1970s and early 1980s these practices were dramatic departures for high schools. Moreover, among efforts to prevent rather than remedy problems, STEP was one of the first to focus on changes in settings that affect entire populations rather than just changing specifically targeted individuals.

The results of the STEP transformation efforts were quite consistent across a large number of replications at both the high school level and, subsequently, the junior high school level. We found clear declines of 40% to 50% or more in the school dropout rate across the high school careers of students in the Project schools [Felner, Ginter & Primavera, 1982; Felner & Adan 1998]. Students in STEP school environments also had more favorable attitudes about school, teachers, and themselves, including higher expectations than students who were not in the initiative [Felner & Adan 1988; Felner et al. 1993]. Importantly for guiding our subsequent efforts, the differences emerged not only because of gains in the STEP group, but also because of declines in the non-STEP groups. It is noteworthy that the larger and "riskier" the high school population, the greater the effects. A significant contributor to the level of risk to students was determined by the number of "feeder schools" and communities that flowed into the building. These are conditions and populations that are not only characteristic of large urban and suburban settings but, as rural communities have increasingly moved to large, consolidated regional middle schools and high schools, have become a cause of concern for rural education as well.

As STEP progressed, our findings were both encouraging and troubling in ways that led to the next generation of our efforts. The reduction in the levels of developmental risk and hazard in the school environment, as well as the enhancement of the positive aspects of school climate, combined to reduce the dropout rate and levels of school violence, enhance safety, and, importantly, stem declines in academic achievement and performance. This was the good news. The bad news was that, although these students were now staying in school, it was not always, or even typically, the case that there were *gains* over time in the performance and achievement of these students. Although students no longer showed significant *declines* in these areas—a nontrivial outcome and a fact that actually increased the average scores for the school as a whole in 9th and 10th grade— neither did they show accelerating levels of achievement and performance. While we were successful in retaining those students who came into the high school or middle school setting already performing at marginal or even below proficient levels, it was simply unacceptable, given the new societal ecology, to just keep these students in school, no matter how positive the experience had become, without also raising their academic skills, performance, and achievement. What was clear was that the modification in the structural and social-development contexts of the school were necessary, but certainly not sufficient elements to obtain these gains for these students.

## Whole-School Change Efforts

As we moved toward efforts to provide for whole-school change models with the capacity to prevent failure and adjustment difficulties, as well as to promote positive levels of academic and performance adjustment, we decided that rather than reinvent the wheel, we would begin by conducting large scale research on existing reform efforts. Here we sought to further understand the adequacy of those conceptually derived models through empirically testing those models of school reform that were consistent with the vision and values of the HiPlaces initiative.

Here we have been very fortunate in the unique opportunities we have had to build on and to integrate the lessons we have learned in conducting the evaluation of and/or providing support to schools in many of the leading "early generation" efforts to enhance the education of adolescents. Under the Project umbrella, with Felner as PI, we have had the opportunity to study and conduct evaluations of most of the major foundation-funded initiatives that have focused on transforming middle grades education—including the Carnegie Corporation's Middle Grades School State Policy Initiative (MGSSPI), the Lilly Endowment's Middle Grades Improvement Project (MGIP) and the related initiative in the Lilly Endowment initiative in the Indianapolis Public Schools, the Ewing Marion Kauffman Foundation's *Successful Schools Project,* and the Kellogg Foundation's *Middle Start* initiative. NCPE has ongoing funding for work on all of these efforts, with the exception of the Kellogg Foundation. In addition, while at the University of Illinois, The Project helped to develop, support, and conduct the evaluation of the Illinois Middle School Network. We have also conducted an evaluation of the Texas Mentor Networks, of the State of Missouri "Outstanding Schools" initiatives (including the RE:Learning High Schools and Accelerated Schools), and evaluated the *Breaking Ranks* [National Association of Secondary School Principals 1996] initiative in Rhode Island. Schools in these initiatives ranged from those in highly urban settings to those in small rural communities, including those in American Indian reservation schools in New Mexico and North Dakota.

Currently, the Project is also extensively involved with coordination, support for, and data collection and analysis with all of the schools in the State of Rhode Island, as part of the State's comprehensive accountability system. Rhode Island's accountability and school change process is heavily grounded in the complimentary strands of using information for school change, standards-based assessments of students, and the provision of HiPlaces assessments to each school in the State for planning and monitoring improvement efforts. As will be seen below, this work, and related efforts on which we are working with a set of states and districts across the country (e.g., Buffalo, New York; Columbus, Ohio; Jefferson County, Colorado), has served to raise new questions and issues for the refinement of the HiPlaces model that we hope to address.

At the core of the study process is a set of assessment instruments completed by teachers, students, other staff, and parents. These assessments, collectively known as the *High Performance Learning Community (HiPlaces) Assessment,* were developed and selected to examine the degree to which a broad range of recommendations for effective school reform are implemented in a school, as well as to examine more fully their impact on students and staff. Initially, in determining the elements of schools on which to focus, we drew from such sources as the work of Sarason [1982, 1992, 1998], the developmental literature on human ecology [Bronfennbrenner 1979], *Turning Points: Preparing American Youth for the 21^{st} Century* [Carnegie Council on Adolescent Development 1989], the work of Comer [1980], the Coalition of Essential Schools [Sizer 1992], the Accelerated Schools Initiative [Finnian, St. John, McCrathy, & Slovacek 1996; Levin 1988], other major reform efforts, the empirical literature, and our previous work. From these sources, we identified a first set of constructs and dimensions of school reform to consider, as they would relate to the outcomes with which we were concerned. Over the last two decades, we have continuously revised and refined these instruments, based on both the emergence of new recommendations and lessons for reform and on the continuous testing of the model and the measures against their ability to predict and account for gains in students' performance, achievement, and adjustment on a broad spectrum of indices (e.g., everything from "standards-based" exams to nationally norm-referenced tests to teacher-provided grades, ratings, and reports of student performance and adjustment). In addition, where funding has allowed, we have selected schools based on patterns of change in student performance, geographic and other sociodemographic conditions, and where schools were more intensively engaged in substudies of the model or implementation issues, we have either conducted our own case studies or collaborated with other research teams working in parallel in the same studies.

Our opportunities have been unusual for their scale, the degree of participation of schools, length of time we have had to follow them (some of these schools are in their seventh year of data collection), and in the diversity of geographic, district, and school settings that were involved. Collectively, during the past eight years alone, we have had more than 1,500 schools, approximately 1 million students, and more than 60,000 teachers participate in this work. For all of these data sets, we have common and longitudinal data elements for the evaluation of the degree to which the HiPlaces model has been implemented and in what ways, as well as both achievement and other adjustment and performance data from students. The *HiPlaces Assessments* obtain survey data from staff, administrators, students, and from teachers about student behavior and performance. The surveys focus on the assessment of the critical elements of the teaching and learning environment that define the implementation of the HiPlaces recommendations, as well as student experiences of school climate, instruction, and student functioning and adjustment. In addition, in most cases we have been able to obtain achievement, performance, and other archival data on participating students.

Figure 1 provides a simplified "logic model" that summarizes the potential pathways of influence and change in educational reform that our evaluation strategy seeks to assess and evaluate. In this model, each of the elements of the pathway has direct influences and/or indirect "mediated" influences—through its influence on other variables and constructs—on the outcomes of concern. To understand the importance of each recommendation, we consider (1) the degree to which the implementation of each recommendation, separately, contributes to the attainment of the processes and impacts depicted in the conceptual and measurement model represented in Figure 1 at its most general level; and (2) the degree to which, as schools implement increasing numbers and levels of the recommendations for HiPlaces schools, the additive and other combination of effects are obtained.

This phase of the model development and evaluation research provided important evidence about the potential viability for produc-

Figure 1. Pathways of Influence Between High Performance Learning Community Implementation Elements and Student Outcomes

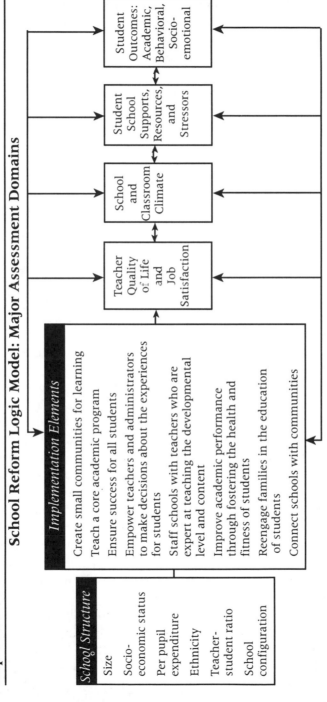

School Reform Logic Model: Major Assessment Domains

ing achievement, performance, and adjustment gains among all students through the implementation of the design elements and framework. In a series of ongoing longitudinal studies we have found that, across projects, initiatives, grade-levels and subject areas, students who were in schools that had more fully implemented the common recommendations and elements (discussed in a later section) for developmentally-focused reform achieved at much higher levels than those in non-implemented schools and substantially better than those in partially implemented schools. This was true both cross-sectionally and longitudinally. Here, as schools made gains in implementation, parallel gains accrued in achievement, although for at-risk students far higher levels of implementation needed to be obtained before significant gains emerged. Still, once these schools reached levels of "sufficiency," small refinement in implementation produced larger and larger gains.

A critical feature of our design has been that we have attempted to obtain multiple convergent measures on aspects of both the implementation of reforms and outcomes across related dimensions. Hence, there were a number of other student outcomes that were considered, including additional indicators of achievement. These indicators included the percentage of students who are performing at grade level and additional student achievement scores in subsets of schools that administer the Iowa Test of Basic Skills, the California Test of Basic Skills and similar nationally norm-referenced assessments. Generally, these additional indicators show strong association with the state-level scores. Illustratively, in one set of analyses we found that as schools move up in their level of implementation of the recommendations of concern, the one-year correlation of such changes with increases in eighth grade reading scores was .51 (p<001) and with increases in eighth grade mathematics scores was .30 (p.<001). Similar patterns were found for two-year changes in implementation level and achievement scores (from 1991–1992 to 1992–1993), with correlations of .53 and .35, respectively (both p<.001). It is encouraging to note that longer-term analyses, if anything, tended to yield findings that were as strong and stable or stronger than did shorter-term change analyses [Felner et al. 1997a].

We also examined different domains of student outcomes as they related to the level of implementation that schools had obtained. These include teacher ratings of student behaviors, as well as student self-reports of behavior, depression (fear, worry), anxiety, and self-esteem. Here the patterns of teacher reports of student behavioral problems, including aggressive, moody/anxious, and learning-related behavior problems, are highly correlated with the patterns noted earlier within achievement data, but in the desired <u>opposite</u> direction. In the most fully implemented schools, teachers report far lower levels of student behavior problems than do teachers in less implemented and nonimplemented schools. Similarly, teachers in the partially implemented schools still perceive students as showing fewer behavioral problems than those in the least implemented schools. Similar patterns were found for student self-reports of a representative set of the domains of socioemotional function that were measured [Felner et. al. 1997a].

## The High Performance Learning Communities Model

The HiPlaces model seeks to provide a well articulated set of principles that, when considered as a comprehensive set, are fully consistent with a developmental ecological approach to school reform [Felner & Felner 1989]. To accomplish this, we seek to continuously evolve a theory-based research model for whole school change that yields clear and testable evaluation research hypotheses, that can be continuously improved and refined, and where each of the elements of that model can also be tested, refined, and evaluated for their contribution to the model and its impact. This approach to evaluation research on school improvement and reform, based on well specified, coherent, and testable theory-derived models, is key to building a cumulative knowledge base for reform and to being able to continuously refine the understandings that are obtained.

That is, we begin with the assumption that further refinements to the model may be possible and required to reach our goals at increasingly high levels. If we have learned anything about the design process from the land grant experience of universities, it is that to be effective, any design process must be, from the beginning, one that is intentionally a *redesign* process. Wilson and Daviss [1994], in their volume on educational redesign, put it this way: If there is to be a Model "A," then an effective redesign process will build in a plan for evolving it to a Model "B" based on hard data that provides feedback from "customers" on efficacy and functioning. Ongoing improvement characterized by this process is intentional, built into the system for change from the outset, and repeated in continuing cycles." One of the appeals of the HiPlaces model and the current initiative is the rigorous, reflective evaluation that has been part of its evolution almost from the start, as well as the degree to which the current initiative allows for us to continue that process.

More than two decades of research have now brought us to the development of a two-level model for the characteristics of High Performing schools that continues to undergo ongoing testing and refinement. In addition to retaining its original focus on modifying the teaching and learning context, our findings have resulted in the addition of several elements of the implementation process that appear to be key to obtaining successful change. We separate these latter features out of the core model as they are a separate set of testable assumptions. The first set pertains to those conditions that may need to be obtained or transformed in the teaching and learning context in order for us to say the model was implemented, and to what degree. The operational/implementation elements, by contrast, represent recommendations, not about what it will take to improve student achievement and performance, but about what it will take to obtain and sustain implementation. Both are testable, but separate models and each can and should undergo continuous testing and refinement.

## Major Dimensions of High Performing Schools

At the first level we have further modified and articulated the common dimensions of high performing schools to include nine major dimensions that are characteristic of such schools. These are:

- Establishing small personalized learning communities

- Integrating standards-based instruction and curricular reform

- A continuing emphasis on literacy and numeracy development

- Holding high expectations and opportunities that promote success for all students

- Empowering decision making at each of the appropriate
  system levels

- Providing professional development to ensure teachers
  are well prepared to teach the subject matter and understand the developmental levels on which they focus

- Fostering health and safety for all student and school-
  community members

- Engaging families in the education of their students

- Creating strong school-community and schoolwork linkages

These nine dimensions are highly consistent with the prior recommendations of *Turning Points* and other reform documents but have a number of key modifications. Some of these reflect changes in the focus and efforts of public education over the last decade. For example, the recommendation to provide for deep, integrative *standards-based* education reflects the emergence and importance of standards as an important element of school reform and integrates into this comprehensive model what had previously been a separate line of reform. For the education of children and youth, this is an important addition to the model in terms of potential impact, but it also represents an important challenge for the design process. Illustratively, in our work we have seen a number of schools move away from some structures and processes that they had put in place as part of implementing *Breaking Ranks* or *Turning Points*. Instead, they attempted to engage what they felt might be more appropriate strategies for providing "standards-focused" instruction. For example, in many of these instances there have been rapid moves away from structures that provided for small learning communities and integrative interdisciplinary instruction, back toward far more traditional secondary structures. The evidence we have on this issue thus far (just over the last two years) suggests, however, that junior/senior high schools and middle schools that have implemented many of the other recommendations and also provide high levels of integrative instruction do, in fact, show greater gains on assessments such as the New American Standards Assessments than do those in more traditional instructional settings for adolescents.

Other recommendations in the HiPlaces set show similar modifications. Professional development has been broadened. Similarly, there is now a recommendation for a continuing focus on instruction and development of literacy and numeracy throughout the k-12 years. Here, for example, although our research shows that at every grade level we have surveyed, continued "integration of reading instruction across the curriculum" is rated by core teachers as the most "essential instructional practice" at their grade level; in fact, the degree to which it occurs drops dramatically after grade five. Some of this is, of course, due to the different preparation of teachers at those latter grade levels. Many of these teachers are less prepared to teach literacy in their subject-based offerings and may not be in team structures that provide access to other teacher resources who can provide assistance. We should also note that in our statistical modeling processes, we have typically included literacy and numeracy in the construct dealing with deep, thematic, standards-based instruction, as statistically and conceptually they do not exist separately. They are broken here as discrete recommendations because of their importance, particularly for disadvantaged students, and because of the tendency to otherwise overlook the focus on literacy and numeracy for all students at the secondary level. Each of the other dimensions is also modified in important ways from those of the prior recommendations of *Turning Points*, *Breaking Ranks*, and other comprehensive efforts at reform, although typically in a generational-evolutionary sense.

Our work and findings have also provided for a critical expansion of the HiPlaces model to a level of the ecology of schooling that has previously been largely ignored in educational reform efforts. This expansion comprises the second level aspects that provide for the further *operationalization* of each of these elements. That is, we have identified five common substratum or crosscutting aspects of the ecology of school settings that shape and define the levels of implementation that schools obtain in their efforts to manifest the nine overarching constructs. This level is key to understanding and creating implementation efforts that are high in fidelity. Understanding these conditions and regularities of school reform provide for articulating far more clearly than has been done previously a common set of research-based conditions that can be considered in assessing the adequacy of implementation of the conceptual recommendations for reform.

The nine dimensions are overarching, concept-level recommendations. So, too, were the recommendations of *Turning Points* [Carnegie Council on Adolescent Development 1989] and other initiatives with which we have been involved. In statistical terms these are known as latent constructs, as they are not directly observable through any one directly measurable variable but, instead, are assessed through some set of observed variables that may be identified as "comprising" that dimension. Through both qualitative procedures and quantitative ones, such as confirmatory factor analyses, the goodness of fit of these operationalizations may then be assessed. In our work, knowing how to get from broad, conceptual recommendations to the necessary elements that should be in place to indicate that they are implemented has been a particularly difficult problem for practitioners.

### Components of Implementation for Each Recommendation

In our evaluation research efforts, we have identified five "components for analysis" that are second level or "crosscutting" common features or elements of the nine dimensions. These need to be considered when assessing the level of implementation of each dimension. Although the specific variable that is of concern under each of these components may only be directly relevant to a subset of the nine dimensions, each of the dimensions is defined by the levels of implementation within each of the five components. The five components that we have identified as key for implementation analysis under each of the nine dimensions include:

- *Structural/organizational characteristics.* These conditions provide the opportunities for other things to change. They may be necessary, but in and of themselves they are typically not sufficient. So, if teachers are provided with common planning time but do not use it to make substantive change in the nature of their practices and interactions, it will be lost. Without such planning time, however, we have found that instructional changes do not occur, or if they do, they are not sustained. Examples of structural/ organizational changes that may impact implementation of the core elements include school and grade enrollment, grade configuration in the building, class size, student-teacher ratios on teams or grades, number of students a teacher is responsible for in one day, instructional tracking and grouping, block scheduling, common planning time for teachers, strategic planning time for staff, bell schedules, length of the day, span of classes covered by a team, length of class periods and school day, number of instructional and professional development days, etc.

- *Attitudes, norms, and beliefs of staff.* Almost all of the existing Comprehensive School Reform Design (CSRD) models focus extensively on staff buy-in, both initially and over time. What appears clear from our research and that of the CSRD teams is that this is yet another necessary but not sufficient element of each dimension. Illustratively, if the staff buys into the professional development offered *and* they have the other necessary structural/organization opportunities and supportive climate, they may implement the practices that are addressed in the professional development. If they do not, however, have buy-in and have negative attitudes about development experience or content, it may do little good.

- *Climate/empowerment/experiential characteristics.* Examples of these conditions include the levels of stress, safety, and support for achievement as well as the degree to which teachers and other staff feel empowered to make necessary decisions for effectively implementing that element. For example, teachers who are overly stressed and feel little opportunity or legitimacy for making instructional changes and improvements are far less likely to make and sustain changes with any degree of fidelity.

- *Capacity/skills.* As should be clear, if people do not know how to do something, they will not do it, or at least not do it well. For each of the dimensions there is a significant skill and knowledge component that is required. For example, teachers who are not well prepared to engage parents, to provide standards-based instruction, or to participate with community agencies will not be able to do any of those things effectively, if at all. They will certainly not do so with the levels of fidelity and skill necessary for adequate implementation to ensure the success of all students.

- *Practice/procedural variables.* These are the practices, processes, and procedures that are used in the building for instruction, decision-making leadership, administration, staff development, parent involvement, community involvement, building and conveying high expectations, and so on through the nine dimensions. Importantly for our work, this is the component that often receives the least amount of attention. What should be clear is that no matter what structural, climate, normative, or professional development conditions obtain for a given dimension, if practice and procedures do not change in the desired directions, schools will fall far short of implementation.

Understanding these five components as they contribute to defining the level of implementation of the dimension in a building can be critical to the school's leaders and staff in assessing the degree to which the decisions they are making are moving them toward necessary levels of implementation of each of the model's dimensions. Attention to each of the five components will serve to increase and strengthen the overall capacity of the entire school. Finally, each of the recommendations at the dimension level and that of the five crosscutting element levels are based on extensive empirical analysis and review. That is, what we <u>can</u> say is that schools that show significant progress in the implementation of these dimensions, comprehensively and with high fidelity, typically also show significant gains in student performance, achievement, and adjustment.

## Implementation Issues

Although the development of a research-based model to guide ever more effective public education efforts is a critical task, it is of little use if we also do not attend to the issues of *"how do we get it to happen?"* In most of our work, we have had a significant number of schools move to relatively higher levels of implementation. But is also the case that they have typically been a minority of schools in any given partnership. For example, a minority of the schools in the major foundation efforts that we have studied have made significant implementation gains, with the exceptions of schools clustered in a few states and districts that had excellent leadership and/or unusual resource conditions. Even fewer have maintained those gains. On the positive side, these patterns of results and change have enabled us to gain extensive understanding of the obstacles, barriers, and resource conditions that may facilitate or impede high levels of implementation. But it is also the case that our most implemented schools are only so in a relative sense.

As we have followed schools during our work we have identified a number of circumstances that either impede or facilitate the implementation of Project HiPlaces' recommendations or similar efforts. The first is the way in which schools organize themselves structurally for change. Many of the schools we work with have a small school improvement team (SIT) that works closely with the administrator while other teachers, staff, and parents are less involved. Progress in these schools has typically been minimal, particularly when the SIT is not effective in continuously engaging other staff. There were many schools where there was a "Carnegie Team" or a "Lilly Team" or an "XYZ" team that made the decisions, met with the outside consultants and, more often than not, was either ignored or the subject of active divisiveness by other staff.

We have found that one effective strategy for helping schools organize for change draws heavily on the work of the Accelerated

Schools. That is, when schools organize into cadres or subcommittees that either parallel the elements of their own school improvement plan or that parallel the dimensions of the recommendations for the high performance learning communities model, and when all teachers and other key staff in the building are on one or more of these committees, there is greater progress made. This is particularly true in schools that attend to a second necessary operational element of the model—the provision of adequate, or at least regular school improvement planning and monitoring time. An important difference here is that we have found that the planning process engaged in by Accelerated Schools is more likely to be ineffective when it does not start with some clear recommendations and reliable, valid data about both student performance and the teaching and learning process. Hence, we would ask schools in a successful initiative to organize according to the HiPlaces model. We would also work toward the development of procedures that facilitated the integration of the school's existing school improvement plan and the model into a research-based approach rather than requiring schools to start from scratch. This strategy can greatly reduce resistance to change.

Third, the HiPlaces design, as currently constructed, requires schools to engage in ongoing information-based school improvement planning and monitoring, which has been called "Empowerment Evaluation" [Fetterman 1996]. We have found in our work that no matter which assessments you have and how high the quality, unless you can directly speak to the association between the Project findings and the local assessments of student achievement, there are difficulties in policy, practice, and implementation discussions.

## Summary and Policy Implications

The findings of Project HiPlaces, only lightly touched on here, demonstrate strongly the potential of a theory-based comprehensive "whole school change" model for effectively promoting student learning, achievement, and school adjustment at levels necessary to enable public schools to address the new challenges and demands of the societal ecology in which they must function and deliver results.

Importantly, the ecologically based model for educational transformation that is offered here appears to be a highly effective one for
guiding the re-engineering and redesign of public school settings, and
for obtaining successful and sustainable implementation when its
recommendations are followed with intensity and fidelity.

Perhaps the most important lesson about implementation from
this ongoing research is that successful reform must be comprehensive and integrative, with careful attention to sequencing and the
establishment of some key elements upon which other elements can
be mounted. There are clear patterns of interdependence among the
implementation elements, which may require additional attention by
those involved in school reform efforts if we are to fully realize the
benefits of middle grade restructuring.

One of the clearest patterns that has emerged in our data is the
difference between a "checklist-based" implementation of structural
changes and implementation that is "idea-driven"—that attempts to
reflect the underlying constructs and issues in the *HiPlaces* recommendations. Consider the recommendation of "Creating Small Communities for Learning" as an example. If one employs a checklist approach
here, as typified in many sets of recommendations for middle grades
reform [c.f., Mergendollar 1993] a school might ask itself whether or
not it has teacher teaming or interdisciplinary instruction. Unfortunately, being able to "check off" these practices becomes an end unto
itself, with little regard to why these practices should be implemented
or in what forms and levels they need to be present in order to
contribute to a more effective teaching and learning process. Across
our samples, schools that say they are "teaming" may have team sizes
ranging from those with 60 to 70 students and 2 to 3 teachers, to those
with over 240 students and from 9 to 12 teachers. Student-to-teacher
ratios on a team may range from below 20 students per teacher to
more than 40 students per teacher. Additionally, levels of common
planning time, which appears to be a critical element of small learning
communities, varies from no common planning time, to the shared
use of individual planning times, to schools that provide daily common planning time in addition to individual planning time, for each
of the teachers on their teams.

There are considerable differences in the costs of these implementation options, and policymakers as well as school administrators who must make decisions about expending resources need to take these differences into account. Our findings reveal a number of patterns that, if they hold, make the case against attempting school restructuring "on the cheap." First, we have found that each of the dimensions of teaming we have considered (e.g., size, student/teacher ratio, amount of common planning time) appear to have a significant association with the degree to which other elements of *HiPlaces* reforms and goals may be accomplished. Our findings indicate that more negative levels of each of these variables are associated with:

- Failure of teams to implement critical teaming activities that focus on curriculum integration, coordination, and collaboration around student needs/assignments, which appears to be true both cross-sectionally and longitudinally, where large team sizes and the absence of sufficient common planning time relate to relatively slow or non-implementation of critical teaming practices;

- More negative school climate as reported by students;

- Self-reports and teacher reports of elevated student mental health and behavior problems; and

- Lags in student achievement.

Indeed, it appears that in cases where schools attempt to implement these practices, but do them poorly (e.g., one or two common planning times per week, interdisciplinary instruction without common planning time, large teams), there may be no effect or even negative effects, especially on teacher attitudes and student performance.

It also appears to be the case that the patterns of gains obtained by reforms are neither linear nor independent. In considering the transition to middle grade schools, Felner and his colleagues [Felner et al. 1997a, 1997b] reported that the patterns of relationships between more positive levels of implementation and student achievement, wellness, mental health, and behaviors, are, at least in part, the result of the preventive and wellness sustaining effects of middle-grades structures. Small teams and teacher-based advisory programming in particular, especially when coupled with keeping those teams in their own areas of the building and away from "older" students, appear to enable students to make the transition into middle schools without the pronounced declines in socioemotional well-being and achievement that have been reported in some studies of students moving into middle schools and junior high schools [Simmons and Blyth 1987].

Hence, the higher scores for achievement and student well-being attained by students in middle grade schools that have created small communities for learning, when compared to those of students in more traditionally structured schools, appear to result more from declines in these indicators among the students in the traditional schools than from gains by students in environments that have only these restructuring elements. This is not a trivial finding. These predictable declines have, in the past, been linked to a full range of socioemotional problems among youth (e.g., school failure, dropping out, crime, depression, substance abuse, and teenage pregnancy and parenthood).

Still, educational reformers have sought not only to avoid the onset of new difficulties, but also to enhance the developmental course of students. In our current samples, we have a growing set of schools that have shown significant levels of implementation across virtually all *HiPlaces* areas. Here, our findings suggest that it is only when schools begin to realize much more complete implementation of the full range of *HiPlaces* recommendations that such enhancement effects accrue.

Illustratively, in the important case of "at-risk" students, our results indicate the majority of "gain" effects are not realized until implementation is quite mature and comprehensive. Previously we have reported the potential importance of high levels of comprehensive school transformation for attaining both preventive and enhancement effects for students at greater risk. The average "effect size" (amount of change in an indicator relative to the standard deviation of that measure) across a set of achievement and adjustment indicators (e.g., classroom behavior, student school attitudes/bonding/climate ratings, sense of efficacy, deviant behavior) for students who are minorities and/or eligible for free/reduced priced lunch exists as a function of the level of implementation of their school. Consistent with much prior work, we found that students in more traditionally structured schools show declines in achievement/adjustment indicators. It is not until substantial transformation had been accomplished (e.g., structural changes that are necessary for creating small learning communities, changes in norms and some instructional practices) that preventive effects (e.g., the absence of declines that would otherwise appear) are found for these at-risk students. Finally, and critically, the findings show that for at-risk students, broad-range enhancements in achievement, adjustment, and overall wellness indicators, are not obtained until implementation is quite mature, comprehensive, and being conducted with a high degree of fidelity.

Assuming that these patterns hold over subsequent analyses as additional data is acquired, our findings should encourage policymakers to move forward rather than decide to stop or move away from restructuring because the results in the early stages are not all that was hoped for. It should not be surprising that it takes fairly comprehensive and intensive levels of implementation for the suggested changes to produce major gains in all spheres of functioning of high-risk students. Often, these students live in community environments that may be high in stress and low in opportunity and resources. However, our findings to date strongly support the view that quality schooling, well implemented, can make profound contributions to the achievement, wellness, and sociobehavioral functioning of students who are often left behind and for whom there is often a sense that school cannot make a difference in their lives. These data also argue for resources to be used effectively in schools with high concentrations of at-risk students, and, in some instances, for resources to be increased significantly in order to create the conditions identified here that are required for all children to be successful in school and in life.

# References

American Psychological Association. (1997, June 26–28). *Bringing to Scale Educational Innovation and School Reform: Partnerships in Urban Education.* Conference Proceedings. Washington, DC: Author.

Bronfennbrenner, U. (1979). *The ecology of human development: Experiments by nature and design.* Cambridge: Harvard University Press.

Carnegie Council on Adolescent Development. (1989). *Turning points: Preparing America's youth for the 21st century.* New York: Carnegie Corporation of New York.

Cowen, E. L. (1977). Baby-steps toward primary prevention. *American Journal of Community Psychology, 5,* 1–22.

Comer, J. P. (1980) *School Power: Implications of an intervention project.* New York: Free Press.

Cowen, E. L. (1985) Person centered approaches to primary prevention in mental health: Situation-focused and competence enhancement. *American Journal of Community Psychology, 13,* 31–48.

Cowen, E. L. (1991). In pursuit of wellness. *American Psychologist, 46,* 404–408.

Cowen, E. L. (1994) The enhancement of psychological wellness: Challenges and opportunities. *American Journal of Community Psychology, 22,*149–179.

Cowen, E. L., Trost, M. A., Lorion, R. P., Dorr, D., Izzo, L. D., & Isaacson, R. V., (1975). *New ways in school mental health.* New York: Human Sciences.

Felner, R. D. & Adan, A. M. (1988). The school transitional environment project: An ecological intervention and evaluation. In R. H. Price, E. L. Cowen, R. P. Lorion, and J. Ramos-McKay (Eds.), *Fourteen ounces of prevention: A casebook for practitioners* (pp. 111–122). Washington, DC: American Psychological Association.

Felner, R. D., Brand, S., Adan, A. M., Mulhall, P. F., Flowers, N., Sartain, B., & DuBois, D. L. (1993). Restructuring the ecology of the school as an approach to prevention during school transitions: Longitudinal follow-ups and extensions of the School Transitional Environment Project (STEP). In L. A. Jason, K. E. Danner, & K. S. Kuralski (Eds.), *Prevention and school transitions* (pp. 103–136). New York: Haworth Press, Inc.

Felner, R. D. & Felner, T. Y. (1989). Prevention programs in the educational context: Transactional-ecological framework for program models. In L. Bond & B. Compas (Eds.), *Primary prevention and promotion in the schools* (pp. 13–48). Beverly Hills: Sage Publications.

Felner, R. D., Jackson, A. W., Kasak, D., Mulhall, P., Brand, S., & Flowers, N. (1997a). *Preparing adolescents for the twenty-first century: Challenges facing Europe and the United States.* Cambridge, U.K.: Cambridge University Press.

Felner, R. D., Jackson, A. W., Kasak, D., Mulhall, P., Brand, S., & Flowers, N. (1997b). The impact of school-reform for the middle years: Longitudinal study of a network engaged in *Turning-Points* based comprehensive school transformation. *Phi Delta Kappan 78*(7), 528–550.

Felner, R. D., Kasak, D., Mulhall, P., & Flowers, N. (1997). The project on high performance learning communities: Applying the land-grant model to school reform. *Phi Delta Kappan, 78*(7), 520–527.

Felner, R. D., Silverman M. M., & Felner, T. Y. (2000). Prevention in mental health and social intervention: Conceptual and methodological issues in the evolution of the science and practice of prevention. In J. Rappaport & E. Seidman, *Handbook of Community Psychology.* New York: Kluwer Academic/Plenum Publishers.

Fetterman, D. M. (1996). Empowerment evaluation: An introduction to theory and practice. In D. M. Fetterman, S. Kaftarian, & A. Wandersan, *Empowerment evaluation: Knowledge and tools for self-assessment and accountability* (pp. 3–49). Thousand Oaks, CA: Sage Publications.

Finnan, C., St. John, E. P., McCarthy, J., Slovacek, S. P. (Eds.). (1996). *Accelerated schools in action: Lessons from the field.* Thousand Oaks, CA: Corwin Press.

Levin, H. M. (1988). Accelerating elementary education for disadvantaged students. In Council of Chief State School Officers (Eds.), *School success for students at-risk* (pp. 209–226). Orlando, FL: Harcourt, Brace, Javonovich.

Lee, V. E. & Smith, J. B. (1994). *Effects of high school restructuring and size on gains in achievement and engagement for early secondary school students.* Madison, WI: University of Wisconsin, Center on Organization and Restructuring of Schools.

Lyon, R. (1999, February). *Literacy in America.* Symposium at the University of Rhode Island, Kingston, R.I.

Mrazek, P. J. & Haggerty, R. J. (Eds). *Reducing risk for mental disorders: Frontiers for prevention research.* Washington, DC: National Academy Press.

Mergendollar, J. R. (1993). Introduction: The role of research on the reform of middle grades education. *The Elementary School Journal, 93,* 443–446.

National Association of Secondary School Principals (1996). Breaking Ranks: Changing an American Institution. Reston, VA: National Association of Secondary School Principals.

Rhode Island Department of Education (1998). *InformationWorks!* Providence, RI: Rhode Island Department of Education.

Sarason, S. B. (1977). *Work, aging, and social change.* New York: Free Press.

Sarason, S. B. (1982). *The culture of the school and the problem of change* (2nd ed.). Boston: Allyn & Bacon.

Sarason, S. B. (1983). Psychology and public policy: Missed opportunity. In R. D. Felner, L. A. Jason., J. N. Moritsugu, and S. S. Farber (Eds.), *Preventive psychology: Theory, research, and practice.* New York: Pergamon Press.

Sarason, S. B. (1992). *The predictable failure of educational reform.* San Francisco: Jossey-Bass

Sarason, S. B. (1998). *Charter schools: Another flawed educational reform?* New York: Teachers' College Press.

Sizer, T. (1992). *Horace's school: Redesigning the American high school.* Boston: Houghton Mifflin.

Simmons, R. & Blyth, D. (1987). *Moving into adolescence.* New York: Aldine De Gruyter.

Wilson, K. G. & Daviss, B. (1994). *Redesigning education: A Nobel prize winner reveals what must be done to reform American education.* New York: Henry Holt.

Wilson, W. J. (1987). *The truly disadvantaged: The inner city, the underclass, and public policy.* Chicago: University of Chicago Press.

# 10

# Interventions to Promote Social Support in Children and Adolescents

*Manuel Barrera, Jr., and Hazel Prelow*

Some children are blessed with those naturally-occurring forces that exist in families, schools, neighborhoods, and other settings to facilitate the development of wellness. Rather than relying exclusively on these natural forces, many are invested in promoting wellness with planned interventions. Interventions to promote wellness include those that are designed to boost competency and positive mental health by mobilizing social support, enriching existing social ties, modifying social networks that are dysfunctional, and introducing new network members such as mentors or support group participants [Gottlieb 1988; Heller et al. 1990]. The ever popular concept of social support that has generated such an enormous volume of epidemiological and other basic research findings, also has been the subject of interventions directed at both adults and children [Bogat et al. 1993; Vaux 1988]. It is apparent from even a superficial reading of this literature that most support interventions are framed as attempts to prevent or treat distress and illness, but some aspects of this research are relevant to our conversation about children's well-being and competencies. The purpose of this chapter is to describe social support interventions that have attempted to alter wellness in children and adolescents. A closely related purpose is to evaluate how well research has established that changing features of children's social networks and social support are effective in changing children's wellness. We also consider directions that future research might take to clarify theory and inform practice.

How might wellness be changed and what is social support's role in this effort? Cowen [1994] proposed five major pathways to wellness:

(a) forming wholesome early attachments; (b) acquiring age- and ability-appropriate competencies; (c) engineering settings that promote adaptive outcomes; (d) acquiring skills needed to cope effectively with life stressors; and (e) fostering empowerment. The concept of social support is not tied equally to each of these pathways, but many of the mechanisms underlying the concept of wellness have some connection to social support.

The concept of social support is aligned closely with attachment, the very first pathway to wellness that Cowen described [Ptacek 1996]. Although the concept of attachment has specialized meaning, it overlaps considerably with the concept of social support when it is applied to a parent's relationship with a child. Interventions that are designed to increase a parent's provisions of social support to a child are contributing to that child's sense of security that the parent is a reliable source of nurturance. This sense of security might be regarded as a component of children's greater sense of well-being, but security is also a feature of intimate social relationships that assist children in coping with stressful events that create upheavals in other areas of their lives [Sandler et al. 1989]. Research suggests that parents' own social support networks influence their parenting, including their ability to establish close relations with their children [Cochran & Brassard 1979; Crittenden 1985; Crnic et al. 1984]. Consequently, some support interventions are designed to increase directly the social support that parents provide to their children while others are designed to increase support to the parents of children.

Another pathway to wellness, children's acquisition of competencies, also takes place in supportive contacts with adults and peers. Mastering social skills, learning and developing talents, creating a sense of competence, and cultivating self-esteem occur in supportive relationships with others [Sandler et al. 1989]. Some social competencies appear to be developed best in relationships with adults, while others, such as conflict resolution and negotiation, benefit from practice with same-aged siblings and friends. There is a role for support interventions that improve social competence through supportive relations with adults as well as peers.

Cowen [1994] pointed out that adaptive outcomes result not only from personal skills, but also from characteristics of the settings where children live. Settings have many features, including supportiveness or what Moos termed the "relationship" dimension in his analysis of environments [e.g., Trickett & Moos 1973]. This point is a reminder that support interventions need not rely exclusively on changing people, such as teaching children and parents new skills, or on instructing members of children's social networks. Intervention efforts also might include modifying settings in ways that facilitate the cultivation of supportive relations and, ultimately, better adaptation.

The pathway concerned with acquiring skills needed to cope effectively with life stressors includes learning how and when to rely on others. Classification schemes of coping activities emphasize cognitive skills such as problem solving and cognitive restructuring [Ayers et al. 1996], yet they also include support seeking. Sandler et al. [1989] discussed several theoretical mechanisms whereby social support might protect children from the effects of stress. These mechanisms include social support's potential ability to enhance children's self-esteem, increase their perceptions of control, and strengthen their sense of security. These largely cognitive mechanisms counteract the negative consequences of negative life events that are also mediated by cognitive events.

Of all the pathways to wellness identified by Cowen, only fostering empowerment has a questionable tie to the concept of social support and its relation to the wellness of children. Definitions of empowerment refer to it as the process of gaining influence over events and outcomes of importance, a definition that incorporates both individuals' perceptions of personal control as well as behaviors to exercise control [Rappaport 1987; Zimmerman 1995]. In her critique of the empowerment construct, Riger [1993] associated empowerment with individualism, competition, and conflict as she contrasted it with opposing concepts of communion and cooperation. However, Perkins and Zimmerman [1995] saw a clear association between empowerment and one of the key social support intervention modalities, mutual help groups. From their perspective, "empowerment is a construct that links individual strengths and competencies, natural helping systems, and proactive behaviors to social policy and social change" [p. 569]. Zimmerman [1995] then illustrated empowerment concepts by describing how mutual help organizations assist their members in developing personal control. Although empowerment emphasizes the concept of personal control, support networks and mutual aid groups are mechanisms through which empowerment can be achieved.

## Social Support Interventions for Children and Adolescents: Definitions and Categorizations

Social support interventions are organized procedures designed to improve individuals' well-being by increasing the quality and/or quantity of tangible, emotional, and informational support. These interventions have been developed to prevent disorders and to ameliorate the effects of risk factors such as child maltreatment, parental alcoholism, divorce, childhood illness, poverty, low birthweight, and other forms of adversity. Researchers have generally used three mechanisms to enhance social support: mentoring, support groups, and interventions designed to change the supportiveness of settings. In many instances, interventions were a combination of two or more of these mechanisms.

### *Mentoring: Adding One Key Support Provider*

According to Blechman [1992], mentoring occurs when a more experienced person transmits knowledge to a less experienced person. This definition does not require an emotional bond between the mentor and protégée for this transmission of knowledge to take place. Mentoring interventions usually have been characterized by "one key person" who provided support. Sometimes this key person has been a professional, such as a nurse. In perhaps the best known and most important experimental evaluation of a support intervention, Olds and his colleagues used nurses to visit mothers during and after their pregnancies to help prevent child abuse and neglect, and to improve pregnancy outcomes [Olds et al. 1986a; Olds et al. 1986b]. Nurses provided emotional support as well as information about pregnancy and child care. They also helped mothers enhance support within their families and connect with resources in the community. In other mentoring interventions the "one key person" was a nonprofessional. LoSciuto et al.'s intervention used older adults as mentors to sixth grade inner city students [LoSciuto et al. 1996]. In this study, older adults helped with homework, attended social activities, and participated in community service activities with their protégées. Big Brothers/Big Sisters programs have been in existence for over 90 years, matching adult mentors with youth from single-parent households. There is now good evidence for the efficacy of these programs that will be described later in this chapter [Tierney et al. 1995].

*Support Groups*

Another category of social support intervention is the support group. Similar to mentoring interventions, support groups often use professionals such as mental health workers or nurses as leaders. Unlike mentoring interventions, which rely on one "key person" to deliver the intervention, group interventions derive their effectiveness from the combination of the group leaders who may provide informational support and from individual group members who provide each other with emotional support.

One example of a support group intervention is Emshoff's [1990] program for children of alcoholics. His 18-session intervention was designed for sixth to eighth grade adolescents affected by familial alcoholism. Sessions were co-led by a psychology graduate student with training in families and substance abuse, and a social worker or counselor. Because children of alcoholics are often isolated from sources of support, some sessions were designed to teach skills that would help students to effectively communicate with peers and parents. Social activities, designed to encourage bonding among group members, also were an integral part of the intervention.

*Changing Settings*

The last category of support intervention involves changing environments so that they are more supportive. Unlike mentoring and support group interventions that focus on creating new contexts for support, environmental interventions focus on changing the structure of an existing setting, such as a school or community, in order to make it more conducive to developing and maintaining consistent sources of social support.

The School Transition Environment Program (STEP), developed by Felner et al. was an example of an environmental intervention [Felner et al. 1982; Felner et al. 1993]. This intervention was designed to facilitate high school freshmen's adjustment to the transition from middle school. One component of the intervention involved changing the role of the homeroom teacher so that students and parents had one consistent person who served as their link to the school's administration. The other focus of the intervention was changing the structure of classes so that program students could take core academic courses with the same group of program students rather than confronting a new group of students each time they moved to a different class.

## The Effectiveness of Mentoring Interventions

*Programs to Influence Child Physical Health During the Prenatal Period*

As previously mentioned, mentoring interventions are interventions designed to enhance emotional, tangible, and informational support of protégées. These interventions differ from other social support interventions, in that social support is changed through the efforts of "one key person." Home visitation is an example of one type of mentoring intervention that has been extensively used to influence child well-being during the critical prenatal period. Improving prenatal care and pregnancy outcomes were goals of the home visitation program by David Olds and his colleagues [Olds et al. 1986]. Their intervention was developed for women with one of three risk factors: under 19 years of age, unmarried, or from a low socioeconomic background. The initial intervention included four treatment conditions: (a) a no treatment control group, (b) free transportation to regular well-child visits, (c) nurse visitation during pregnancy, and (d) nurse visitation that began in pregnancy and continued through the first two years of the child's life. Nurses provided informal support and prenatal care information. Another important objective of the intervention was to improve the mother's support system and her connections to community services.

Olds and his colleagues found support for the beneficial effects of the nurse visitation mentoring relationship. Nurse visitation had a positive impact on the mothers' immediate support system, her use of other community resources, and the health of their children. Compared to controls, nurse-visited mothers reported that they had more conversations with support network members about their pregnancies and personal problems, and were accompanied more often by support persons to the hospital when giving birth [Olds et al. 1986]. Nurse-visited mothers under the age of 17 had higher birthweight babies than similarly aged mothers in the comparison group; nurse-visited mothers who were smokers had fewer preterm deliveries than mothers in the comparison group. It also appeared that the nurse-mother mentoring relationship had some long-term beneficial effects on children's well-being [Olds et al. 1994; Olds et al. 1998]. Assessment of mothers and children at 46 and 48 months revealed that nurse-visited children had fewer injuries, ingestions, and emergency room visits than comparison group children [Olds, Henderson, & Kitzman 1994]. The authors also noted that nurse-visited mothers were more involved with their children and punished them more than comparison group mothers. However, punishment did not function in the same way in the nurse-visited and comparison group. For nurse-visited mothers, higher punishment was associated with fewer injuries and ingestions. In contrast, higher punishment was associated with more injuries and ingestions in the comparison group.

## Mentoring in the Prenatal and Infancy Period to Influence Mother-Child Attachment

The mentoring approach also has been used to improve child well-being by enhancing mothers' social competencies [e.g., Booth et al. 1989]. Booth et al. [1989] posited that social skills were necessary for establishing and maintaining supportive relationships. Supportive relationships increased mothers' feelings of efficacy and self-esteem which, in turn, positively influenced the mother-child relationship.

Nurse visitors developed a therapeutic relationship with mothers and through this relationship helped mothers acquire interpersonal competencies. These researchers intended to test two treatment conditions, (a) a Mental Health Model in which the nurse "fostered an explicitly therapeutic relationship" [p. 405] to develop interpersonal competencies and (b) an Information/Resource model, which was intended to include information and referrals, but no therapeutic transactions, between nurses and mothers. However, subsequent review of the treatment process revealed that both groups had received a majority of nursing acts that were classified as providing therapy. That is, a majority of the Information/Resource group received therapy that was to have been given to the Mental Health group only. Subsequently, the researchers combined these two groups in analyses. Results of their analyses indicated that for those mothers who began the intervention with low social skill and who reached treatment goals (i.e., improved social skills), goal attainment was positively related to mother-child interaction. Furthermore, social skills at posttreatment had an indirect positive effect on mother-child interaction such that treatment goal attainment was positively related to social skills at posttreatment, and social skills at posttreatment, in turn, was positively related to mother-child interaction.

## Other Mentoring Programs

Unlike the home visitor interventions, which tend to focus on child well-being by helping mothers, the mentor-protégée approach focuses directly on the child. Similar to some of the home visitor interventions [Booth et al. 1989; Dawson 1989], mentor-protégée relationships tend to be characterized by a strong emotional bond between the mentor and protégée. It is through this relationship of mutual trust and understanding that emotional, tangible, and informational support are provided from the more experienced mentor to the protégée.

The program entitled Across Ages is a good example of a mentor-protégée intervention [LoSciuto et al. 1996]. According to LoSciuto et al., the intervention was designed to increase protective factors in an ethnically and racially diverse group of sixth-grade urban adolescents from low socioeconomic backgrounds. Among the factors targeted for change were coping skills; self-esteem; and attitudes toward school, elders, and the future. They also wanted to increase knowledge about drug use and decrease the frequency of drug use. Students were randomly assigned to one of three conditions: no treatment control, Public Service, or Mentoring Public Service. Pre- and postprogram tests were administered to the students. The Public Service group received a treatment which consisted of performing public service, a support group for parents, and a school-based life skills curriculum. Participants in the Mentoring Public Service group received the same treatment as the Public Service group plus mentoring from older adults. Mentors spent at least four hours per week with students in activities such as helping with homework or attending social and cultural events. In general, the group that received mentoring in addition to the other program components showed more treatment gains than the Public Service group at the post-program test. The Mentoring group scored better than the Public Service group on school absences and attitudes toward school, future, and elders. In addition, the mentoring group was marginally better than the Public Service group on knowledge of older people and frequency of substance use. In summary, it appears that the mentoring intervention may have had an additional effect over and above that of the Public Service intervention.

An experimental test of a home visitation program for bereaved children was a rare example of research which assessed changes in support that resulted from the intervention and the role of support as a mediator of intervention effects [Sandler et al. 1992]. Home visitors (called "family advisers" in this project) were college-educated adults who had personally experienced the death of a close family member. They conducted 12 sessions with families that had experienced the death of a parent. Five of the 12 sessions were devoted to skills for improving the warmth of the parent-child relationship. Results showed that the intervention was successful in increasing parent-child warmth and parents' satisfaction with the support they received. Furthermore, parent-child warmth mediated the intervention's effects on parents' reports of their children's psychological distress. Conventional measures of well-being were not featured in this project, but it was significant that this mentoring intervention improved support from parents, and that this effect was related to changes in their perceptions of their children.

Have mentoring interventions been successful in positively influencing child well-being? While mentoring interventions appear to positively affect child well-being [Booth et al. 1989; Dawson et al. 1989; LoSciuto et al 1996; Olds et al. 1986], it is difficult to attribute these effects solely to the mentoring component because many mentoring interventions include several components. For example, LoScuito et al.'s mentoring intervention included mentoring, community service, parents' workshops, and a classroom-based life skills curriculum. Individual components of multifaceted mentoring interventions are rarely tested to determine whether mentoring had an significant effect on child well-being.

A critical piece of research on a pure mentoring intervention was a national study of Big Brothers/Big Sisters (BBBS) programs [Tierney et al. 1995]. This experimental trial involved 959 10- to 16-year-olds who were randomly assigned to BBBS or to a waiting list. Youth were from single-parent households; 57% of the sample consisted of ethnic minority boys and girls. BBBS programs match youth with adult volunteers who agree to meet two to four times each month for at least a year. In this study, 70% of mentors and mentees met three to four times each month, with the typical meeting lasting at least four hours. The experiment covered an 18-month period, but two to six months of this period was devoted to finding matches for children assigned to the BBBS program. Results showed that youth in BBBS were significantly less likely than controls to report the initiation of drug use, hitting someone, skipping classes, skipping days of school, and lying to parents. BBBS children were significantly more likely than controls to report competence in completing schoolwork and a positive relationship with parents. BBBS organizations have been operating for 90 years, but this was the first convincing demonstration of their effectiveness. Unlike other mentoring programs, BBBS does not combine mentoring with a host of behavior-change techniques; it focuses on the relationship between the mentor and the protégée.

Olds and Kitzman [1993] did a comprehensive review of 31 randomized trials of home visiting programs that were directed at decreasing the occurrence of adverse birth outcomes, and increasing health of parents and young children under age three. Overall, these studies did not show that home visiting decreased rates of preterm delivery or low birthweight. Very few of the studies assessed the impact of the intervention on health-related behaviors (e.g., reductions in smoking) or psychosocial functioning (e.g., provision of emotional support by the home visitor, involvement of family and friends). On the other hand, home visiting programs were effective in improving the cognitive development of preterm and low birthweight infants, and in improving maternal caregiving and stimulation in the home. Olds and Kitzman speculated that the success of home visiting programs depended on the content and intensity of the intervention, the training of the home visitors, and the program's flexibility in responding to the needs of families. They asserted that low-intensity interventions or home visitor interventions that focused exclusively on social support without an emphasis on health-related behaviors would not produce positive outcomes, particularly outcomes concerned with physical well-being.

Does the mentoring relationship, which is the essential feature of mentoring interventions, enhance social support? If so, does this social support lead to child well-being? These questions have not been addressed adequately. Most mentoring interventions rely on the mentor to build a therapeutic or personal relationship with the participants. It is through this relationship that participants acquire social skills, receive health information, increase social support, develop strategies for behavioral change, or become linked with community resources. The mentoring relationship itself constitutes a supportive relationship, however, this relationship is rarely assessed and the process by which this relationship influences child well-being has not been explored adequately.

## Support Group Interventions

Groups have many attractive features as a format for improving children's social support. In practice, children's support groups almost always have an adult leader who is a professional such as a counselor or teacher. Similar to the mentoring interventions, this adds at least one new adult to children's networks of responsible adults who teach new skills, offer advice, or engage the child in positive activities. Obviously, support groups also consist of children's peers who sometimes are selected for participation because they share salient background characteristics such parental substance use [Emshoff 1990 ; Gross & McCaul 1992], parental divorce [Alpert-Gillis et al. 1989; Kalter et al. 1984; Kalter et al. 1988; Pedro-Carroll & Cowen 1985; Stolberg & Garrison 1985; Stolberg & Maher 1994] or school difficulties [Eggert et al. 1990]. Shared background characteristics and planned group activities can assist in building cohesion among group members. Groups can be structured with the explicit goal of increasing the social integration of group members within the larger social setting [Haring & Breen 1992]. Such groups create the opportunity for participants to add social network members while they acquire social skills that might be used to add nongroup members to their larger networks of friends.

There have been two broad applications of social support principles in groups to affect the well-being of children. First, there are approaches that involve children as participants in groups. Similar to others, we will refer to these applications as "support groups," but we recognize that there is some danger in confusing these groups with self-help support groups that are often directed by and to adults. If it was not such an awkward term, children's support groups might be more accurately called "support in groups" to convey the kind of interactions that are desired but achieved by methods that differ from information-and-discussion-oriented adult support groups. It is understandable that children's support groups involve some discussion, but also include instruction and activities such as games, drawing, and writing that engage children in collaborative tasks [e.g., Stolberg & Mahler 1994]. Second, there are group approaches that offer support to the caregivers of children, particularly mothers, in hopes of improving the lives of children. These groups more closely fit the model of support groups for adults who assemble around other foci such as chronic illness or addictions. Some parent support groups are deliberately nonprescriptive in setting any agenda for meetings [e.g.,

Broussard 1989], while others follow a plan that identifies specific topics [e.g., Lovell & Hawkins 1988].

## Children's Support Groups

There are several common features to group approaches for changing the social support of children and adolescents. Children's support groups are usually led by an adult professional such as a teacher, school counselor, or specially-trained adult. These support groups are often multifaceted due to a variety of components that go well beyond support to include activities such as supervised study and academic tutoring [Eggert et al. 1990], decision making and personal control [Eggert et al. 1995], problem solving, communication, anger control [Pedro-Carroll & Cowen 1985], and other skill-building topics. Those groups that have been evaluated have been of fixed duration, ranging from 11 weekly sessions [Pedro-Carroll et al. 1986] to 18 sessions once or twice a week [Emshoff 1990]. As previously noted, children's support groups are often structured by including exercises or games that are designed to engage participants in interacting with their peers. This is unlike the emphasis on verbal discussion that characterizes adult support groups.

Have support groups been successful in increasing children's well-being? There is only very modest support of their effectiveness in changing well-being. The literature provides some isolated examples of evaluated support group interventions, but there is not a consistent pattern of findings. One of the strongest demonstrations of support group effectiveness was reported by Stolberg and Garrison [1985] in evaluating components of their Divorce Adjustment Project for children of divorce and their mothers. Stolberg and Garrison [1985] designed their study to compare the effects of their Children's Support Group (CSG), Single Parents' Support Group, the combination of the two support groups, and a no-intervention control. The CSG actively taught participants cognitive-behavioral skills along with providing them emotional support, but this intervention was still less heterogeneous than others that have incorporated social support into their larger intervention. Participants were assessed at pre-, post-and 5-month follow-ups on measures of self-concept, child behavior, parent's adjustment, parenting behaviors, and life events. Children in the CSG showed greater pre-post change on the self-concept measure than children in the combined intervention or the control group. The CSG condition also showed greater improvement from posttest to follow-up on adaptive social skills than the combined CSG and parent support group. The authors explained that the failure of the combined CSG and parent support group to show beneficial effects might have been due to demographic differences between groups (e.g., duration of separation). Because participants had not been randomly assigned to groups, between-group differences (and the lack of differences) following intervention could not be interpreted with complete confidence.

Because the CSG condition in the Stolberg and Garrison study combined skill training with group social support, the effectiveness of the support alone was not evaluated. A subsequent study evaluated the effectiveness of group support without the skill training elements [Stolberg & Mahler 1994]. Stolberg and Mahler [1994] did not find that the support group intervention for children of divorce (in isolation of skill-building components such as labeling feelings, problem solving, and anger control) was more effective than a no-intervention control condition in reducing psychological distress or boosting competence. However, the support group elements in combination with skill building components were effective in reducing internalizing and externalizing behaviors. This combination of skill development and support was similar to the effective intervention used in Stolberg and Garrison [1985].

Another children's support group intervention showed positive effects on school attendance, grades, credits earned, and substance use, but it used a quasi-experimental design, and the intervention included many strategies in addition to social support such as visits to community agencies, recreation, supervised study, tutoring, and school attendance monitoring [Eggert et al. 1990]. The support group elements occurred in the form of a semester-long counseling class that met daily. Classes of about 10 students met with a specially trained teacher to allow students to express problems that could be discussed by the group and provided a framework for teaching communication, problem solving, decision making and self-management. Participants were students who had truancy records, poor grades, or insufficient credit hours. Similar to many of the other support group interventions, skill building was combined with the group support to form an intervention that appeared to be effective in assisting these at-risk students in staying in school, improving grades, reducing truancy, and avoiding drug involvement.

Evidence of the effectiveness of support group interventions in elevating children's well-being is modest because of many factors. A focus on psychological distress still predominates in evaluations of these interventions. Outcomes such as depression, anxiety, conduct problems [e.g., Stolberg & Mahler 1994]; drug use [Eggert et al 1990; Emshoff 1990; Gross & McCaul 1992] and school dropout [Eggert et al. 1990] are much more common than indicators of positive mental health or competence. Measures of well-being that have been used are self-esteem [Eggert et al. 1995; Gross & McCaul 1992; Stolberg & Garrison 1985], competence [Stolberg & Mahler 1994], and adaptive social skills [Stolberg & Garrison 1985], but they are not primary foci. When measures of well-being are included, support group interventions do not always affect them [Eggert et al. 1995; Kalter et al. 1984]. Support interventions usually are multifaceted, precluding firm conclusions that support was the effective ingredient [Alpert-Gillis et al. 1989; Eggert et al. 1990; Eggert & Herting 1991; Emshoff 1990; Pedro-Carroll et al. 1986]. In the one study that isolated the effects of support, the support group without skill building was not more effective than a no-intervention control group [Stolberg & Mahler 1994].

Social support intervention studies almost never include measures of social support. Are support groups effective in increasing children's social support? Can effects of support group interventions be attributed to changes in social support? Answers to these questions are not apparent in the literature on children's support groups. A rather consistent characteristic of research on children's support groups is that they do not directly assess changes in social support that might result from participation in groups. The failure to assess the effects of support group interventions on social support does not allow us to determine if social support mediates the effect that interventions have on measures of well-being. Finally, even well conceived interventions designed to improve social support are not always effective [e.g., Eggert et al. 1995]. A starting point for evaluations of children's support group interventions should be a greater understanding of how they might effectively improve children's social support.

## Parenting Support Groups

Parenting support groups have the dual goals of assisting parents, particularly new parents, with the challenges of child rearing and improving the lives of their children. Part of the rationale for parenting groups is based on developmental research [Cochran & Brassard 1979; Crittenden 1985; Crnic et al. 1983] and Wahler's [1980] observations about "insular" parents. Parents who lack contact with other parents and their own family are cut off from people who could assist in reducing the burdens associated with parenting and who could be the source of useful information about child rearing. Research points to the beneficial effects of naturally occurring support networks for parents, but when this support is absent in the environment, parenting groups are seen as one possible way to fill the void.

Most parent support groups have the immediate goal of bolstering parents' resources in the face of stress that comes from child rearing; benefits to children are more distal goals. For example, a 30-week support group for parents of abused or neglected children included stress management, anger control, positive self-talk, assertiveness, and child management [Lovell & Hawkins 1988]. Some parenting groups [e.g., Broussard 1989] are explicit about their goal of promoting parents' attachment to their children, one of the pathways to wellness that Cowen [1994] described. Broussard [1989] sought to accomplish this with unstructured, nondirective support groups in which mothers met for 1-1/2 hours, every other week, during the critical period in their infants' lives between 2 months and 3-1/2 years old. Wolchik et al. [1993] conducted groups for divorced mothers with the goal of affecting children's mental health through a variety of mediators including the quality of the mother-child relationship, contact with the noncustodial father, and support from nonparental adults. Five of the group sessions were devoted to methods for elevating the quality of the mother-child relationship, such as engaging in joint positive activities, improving listening skills, and giving positive attention for desirable child behaviors. Compared to a no-intervention control condition, the intervention was successful in improving the quality of the mother-child relationship, which also mediated the intervention's reduction of children's behavior problems.

Other groups are specifically directed at preventing postpartum depression in the mothers, and only indirectly concerned with promoting parent-child attachment or children's well-being [Elliott, Sanjack, & Leverton 1988]. Because the emphasis is on support to parents, changes in well-being of children and infants are rarely reported.

Do parent support groups change the social support that is available to parents? The results are somewhat mixed, but some studies suggest that parents who participate in parenting groups do increase their available support. A one-year prospective study of 150 mothers who had children with disabilities assessed the extent to which these mothers participated in parent support groups, characteristics of parents' social support networks, adversity experienced by the family, and other factors [Krauss et al. 1993]. The study found that mothers who participated in parent support groups showed greater increases in the size of their networks and perceived their peers to be more helpful than mothers who did not participate. The study was also an important reminder of how support receipt can be positively related to adversity. Mothers who had children with more severe impairments, who experienced more parenting strain, and who reported more adverse impacts on the family also reported more participation in parent support groups. In a controlled experiment with a sample of 24 couples, McGuire and Gottlieb [1979] found that those who participated in the parenting groups discussed child-rearing issues with network members more often than those who were in the control condition (written information only). Parents in one of the two parenting groups also reported increasing the size of their support networks more than parents in the other groups, at least a modest indication that the intervention was successful in helping couples expand their network members. Unfortunately, the study did not find that the intervention was successful in changing parents' stress, well-being, and overall health. Finally, a quasi-experimental study of 79 adolescent mothers showed that groups for teaching coping skills, particularly skills involved in conflict management and improving social networks, were effective in increasing mothers' social support and social competence at the end of a 12-session intervention [Schinke, Barth, et al. 1986]. At the end of a three-month follow-up, teen mothers who received the intervention scored better than the control condition on measures of social support, cognitive performance, parenting ability, child-care self-efficacy, and psychological well-being. A similar intervention with a similar design showed similar results [Schinke, Schilling, et al. 1986].

Whereas there was some suggestion from these studies that parenting groups were successful in increasing the support available to participants, Lovell and Hawkins [1988] found that members of their parenting support groups did not become part of parents' social networks. In their study, the largest changes in participants' social networks were additions of formal service providers and individuals who were known to mothers prior to intervention. Other well-conceived efforts to increase support to parents have also been unsuccessful, but in one case the intervention was brief [Dadds & McHugh 1992] and in another there were trends in the data, but the sample size was relatively small [Ireys et al. 1996]. Despite anecdotal evidence that parent support groups can be popular and useful for new parents and parents facing adversity, there is a disappointing lack of experimental data showing that parents who participate in support groups increase their social support and pass on benefits to their children's well-being as a result of their participation.

## Changing the Supportiveness of Settings

Engineering settings that promote adaptive outcomes was one of the pathways Cowen [1994] identified as leading to wellness. As previously noted, Felner et al.'s [1982, 1993] School Transitional Environment Project (STEP) stands out as the best example of changing the social support in an environment to promote the wellness of adolescents. Transitions from middle school to high school can be marked by adverse changes in school achievement, increased classroom behavior problems, and elevated anxiety. The negative consequences of school transitions were attributed to the "flux" of the social setting—a new school combined with a structure of constantly changing peer groups as students move from class to class throughout the school day. The initial STEP intervention involved 59 students in an effort that was designed to ease the school transition by enhancing the homeroom teacher's role and clustering project students into the same classes. Homeroom teachers accepted responsibility for administrative and counseling functions, thereby becoming the prime link between project students, their families, and the school. Rather than constantly changing classmates, project students took their four primary academic subjects with the other project students.

In evaluating the intervention, project students were contrasted with a matched control sample of 113 freshmen from the same high school. At the end of the school year, project students reported more teacher support, better grades, better self-concept, and less absenteeism than the control students. Control students' scores declined over the school year, while intervention students' scores improved or stayed the same. The authors interpreted their results as evidence that modifying the social ecology of the school improved the social support provided to students and reduced confusion associated with the transition. The five-year follow-up evaluation of this initial intervention showed that STEP students experienced half of the school dropout rate and less absenteeism compared to students in the control condition [Felner et al. 1993].

Although the initial STEP demonstrated many positive effects, this study missed the opportunity to show that changes in social support mediated the relationship between the intervention and wellness outcomes. The intervention appeared to lead to changes in teacher support, but we do not know with certainty that better grades, self-concept, and absenteeism were affected by improved teacher support. Analytic procedures such as those used by Wolchik et al. [1993] would have been needed to show that teacher support mediated the intervention effects. It is possible that the intervention could have affected peer support because the Transition Project was structured to build cohesion among project participants. However, peer support could not be evaluated as a mediator because it was not assessed.

Replication and extension of STEP focused on the transition from elementary grades to middle school and included the assessment of perceived school climate factors such as student affiliation, negative interactions between students, and positive teacher-student interactions. Comparisons between STEP students and students in nonparticipating schools showed that STEP students had fewer negative interactions in school, greater peer affiliation, and greater teacher support. Formal mediational analyses were not done, but the authors indicated that they computed correlations between the school climate variables and outcomes such as self-esteem, depression, anxiety, behavior problems, classroom behavior, and academic adjustment. These correlational analyses (112 analyses) were not reported in Felner et al. [1993]; the authors noted that because all but 11 were significant, there was some evidence that the program's influence on school climate was associated with positive student outcomes.

A separate environmental intervention was also school-based and attempted to influence high school students' social support through constructive conflict resolution and cooperative learning [Zhang,1994]. This study was designed to test the theory that constructive conflict resolution and cooperative learning would exert their effects on self-esteem, mental health, sense of self-control, and academic achievement through changes in high school students' social support. Students and teachers from three alternative high schools in New York participated in the project. This quasi-experimental research made effective use of structural equation modeling to show that constructive conflict resolution increased social support (from a variety of sources) and decreased victimization (e.g., victim of theft or assault) to lead to several important wellness outcomes: increased self-esteem, more positive attitudes toward life, greater internal locus of control, and improved academic achievement.

Ambitious interventions sought to change the supportiveness of neighborhoods for parents [Cochran & Henderson 1990; Powell 1979, 1987]. Cochran's Family Matters intervention began in 1975 with 160 families in 10 different neighborhoods in Syracuse, New York. Family Matters was originally designed to compare a home-visitor intervention with a cluster-group intervention in which participating families met in neighborhood groups, but after the first nine months of this two-year program, these two intervention methods were combined. The results of this study are difficult to summarize succinctly because the data were presented separately for African American and Caucasian families, and for single and married parents. Furthermore, many distinctions were drawn in the assessment of social support, including the distinction between kin and nonkin social network members. Among a number of changes that occurred, AfricanAmerican and Caucasian single mothers in the intervention group had greater increases in the number of nonkin functional network members than control group mothers. For African American parents, increases in support network membership were related to parents' involvement in parent-child activities and positive school outcomes. The pattern of results were different for Caucasian families, but still offered some support for the ability of the intervention to alter dimensions of mothers' social networks, their perceptions of themselves as parents, and the school outcomes of their young children.

The design of Family Matters, like the intervention methods used by Olds and his collaborators, recognized the potential value of combining the support from a mentor with peer support or even support from community organizations. Despite its effectiveness, there is a recognition that a mentor in the form of a home visitor is a contrived intervention that increases a person's network by one, and only for a specific period of time. There is the hope and the expectation that developing supportive ties among neighbors or facilitating the use of formal supports found in available community organizations could have the effect of sustaining the beneficial effects of support long after the relationship with a mentor has passed. Building natural supportive ties to existing community resources while introducing an effective change agent is having the best of both worlds—the world of natural support and the world of trained helpers.

## Directions for Practice and Theory

With the possible exception of mentoring programs such as home visitation, there is not extensive research on any category of social support interventions directed at children's wellness. What we have are many examples of promising intervention programs that have been put into practice and evaluated with various levels of sophistication. Encouraging the continued development of effective social support interventions has importance for both practice and theory. Because much of the literature on social support is based on nonexperimental research, there are persistent questions about social support's true relation to outcomes such as psychological distress, health, and well-being. A potential contribution of intervention research is when it provides experimental tests of theoretical models that are based on intuition, observations, and correlational data [Sandler et al. 1997]. From our review of this specialized literature on support interventions for children, we draw a conclusion that is very similar to that of Bogat et al. [1993] who observed that most prevention researchers who used support interventions did not posit or test a theoretical model of social support when they set out to evaluate the efficacy of their interventions. Not only have models such as the stress-buffer model not been tested with experimental trials of interventions, but there continues to be a distinct need for research to establish the basic theoretical premise that children's social support affects changes in wellness and other outcomes.

To test this basic question which underlies both theory and practice, research must demonstrate that (a) interventions can change both social support and wellness, and (b) that the changes in social support are at least partially responsible for the changes in wellness. We were unable to identify a single study that used experimental trials to demonstrate both features. Although some studies offered suggestive evidence [e.g., Booth et al. 1989; Cochran & Henderson 1990; Felner et al. 1982; Zhang 1994], research was either quasi-experimental or failed to use optimal data analytic procedures for testing mediation. For example, Booth et al. [1989] tested mediation, but what had started as an experimental evaluation of a support intervention turned out to be a nonexperimental study. The two intervention conditions could not be differentiated and did not result in between-group differences on the hypothesized mediator—mothers' social skill improvements. When intervention conditions were disregarded, path analyses offered some support for the authors' hypotheses that mothers' attainment of intervention goals led to improvements in mother-child interactions and that this effect was partially mediated by mothers' social skills.

Establishing that interventions can reliably change features of social support is far from trivial. As noted, there have been well-designed interventions that failed to increase social support [e.g., Ireys et al. 1996]. Those that have been successful in changing social support and social networks have redesigned social environments to more effectively promote social support [Felner et al. 1982], used teaching methods that required students to work together cooperatively [Zhang 1994], implemented very active interventions for teaching social skills [Schinke et al. 1986; Varni et al. 1993] or were protracted interventions that extended over several months or years [Cochran & Henderson 1990; Felner et al. 1982; Olds et al. 1996]. These studies contained descriptions of procedures that could be followed to manipulate children's social support and that of their parents. It is important to note that a large number of support intervention studies could not determine if they were successful in changing social support because they contained no direct measure of support.

Evaluations of support interventions have not provided extensive evidence that they result in improvements in children's wellness. Again, we have isolated examples that show the promise of such interventions, but measures of wellness are not always included in support intervention studies. For example, many studies of parent support groups do not assess for potential changes in children's well-being even though they were implemented with the expectation that children as well as parents would benefit from the programs. The studies by Sandler et al. [1992] and Wolchik et al. [1993] were rare experimental demonstrations that an intervention was effective in changing social support (from a parent) and that support mediated changes observed in child outcomes. In those studies, the outcomes were aspects of psychological distress such as anxiety, depression, and behavior problems, but it is quite conceivable that these intervention might have affected measures of well-being if they had been assessed.

Once it can be established that interventions affect both social support and wellness outcomes, then it is critical to use data analytic methods for assessing social support as a mediator. Sandler et al. [1997] discussed considerations in theory, research design, and statistical analyses for testing mediation with experimental intervention trials. These procedures and those proposed by West and Aiken [1997] for evaluating specific program components have exciting applications for testing support interventions in ways that will inform theory and provide practitioners with valuable information about the effectiveness of programs.

Future research also should attend to methodological features that could increase our understanding of social support interventions. Untangling the effects of multicomponent interventions is one such need because prominent interventions include elements that extend well beyond the social support construct. For example, it is difficult to interpret the results of some "family support" programs as evidence that social support is an effective change agent because these interventions include components such as pediatric care, day care, developmental evaluations, as well as home visitation [Seitz & Apfel 1994; Seitz et al. 1985]. Children support groups as well as home visitation interventions are likely to be multifaceted. The challenge, then, for outcome research is to design evaluations in ways that will allow us to attribute experimental effects to the support components.

In a somewhat related point, Booth et al. [1989] pointed out that some social support interventions such as home visitation by mentors present a challenge for maintaining treatment fidelity. Because these interventions are provided in individuals' homes, little monitoring of fidelity to the treatment protocol is done. When methods for evaluating treatment delivery was included in one study, the authors showed that treatment was not be carried out as planned, which blurred the distinctions between different intervention conditions [Booth et al. 1989]. Failure to differentiate treatment conditions compromises the internal validity of studies and the conclusions that can be made about the effectiveness of social support interventions.

Beyond the fundamental question of determining that the manipulation of support results in changes in wellness, there are a multitude of more refined questions that concern specific mechanisms of change. For example, Sandler et al. [1989] identified a number of cognitive mechanisms whereby stressful events might result in psychological distress and how social support might prevent deterioration or restore a child's sense of predictability and control in the wake of adversity. Also, the process by which mentoring relationships might promote well-being could be explored with variations of mediational analyses. Whether mentoring relationships are effective because they influence cognitive mechanisms, social competencies, access to resources, or a combination of mechanisms has not been determined.

An important direction for future research would be to investigate how support <u>provision</u> affects the well-being of the support provider (e.g., a mentor). Support provision takes place in the context of children's support groups, mentor-protégée relationships, and community service activities that are components of some comprehensive interventions [Allen et al. 1994; LoSciuto et al. 1996]. The well-known helper-therapy principle would suggest that the benefits for support providers are at least as great as the benefits for the support recipients [Gartner & Reissman 1977]. While there has been much research investigating the impact of mentoring on protégées, few studies have examined the effects of mentoring on the mentor. There is some qualitative research that suggests that mentoring may have positive effects on the mentor's well-being [Wright & Borland 1992]. While it is certainly worthwhile to understand the positive consequences of providing support to children and their parents, we should not ignore the possibility that children's competence and well-being might benefit the most from opportunities to provide support to others.

# References

Allen, J. P., Kuperminc, G., Philliber, S., & Herre, K. (1994). Programmatic prevention of adolescent problem behaviors: The role of autonomy, relatedness, and volunteer service in the teen outreach program. *American Journal of Community Psychology, 22,* 617–638.

Alpert-Gillis, L. J., Pedro-Carroll, J. L., & Cowen, E. L. (1989). The children of divorce intervention program: Development, implementation, and evaluation of a program for young urban children. *Journal of Consulting and Clinical Psychology, 57,* 583–589.

Ayers, T. A., Sandler, I. N., West, S. G., & Roosa, M. W. (1996). A dispositional and situational assessment of children's coping: Testing alternative models of coping. *Journal of Personality, 64,* 923–956.

Blechman, E. A. (1992). Mentors for high-risk minority youth: From effective communication to bicultural competence. *Journal of Child Clinical Psychology, 21,* 160–169.

Bogat, G. A., Sullivan, L. A., & Grober, J. (1993). Applications of social support to preventive interventions. In D. S. Glenwick & Jason, L. A. (Eds.), *Promoting health and mental health in children, youth, and families* (pp. 205–232). New York: Springer.

Booth, C. L., Mitchell, S. K., Barnard, K. E., & Spieker, S. J. (1989). Development of maternal social skills in multiproblem families: Effects on mother-child relationship. *Developmental Psychology, 25,* 403–412.

Broussard, E. R. (1989). The Infant-Family Resource Program: Facilitating optimal development. In R. E. Hess & J. DeLeon (Eds.), *The National Mental Health Association: 80 years of involvement in the field of prevention* (pp. 179–224). New York: Haworth.

Cochran, M. & Brassard, J. (1979). Child development and personal social networks. *Child Development, 50,* 609–616.

Cochran, M. & Henderson, C. R., Jr. (1990). Formal supports and informal social ties: A case study. In M. Cochran, M. Larner, D. Riley, L. Gunnarsson, & C. Henderson, Jr. *Extending families: The social network of parents and their children* (pp. 230–261). New York: Cambridge University Press.

Cowen, E. L. (1994). The enhancement of psychological wellness: Challenges and opportunities. *American Journal of Community Psychology, 22,* 149–179.

Crittenden, P. M. (1985). Social networks, quality of child rearing, and child development. *Child Development, 56,* 1299–1313.

Crnic, K. A., Greenberg, M. T., Ragozin, A. S., Robinson, N. M., & Basham, R. B. (1983). Effects of stress and social support on mothers and premature and full-term infants. *Child Development, 54,* 209–217.

Dadds, M. R. & McHugh, T. A. (1992). Social support and treatment outcome in behavioral family therapy for child conduct problems. *Journal of Consulting and Clinical Psychology, 60,* 252–259.

Dawson, P., van Doornick, W. J., & Robinson, J. L. (1989). Effects of home-based, informal social support on child health. *Journal of Developmental and Behavioral Pediatrics, 10,* 63–67.

Eggert, L. L. & Herting, J. R. (1991). Preventing teenage drug abuse: Exploratory effects of network social support. *Youth and Society, 22*, 482–524.

Eggert, L. L., Thompson, E. A., Herting, J. R., & Nicholas, L. J. (1995). Reducing suicide potential among high-risk youth: Tests of a school-based prevention program. *Suicide and Life-Threatening Behavior, 23*, 276–296.

Eggert, L. L., Seyl, C. D., & Nicholas, L. J. (1990). Effects of a school-based prevention program for potential high school dropouts and drug abusers. *International Journal of the Addictions, 25*, 773–801.

Elliott, S. A., Sanjack, M., & Leverton, T. J. (1988). Parents groups in pregnancy: A preventive intervention for postnatal depression? In B. H. Gottlieb (Ed.), *Marshaling social support: Formats, processes, and effects* (pp. 87–110). Beverly Hills: Sage Publications.

Emshoff, J. G. (1990). A preventive intervention with children of alcoholics. *Prevention in Human Services, 7*, 225–253.

Felner, R. D., Ginter, M., & Primavera, J. (1982). Primary prevention during school transition: Social support and environmental structure. *American Journal of Community Psychology, 10*, 277–290.

Felner, R. D., Brand, S., Adan, A. M., Mulhall, P. F., Flowers, N., Sartain, B., & DuBois, D. L. (1993). Restructuring the ecology of the school as an approach to prevention during school transitions: Longitudinal follow-ups and extensions of the school transitional environment project (STEP). *Prevention in Human Services, 10*, 103–136.

Gartner, A. & Reissman, F. (1977). *Self-help and the human services.* San Francisco: Jossey-Bass.

Gottlieb, B. H. (1988). Support interventions: A typology and agenda for research. In S. W. Duck (Ed.), *Handbook of personal relationships* (pp. 519–541). New York: Wiley.

Gross, J. & McCaul, M. E. (1992). An evaluation of a psychoeducational and substance abuse risk reduction intervention for children of substance abusers. *Journal of Community Psychology* (Office for Substance Abuse Prevention special issue), 75–87.

Haring, T. G. & Breen, C. G. (1992). A peer-mediated social network intervention to enhance the social integration of persons with moderate and severe disabilities. *Journal of Applied Behavior Analysis, 25*, 319–333.

Heller, K., Price, R. H., & Hogg, J. R. (1990). The role of social support in community and clinical interventions. In B. S. Sarason, I. G. Sarason, & G. R. Pierce (Eds.), *Social support: An interactional view* (pp. 482–507). New York: Wiley.

Ireys, H. T., Sills, E. M., Kolodner, K. B., & Walsh, B. B. (1996). A social support intervention for parents with juvenile rheumatoid arthritis: Results of a randomized trial. *Journal of Pediatric Psychology, 21,* 633–641.

Kalter, N., Pickar, J., & Lesowitz, M. (1984). School-based developmental facilitation groups for children of divorce: A preventive intervention. *American Journal of Orthopsychiatry, 54,* 613–623.

Kalter, N., Schaefer, M., Lesowitz, M., Alpern, D., & Pickar, J. (1988). School-based support groups for children of divorce. In B. H. Gottlieb (Ed.), *Marshaling social support: Formats, processes and effects* (pp. 165–185). Newbury Park, CA: Sage Publications.

Krauss, M. W., Upshur, C. C., Shonkoff, J. P., & Hauser-Cram, P. (1993). The impact of parent groups on mothers of infants with disabilities. *Journal of Early Intervention, 17,* 8–20.

LoSciuto, L., Rajala, A. K., Townsend, T. N., & Taylor, A. S. (1996). An outcome evaluation of Across Ages: An intergenerational mentoring approach to drug prevention. Special Issue: Preventing adolescent substance abuse. *Journal of Adolescent Research, 11,* 116–129.

Lovell, M. L. & Hawkins, J. D. (1988). An evaluation of a group intervention to increase the personal social networks of abusive mothers. *Children and Youth Services Review, 10,* 175–188.

McGuire, J. C., & Gottlieb, B. H. (1979). Social support groups among new parents: An experimental study in primary prevention. *Journal of Clinical Child Psychology, 8,* 111–116.

Olds, D. L., Henderson, C. R., Chamberlin, R., & Tatelbaum, R. (1986a). Preventing child abuse and neglect: A randomized trial of nurse home visitation. *Pediatrics, 78,* 65–78.

Olds, D., Henderson, C. R., Cole, R., Eckenrode, J., Kitzman, H., Luckey, D., Pettitt, L., Sidora, K., Morris, P., & Powers, J. (1998). Long-term effects of nurse home visitation on children's criminal and antisocial behavior: 15 year follow-up of a randomized control trial. *Journal of the American Medical Association, 280,* 1238–44.

Olds, D. L., Henderson, C. R., & Kitzman, H. (1994). Does prenatal and infancy nurse home visitation have enduring effects on qualities of parental care giving and child health at 25 to 50 months of life? *Pediatrics, 93,* 89–98.

Olds, D. L., Henderson, C. R., Tatelbaum, R., & Chamberlin, R. (1986b). Improving the delivery of prenatal care and outcomes of pregnancy: A randomized trail of nurse home visitation. *Pediatrics, 77,* 16–28.

Olds, D. L. & Kitzman, H. (1993). Review of research on home visiting for pregnant women and parents of young children. *The Future of Children, 3*, 53–92.

Pedro-Carroll, J. L. & Cowen, E. L. (1985). The children of divorce intervention program: An intervention of the efficacy of a school-based prevention program. *Journal of Consulting and Clinical Psychology, 53*, 603–611.

Pedro-Carroll, J. L., Cowen, E. L., Hightower, D., & Guare, J. C. (1986). Preventive intervention with latency-aged children of divorce: A replication study. *American Journal of Community Psychology, 14*, 277–290.

Perkins, D. D. & Zimmerman, M. A. (1995). Empowerment theory, research, and application. *American Journal of Community Psychology, 23*, 569–579.

Powell, D. (1979). Family environment relations and early childbearing: The role of social networks and neighborhood. *Journal of Research and Development in Education, 13*, 1–11.

Powell, D. (1987). A neighborhood approach to parent support groups. *Journal of Community Psychology, 15*, 51–62.

Ptacek, J. T. (1996). The role of attachment in perceived support and the stress and coping process. In G. R. Pierce, B. R. Sarason, & I. G. Sarason (Eds.), *Handbook of social support and the family* (pp. 495–520). New York: Plenum.

Rappaport, J. (1987). Terms of empowerment/exemplars of prevention: Toward a theory for community psychology. *American Journal of Community Psychology, 15*, 121–148.

Riger, S. (1993). What's wrong with empowerment? *American Journal of Community Psychology, 21*, 279–292.

Sandler, I. N., Miller, P., Short, J., & Wolchik, S. A. (1989). Social support as a protective factor for children in stress. In D. Belle (Ed.), *Children's social networks and social supports* (pp. 277–307). New York: Wiley.

Sandler, I. N., West, S. G., Baca, L., Pillow, D. R., Gersten, J. C., Rogosch, F., Virdin, L., Beals, J., Reynolds, K. D., Kallgren, C., Tein, J. Y., Kriege, G., Cole, E., & Ramirez, R. (1992). Linking empirically-based theory and evaluation: The Family Bereavement Program. *American Journal of Community Psychology, 20*, 491–521.

Sandler, I. N., Wolchik, S. A., MacKinnon, D., Ayers, T. S., & Roosa, M. W. (1997). Developing linkages between theory and intervention in stress and coping processes. In S. A. Wolchik & I. N. Sandler (Eds.), *Handbook of children's coping: Linking theory and intervention* (pp. 3–40). New York: Plenum.

Schinke, S. P., Barth, R. P., Gilchrist, L. D., Maxwell, J. S. (1986). Adolescent mothers, stress, and prevention. *Journal of Human Stress, 12*, 162–167.

Schinke, S. P., Schilling, R. F., Barth, R. P., & Gilchrist, L. D. (1986). Stress management intervention to prevent family violence. *Journal of Family Violence, 1*, 13–26.

Seitz, V. & Apfel, N. H. (1994). Parent focused intervention: Diffusion effects on siblings. *Child Development, 65*, 677–683.

Seitz, V., Rosenbaum, N. K., & Apfel, N. H. (1985). Effects of family support intervention: A ten-year follow-up. *Child Development, 56*, 376–391.

Stolberg, A. L. & Garrison, K. M. (1985). Evaluating a primary prevention program for children of divorce. *American Journal of Community Psychology, 13*, 111–124.

Stolberg, A. L. & Mahler, J. (1994). Enhancing treatment gains in a school-based intervention for children of divorce through skill training, parental involvement, and transfer procedures. *Journal of Consulting and Clinical Psychology, 62*(1) 147–156.

Tierney, J. P., Grossman, J. B., & Resch, N. L. (1995). *Making a difference: An impact study of Big Brothers/Big Sisters*. Philadelphia: Public/Private Ventures.

Trickett, E. J. & Moos, R. H. (1973). The social environment of junior and senior high school classrooms. *Journal of Educational Psychology, 65*, 93–102.

Varni, J. W., Katz, E. R., Colegrove, R., & Dolgin, M. (1993). The impact of social skills training on the adjustment of children with newly diagnosed cancer. Special issue: Interventions in pediatric psychology, *Journal of Pediatric Psychology, 18*, 751–767.

Vaux, A. (1988). *Social support: Theory, research, and intervention*. New York: Praeger.

Wahler, R. G. (1980). The insular mother: Her problems in parent/child treatment. *Journal of Applied Behavior Analysis, 13*, 207–219.

West, S. & Aiken, L. (1997). Toward understanding individual effects in multiple component prevention programs: Design and analysis strategies. In K. Bryant, M. Windle, & S. West (Eds.), *New methodological approaches to prevention research*. Washington, DC: American Psychological Association.

Wolchik, S. A., West, S. G., Westover, S., Sandler, I. N., Martin, A., Lustig, J., Tein, J. Y., & Fisher, J. (1993). The children of divorce parenting intervention: Outcome evaluation of an empirically based program. *American Journal of Community Psychology, 21,* 293–331.

Wright, L. & Borland, J. H. (1992). A special friend: Adolescent mentors for young, economically disadvantaged, potentially gifted students. *Roeper-Review, 14,* 124–129.

Zhang, Q. (1994). An intervention model of constructive conflict resolution and cooperative learning. *Journal of Social Issues, 50,* 99–116.

Zimmerman, M. A. (1995). Psychological empowerment: Issues and illustrations. *American Journal of Community Psychology, 23,* 581–599.

# Acknowledgments

Preparation of this chapter was supported by NIMH grant 5-P30-MH39246-13. The second author was funded by a postdoctoral fellowship through NIMH grant 5-T32-MH1837.

# 11

## Pursuit of Wellness in Head Start: Making Beneficial Connections for Children and Families

*John W. Fantuzzo and Wanda K. Mohr*

The readiness of young children for school is a national priority. Unfortunately, a disproportionate number of hardships threaten the well-being of young children in large cities in the United States. Unprecedented levels of poverty and menacing urban social problems adversely affect the development of children ages zero to five. The prevalence and intensity of these social toxins have significantly damaged community organization and vital social and family networks [Garbarino 1995]. Not surprisingly, the cumulative impact of these difficulties is associated with emotional and behavioral problems and poor school adjustment [Campbell 1997].

According to the latest epidemiological statistics, during the course of a single year, approximately one in five children and youth experience signs and symptoms of emotional distress that are sufficiently severe to warrant a DSM-IV diagnoses. Five percent of all children experience what professionals term "extreme emotional disturbance" [U.S. Department of Health and Human Services 1999]. Irrespective of this number of children in need of mental health services, the use of such services is significantly lower than expected, with only 2% of these children currently receiving treatment [Burns 1991]. Moreover, between 70% and 90% of all children classified as having severe disorders are not currently receiving mental health services [Costello et al. 1993].

Among other important circumstances responsible for this state of affairs are structural barriers to care that include the lack of early identification and intervention efforts for emotional disorders, and the scarcity and inappropriateness of existing services. These barriers are in part grounded in an overreliance on tertiary care provision. This predominant focus on tertiary care creates serious gaps in primary and secondary mental health service provision that impede least restrictive, prevention efforts. For children and families, this translates into a service system devoid of home and community options and treatment separated from the natural settings where the problems occur.

Community-based early childhood intervention programs have shown great promise as a means of promoting healthy and adaptive psychological development for vulnerable children and families. However, the quality of these programs must improve to respond to the increasing amount of adversity that families experience in high-risk environments. Head Start is the nation's largest community-based program for young, low-income children. Embracing life span and ecological perspectives of development, Head Start has delivered a comprehensive array of educational, psychological, health, and social services to children and families in need [Zigler & Styfco 1994]. But, the challenges to provide quality services have grown as economic and social conditions in the United States have worsened for young children and families. Demographic and socioeconomic changes have placed a tremendous burden on Head Start programs to keep up with the growing needs of a very diverse and stressed low-income population [HHS 1993].

Head Start leadership is faced with the necessity of expanding its educational and family support mandates to address these major risk factors and their negative consequences. At this critical juncture, Head Start must formulate a substantive mental health agenda and forge closer ties with mental health professionals to seek solutions to these complex and daunting problems. Mindful of the words of the poet William Cowper—"Beware of desperate steps!"—Head Start must carefully select a model to guide the redesign and reconceptualization of its mental health services. Moreover, it must examine existing alternatives to determine which one is most consistent with its mission and most likely to maximize the well-being of Head Start children and families. Two distinctive paths lie before the Head Start leadership: the traditional "Illness" path of mental health or the less traveled "Wellness" path.

In this chapter we discuss how the dominant illness, deficiency-based system of care in child psychology and psychiatry perpetuates unhealthy "disconnections." We argue for an alternative "pursuit of wellness" model based on individual and community strengths and contend that this model nurtures hope by establishing vital connections. Using this model, we illustrate the capacity of this approach to inform the development of needed Head Start-based assessment, intervention, and training methods. A core assumption of this chapter is that wellness mental health methods establish multiple worthwhile connections for children and their families and that these connections hold the greatest promise for beneficial and enduring outcomes for Head Start children.

## Illness Model: Dead Ends and Disconnections

The identification of disorders and the treatment of pathology have been primary concerns in the illness model of mental health. This perspective is represented by its system of classifying symptoms of mental disorders and by its formalized methods to treat these symptoms. Although these methods of classification and treatment currently dominate the child mental health system, dead ends and critical disconnections associated with this approach raise questions about the adequacy and appropriateness of this approach for Head Start.

Foundational to the present mental health care system is an underlying assumption that disability has already occurred. Research, assessment, diagnosis, and treatment of children focus on the cause of maladaptive symptoms and their management. The logical consequence of this assumption is an approach to mental health service delivery that is illness or deficiency driven. These deficiencies are categorized into diagnostic entities determined by the consensus of the American Psychiatric Association [1994] and contained within the Diagnostic and Statistical Manual of Mental Disorders (DSM). When a child's behavior comes to the attention of clinicians by its disruption of social institutions, the DSM serves as their key reference guide. Children are observed and interviewed against its criteria for evidence of the signs and symptoms of disorders and discrete categories——the DSM diagnoses—are applied by clinicians based on the data they collect. The present mental health care system views behaviors warranting a DSM diagnosis as "disorders," the etiology of which are presumed to be within the child and resulting from some process of pathogenesis [Sroufe 1997].

The DSM system has been questioned from the time it was developed. Major shortcomings include: (a) Lack of theoretical foundation, (b) failure to consider context, and (c) lack of consequential validity. Scholars in child development posit that the DSM is a collection of symptoms devoid of theory [Jensen & Hoagwood 1997; Richters & Cicchetti 1993]. These symptoms are not grounded in an understanding of human development as it informs children's functioning; instead, they are typically derivative of adult deviancy. Therefore, for the most part, DSM terminology is inappropriate for children and negatively oriented (e.g. disorder, dysfunction, disturbance, and deficit).

The DSM categories are fixed tags that fail to consider peoples' capacity to grow, adapt, regenerate, differentiate, or reorganize. The system tacitly assumes that human beings possess the same values, attitudes, experiences, and developmental trajectories. Because the DSM labels are devoid of context, they are unidimensional, isolated conglomerates of behaviors that fail to consider human beings as open systems contiguous with their environment [Jensen & Hoagwood 1997]. Despite its attempt to give the categories more dimensionality through its multiaxial system of diagnostics, the axial approach fails to provide clinicians with information regarding key sources of competence and support within the environment. Moreover, the system's acontextual and cross-sectional nature precludes consideration of the human capacity to exhibit similar patterns of functioning resulting from qualitatively different structures (equifinality) and for different patterns of overt functioning that stem from similar processes (multifinality). Ignoring these capacities means that people are presumed to react in similar ways for similar reasons, whereas the similarity of their patterns of functioning may be the result of very different objectives. For example, "psychopathology" may actually reflect individuals' attempt at adapting to noxious environmental influences. Thus DSM criteria such as "often initiates physical fights," "runs away from home," or "often fidgets with hands or squirms in seat" may result from abusive and unstable environments, rather than from presumed, intrapsychic pathology [Richters & Cicchetti 1993].

Using the DSM system to underpin assessment and treatment is inadequate because it is not geared toward the planning of prevention or interventions [Sroufe 1997]. While maladaptive behavior is seen as symptomatic of disturbance within the individual, however, the DSM system does not specify what pathogenic processes contribute to maladaptation . Thus treatment is not focused on processes but on symptom reduction. Choice of treatment is left solely in the hands of the mental health experts. Therefore, because there is no way to scientifically link the presumed benefits of psychotherapy to any underlying psychopathological processes, the DSM lacks consequential validity [Messick 1995].

The present system represents a failure to integrate children and the relational aspects and elements of their environment. It contributes to a constricted approach to children and their special needs in both research and intervention initiatives. It makes it possible to conceptualize their lives and their worlds in isolation from researchers and service providers, and it further separates children from the situations that shape their identities. This compartmentalization too often contains a bias that blames the child and family. Isolating problems using individual problem lists or diagnostic categories calls attention from social, economic, and interpersonal causal factors that may heavily impede healthy functioning for those children who live in a particular set of circumstances. This is not to suggest that people are ruled by their circumstances; rather, the present rendering of an individuals as diagnostic categories presents an overly deterministic and fatalistic conception that impedes attention to children and their special needs. Such an approach is not informative because it does not capture the rich and complex transactions that occur between children and the dynamic systems in which they exist.

Resistance to being negatively categorized is an inevitable by-product of this deficiency driven system. Studies indicate that both early childhood educators [Mallory & Kerns 1988; Piotrowski et al. 1994] and low-income minority families [Boyd-Franklin 1989] are reluctant to comply fully with assessment and treatment regimens derived from this illness approach. This resistance suggests that this model is not the best fit for Head Start.

A system dependent on outside experts, who prescribe culturally and ecologically irrelevant mental health services, has more risks than benefits for vulnerable children. Kohler [as cited in Viney & King 1998] in his evaluation of models of psychology simply stated, "A method is good if it is adapted to the given subject matter; and it is bad if it lacks regard for this material and misdirects research" [p. 353]. In other words, appropriate models are shaped by the realities of low-income children and families and designed to optimize their well-being; inappropriate models disregard these realities and force poor families to fit into existing systems, which are already failing to meet their needs.

New models are needed that can foster constructive developments in theory, research, and practice that are tailored to the needs of Head Start children. A Wellness approach to mental health based on child, family, and community strengths offers a more positive alternative to the traditional deficiency-driven model as a guide to mental health research and services.

## Wellness Model: The Resiliency, Partnership-directed Approach

The Resiliency, Partnership-directed approach, developed by Fantuzzo and his associates [Fantuzzo, Coolahan, et al. 1997], offers a competency-based framework for developing measurement, intervention, and training strategies for Head Start. This approach was informed by the work of Emory Cowen, a pioneer in wellness methods. In a seminal article entitled, "In Pursuit of Wellness," Emory Cowen identified four concepts that are fundamental to an understanding of wellness: competence, resilience, empowerment, and social system modification [Cowen 1991]. These concepts are incorporated into the four stages of the Resiliency, Partnership-directed approach. The four stages involve: (1) partnering with resistance, (2) identifying resilience, (3) engaging and empowering resilient natural helpers to develop effective methods, and (4) enhancing Head Start service delivery systems based on methods developed in partnership. This approach has been empirically tested in large, urban Head Start programs and has evolved out of several years of experience in partnering with Head Start parents and staff.

## Stage 1: Partnering with Resistance

Unfortunately, cultural, socioeconomic, and political gaps often separate researchers, practitioners, and citizens. These gaps can be sources of mistrust and tension that impede or block the conduct of research in community settings, as well as the use of research findings by educators, clinicians, and parents. This reality is most acute when the research participants represent economically disadvantaged and politically marginalized groups in our society. The greater the gaps are between researchers and other stakeholders, the higher the likelihood is that the efforts from "outside" investigators will be mistrusted and rejected in various overt and covert ways.

Recognizing the reality of resistance, Head Start researchers must establish a foundation of trust from which to build a "collaborative" research agenda. Genuine partnership is possible only when trust is established among all of the stakeholders in the partnership process—researchers, administrators, front-line staff (i.e., teachers and caseworkers), and the recipients of services (i.e., parents). When researchers are willing to bracket their research agenda and make partnership their prime objective, there is hope for mutual and honest involvement. To accomplish this, researchers must reframe stakeholders' resistance and view it not as a threat to the research process, but as an opportunity to initiate a partnership dialogue. In our experience, the most visible forms of resistance from Head Start parents and staff were related to protecting children and families from being exploited by outside data collectors. Practitioners and parents most feared that research would produce just negative statistics that unjustly characterize minority, low-income, urban families as disadvantaged and deficient. The flipside of these fears was their strong desires to see research surface and showcase the strengths of children and families who function well in the face of many hardships. Rather than trying to avoid these strong feelings, these emotions should be

carefully considered. Honest communication about fears and expectations for research provides potential research partners with an
opportunity to identify the shared commitments that will inform and
guide their study of competence and resilience.

## Stage 2: Identifying Competence and Resilience

A developmental perspective provides a theoretical framework for
Head Start research partners to identify and develop competence. This
perspective emphasizes the importance of human development in the
context in which the development occurs, and seeks to understand
human development in terms of changes in the multifaceted nature
of functions over time. Development is multifaceted in that it is
understood by looking at the central tasks that children are expected
to perform involving their physiological, cognitive, emotional, and
social capacities [Cicchetti & Lynch 1993]. Studying *what* constitutes
competent, normal performance in these areas of functioning and
understanding *how* this development occurs along various courses or
pathways across time is the major focus of this approach.

Understanding the role that context plays in development is an
essential feature of this model. In this approach, context is the larger
sphere in which development takes place. Interaction with context is
what affects how and when persons manifest psychological competencies. Context includes spheres of influence that create the expectations for performance, and hence, impact that person throughout
development. Various influences can alter the course of development
creating different pathways for children attempting to adapt within
their context. These systems or spheres of influence can enhance or
impede development in various ways. Overall, multiple influences
and multiple areas of functioning combine to shape the path a child
travels upon as well as the child's outcomes. In this model, current
and historical data about a child's functioning in multiple areas and
an appreciation for the multiple influences in the child's life are
crucial to obtaining a comprehensive understanding of the child
[Cicchetti & Lynch 1993]. Furthermore, from this perspective, resiliency is understood as the display of competence in an adverse
context. Resilient children and family members are those who exhibit

competencies to cope with very negative environmental influences that are associated with negative outcomes. In this model, resiliency is understood as human functioning in context, that is, resilient functioning is competency in context [Fantuzzo, Childs, et al. 1997]. Therefore, ignorance of the nature and extent of the adverse context within which individuals are expected to function diminishes the likelihood that the competencies of resilient individuals will be detected.

## Stage 3: Empowering Resilient Natural Helpers

Shared commitments and methods to identify resilient natural helpers in Head Start are necessary but not sufficient to a wellness approach. Disproportionate risk factors and social problems associated with large urban settings increase the likelihood that resilient functioning will go undetected. Resilient individuals who are struggling against formidable odds are less apt to recognize their coping behaviors as competencies, being more likely to see themselves as survivors and not resilient exemplars. Second, socially toxic environments significantly erode social networks and breakdown community support. Therefore, reduced community organization and support lessen the likelihood that resilient members will be recognized by their community and that their effective strategies will be investigated and disseminated within their community. The antidote to these toxins is to establish a process in Head Start that recognizes exemplars and *empowers* them by employing their knowledge and talents to bring about positive change for children and families that are adversely effected by risk factors. In other words, a process that gives them power to realize that they can *"make a difference!"*

The Resiliency, Partnership-Directed Approach applies four major principles to empower resilient Head Start parents and staff: partnership, critique, co-construction, and mastery. The first two stages described above provide the partnership foundation. They involve the decentralization of authority and the recognition that resilient natural helpers have unique knowledge and experiences to contribute to research. Critique refers to the process of having these helpers share their perspectives on existing or proposed research objectives and methods and identify those that are most relevant and appropriate for Head Start. Co-construction actualizes partnership and critique as natural helpers work with university researchers to see how their input shapes the research. Finally, mastery pulls it all together. Mastery involves participation in the successful completion of research that is based on partnership, critique, and co-construction. The Resiliency, Partnership-Directed Approach dictates that co-construction of the research agenda must be followed by co-implementation of research activities. Involving Head Start partners in the design and implementation of research strategies maximizes their contributions to the process and helps to ensure the social validity of research products. In sum, shared commitments form the basis for the co-construction of a plan of shared action. In other words, genuine partnership = *shared commitments* + *shared ideas* + *shared actions*.

## Stage 4: Enhancing Systems with Knowledge Gained from Partnership-based Inquiry

To fully realize the benefit of Head Start research partnerships, an additional essential connection must be made. This is the connection between the effective competency-based methods produced in partnership and the daily operations of the Head Start service delivery system. In order for research products to have an enduring and comprehensive impact on Head Start, they must be translated into routine practice. Just as it is critical to understand the realities of individual partners and demonstrate a willingness to be responsive to these realities in establishing effective collaborations, it is critical to understand the realities of a system and address its high priority needs.

All service systems have mandates and requirements to collect information, deliver services, supervise personnel, and give an account of their operations to superiors or funding agencies. As a result, they use methods to assess, intervene, train staff, and evaluate their activities. Therefore in order to have the greatest impact, researchers must have an understanding of the system's needs in these areas and be able to articulate how the research agenda transacts with these needs. In the ideal situation, the research process and the resulting products are directly associated with building capacity for enhanced

Head Start programming. The Resiliency, Partnership-Directed Approach seeks to achieve this ideal by connecting research partnership objectives with Head Start mandates and requirements. The eventual aim of this approach is to make beneficial system modifications by bringing state-of-the-art technology from the periphery to the center of Head Start operations.

## The Resiliency, Partnership-Directed Approach and Head Start

The competence and partnership emphasis of the Resiliency, Partnership-Directed Approach (RPDA) is congruent with Head Start's mission and standards. The minimum requirements for the entire range of Head Start services are set forth in the Head Start Performance Standards [HHS 1997]. This document, better than any other document, explicitly defines Head Start's early childhood intervention approach to promote the social and emotional adjustment of low-income children. It presents two superordinate mandates that guide all of Head Start's operations: first, enhance children's developmental competencies to prepare them to succeed in their present environment and with later responsibilities in school and life; second, partner with families and the community to enable, empower, and support families' efforts to enhance their children's developmental competencies. To address these mandates, the standards call for Head Start programs to:

- Identify children's unique strengths and needs and the services appropriate to meet those needs with developmentally and linguistically appropriate measures that are sensitive to each child's individual cultural background. [HHS 1997, Standard 1304.3].

- Engage in a process of collaborative partnership building with parents to establish mutual trust and to identify family goals, strengths, and supports necessary to enhance the family's capacity to meet the developmental needs of their child. [HHS 1997, Standard 1304.4].

- Provide opportunity for parents to increase their child observation skills and to share assessments with staff that will help plan learning experiences and contribute to the program's curriculum. [HHS 1997, Standard 1304.21].

- Develop program experiences responsive to children's developmental and learning needs, which specify what staff and parents do to help children meet these needs. [HHS 1997, Standard 1304.3].

- Strengthen nurturing, supportive environments and relationships that foster development of children's competencies. [HHS 1997, Standard 1304.24].

Unfortunately, the mandates to pursue wellness for Head Start's ethnically diverse populations are more plentiful than are carefully developed and empirically validated methods to implement them. We have few examples of methods that were designed explicitly for Head Start, which fully embody a commitment to actualize strengths and respond to the partnership challenges posed by the Performance Standards. The purpose of the following section is to illustrate three research projects guided by the RPDA to promote children's social competency in Head Start. These studies apply the RPDA stages to the development and validation of assessment, intervention, and training methods, respectively. These illustrations represent products from large-scale Head Start research projects that are directed by John Fantuzzo of the University of Pennsylvania in partnership with the School District of Philadelphia's Head Start Program.

### Parent and Teacher Assessment of Peer Play Competency

Although children's play is often thought of as light and frivolous activity, it is actually a medium in which children conduct the serious business of defining and refining the traditions, rules, and politics of child culture [Sutton-Smith 1997]. A leading source of social development during the preschool years, play is a primary context in which children acquire essential social knowledge and interactive skills with peers [NAEYC 1994; Pellegrini 1992]. In play, young children develop the capacity to consider others' perspectives, interpret others' behavior, and adjust individual beliefs or desires to create mutually determined rules and outcomes. These newfound abilities are reflected in an expanded behavioral repertoire for preschool children that includes problem solving, communication, and perspective taking [Fisher 1992]. Successful attainment of these competencies represents a primary developmental task for preschool children and is associated with successful school adaptation and psychological adjustment [Ladd & Profilet 1996; Raver & Zigler 1997].

Head Start's Performance Standards require social competency assessment instruments that describe effective peer play interaction skills and build parent-staff partnerships related to children's skill attainment. Therefore, we partnered with resilient parents and teachers to learn about the qualities of interactive peer play in resilient African American Head Start children and to develop assessment methods that could inform classroom interventions. The following presents a summary of the partnership process, development, and research findings.

*Partnership.* In the early stages of the research project, measurement issues provoked intense resistance from teachers and parents. The research team set up meetings with an advisory committee of teachers and parent representatives. The committee reviewed a battery of measures that were proposed in an initial Head Start research grant application. The committee had strong negative reactions to clinically oriented measures (e.g., Child Behavior Checklist, Conflict Tactics Scale, Beck Depression Inventory) and they refused to permit these measures to be used.

Dialogue between researchers and Head Start teachers and parents about the measures brought to the surface many negative feelings about assessment in minority communities. Through these dialogues, we became aware of their resistance to conventional research practices and the potential risks they posed to the community. Basically, parents and teachers detailed how *not* to pursue wellness in low-income, urban Head Start settings. They protested against the deficiency-oriented nature of research, noting researchers' almost exclusive focus on identifying and "fixing" deficiencies and problems in the community. They viewed this focus as entailing the measurement of pathology while ignoring signs of individuals' successful adaptation to stressful environments. Parents expressed resentment toward researchers' use of measures that portray deviance in minority children by focusing on negative behaviors and judging normality by white, middle-class standards. Parents identified the cultural mismatch between test content and their cultural values by pointing to test items that were incongruent with the normative, adaptive behavior of children and families living in urban neighborhoods. Furthermore, parents and teachers objected to the use of these measures for formally labeling their children as deficient within the school or social service systems.

This exchange resulted in the formation of a research team composed of university researchers, teachers, and parents. This team's objective was to develop culturally appropriate measures that would accurately reflect the abilities of African American Head Start children. Head Start partners were invited to help shape a research agenda that was responsive to their passions and that incorporated their ideas. The aim was to develop a measure that would sensitively reveal the variability of interactive peer play among urban African American Head Start children to identify relative levels of strength and need within this group of children.

*Development*. Partnering with resistance produced a hopeful context for conjoint research. At the end of this process, the research team faced the empirical challenge of putting this approach to the test. The team set its sights on the study of preschool children's play. Focusing exclusively on Head Start children in high-risk environments, the team used ethological research methods to study the play behaviors of resilient and vulnerable children.

The utility of using an ethological approach to study children's play derives from its reliance upon detailed, inductively-derived descriptions of children's behavior in their natural context [Pellegrini 1992]. This methodology calls for a preliminary phase of unstructured observation, during which typical behavior patterns are identified and a descriptive base is compiled. This phase is necessary because accurately characterizing interactional behavior depends upon prior intimate knowledge of it. As a result, successful investigators necessarily spend a considerable time studying the nature of the phenomena before making decisions about how to categorize it [Pellegrini 1992]. Once a thorough descriptive base of the phenomena of interest is catalogued, ethological researchers employ factor analytic and sequential analytic techniques to form behavioral categories. Ethological methods help ensure the ecological validity of research findings, a consideration which is especially important in research with understudied groups who are, to some extent, socioculturally unfamiliar to researchers. Across a two-year period, the research partnership team undertook these tasks.

The first phase of this study required the team to identify boys and girls who were the most resilient and the most vulnerable from a population of approximately 800 children in central city Head Start centers. By definition, resilient children were children in these high-risk environments who displayed high levels of prosocial, interactive peer play. Vulnerable children, on the other hand, were children who were evidencing relatively low levels of peer play interactions. The team worked with Head Start staff to identify these two groups of children and conducted classroom observations of all children who were nominated. From these observations, 25 of the most resilient and 25 of the most vulnerable children were selected for more extensive observation. Teams videotaped the free play behaviors of these children across numerous play sessions in their natural classroom settings. Next, the team consulted with teachers and parents to gain contextual information about children's play activities. Teachers and parents interpreted the meaning of songs and games that children were integrating into their play in Head Start classrooms, at home, and in their neighborhood. Without their contributions to this process, the university researchers would have missed the significance of meaningful social exchanges.

After hours of tapes were reviewed, the team was ready to sort through the behavioral descriptions and identify the most frequent descriptors of the most and least effective peer interaction behaviors. This process resulted in 36 descriptors. Effective interaction behaviors involved behaviors related to initiating and maintaining interactive play and displaying positive affective characteristics. Ineffective behaviors blocked or impeded peer play interaction.

At this point, the team was ready to determine if these behaviors could be classified empirically and reveal important interaction categories related to adaptive social functioning and school readiness. To accomplish this goal, the team took the 36 behavioral descriptors and developed a rating scale. This process involved developing items and a questionnaire format. Capturing the behavioral descriptors in language that would be straightforward and not sound unnatural or overly scientific was a foremost concern. It was also important to write items in a manner that would be both easily understood and interesting to respondents of varying educational and reading levels. Finally, the team wanted to make sure that the format for responding to the rating scale was clear and nonthreatening. Once again, teacher and parent input was essential to accomplish these objectives. Parent and teacher team members helped to design drafts of the rating scales and obtained input from various groups of parents and teachers for the purpose of revising the drafts.

The resulting scale was called the Penn Interactive Peer Play Scale (PIPPS). First, the teacher version of the PIPPS was piloted [Fantuzzo et al. 1995]. Analyses of the preliminary teacher version indicated ways in which the rating scale could be improved. The team made minor adjustments and had a revised 32-item version of the PIPPS ready for extensive psychometric evaluation. In addition to preparing the teacher PIPPS, parents and researchers worked together to establish a complementary version of the PIPPS for parents. Since parents were coparticipants in the entire process up to this point, the 32 items did not need to be altered. The only difference in the parent version was the context for parent ratings of their children's peer play behavior. Whereas the teachers were asked to rate the frequency of play behaviors observed in the classroom in a two-month period, parents were asked to indicate the frequency of play behaviors observed at home or in the neighborhood during the same time period.

***Research Findings.*** Evidence of the fruits of this partnership-directed research process was found in the empirical support obtained for the PIPPS. A series of studies were undertaken to address three major questions. First, does this collection of behavioral descriptors yield psychologically meaningful categories of interactive peer play behavior for African American Head Start children? Second, do other established measures of preschool social competence provide concurrent validity for empirically derived constructs of interactive play? Third, do parent evaluations of home and neighborhood preschool play yield constructs of peer play that are congruent with teacher ratings of classroom peer play?

We found that construct validity analyses of the teacher version of the PIPPS repeatedly revealed a three-factor solution across multiple cohorts of urban Head Start children. These analyses provided support for the following constructs of interactive peer play: Play Interaction, Play Disruption, and Play Disconnection. Play Interaction describes creative, cooperative, and helpful behaviors that facilitate successful peer play interactions. Play Disruption describes children's aggressive, antisocial play behaviors that interfere with maintaining ongoing peer interactions. Play Disconnection reflects withdrawn and avoidant behaviors that impede access and active involvement in peer play. Our analyses showed that these constructs were highly reliable with 94% of the items loading appreciably on only one factor.

Upon obtaining three reliable constructs of interactive peer play, our major effort was to discover if these constructs were indeed valid for this population of preschool children. Since our intent was to develop an assessment tool that was oriented primarily toward measuring social competencies, our validity assessment strategy included multiple methods of measuring effective peer interactions and school readiness constructs related to classroom peer interaction. The PIPPS measure captured positive play interaction behavior among preschool children. Play strengths, represented by the Play Interaction factor of the PIPPS, accounted for the majority of overlapping variance in concurrent validity analyses, confirming the competency orientation that guided the development of this measure.

Findings from these studies revealed meaningful relationships across measures that inform our understanding of how children's peer play behaviors comport with other data regarding preschool classroom functioning. Children who demonstrated high levels of interactive play behaviors on the PIPPS, such as directing play activity and helping other children, also received high teacher ratings for social skills and were reported to be actively engaged in classroom learning activities. Observational data showed that these children also exhibited competencies in peer play, validating the PIPPS, and received high ratings of peer acceptability.

While the PIPPS is capable of capturing children's play strengths, this measure also provides information about needs regarding preschool children's peer-related social competence. For example, our investigations showed that children who received high ratings for disruptive peer play on the Play Disruption factor also received high teacher ratings of conduct problems and hyperactivity. According to the teachers, these children lacked self-control and their activity level was not positively directed toward classroom learning. Children who were disruptive in their play with peers tended to display an aggressive attitude toward the teacher, an unwillingness to receive help, solitary play behavior, and low sociometric ratings. Children who received high ratings for disconnected peer play on the PIPPS were also reported to be inattentive and passive and disengaged in classroom learning activities.

Investigations of the parent version of the PIPPS for the assessment of preschool children's peer play behaviors supported it use. A reliable three-factor solution was obtained with African American Head Start children that was identical to those obtained from prior studies investigating the reliability and validity of the teacher version of the PIPPS [Coolahan et al. 1998; Fantuzzo et al. 1995; Fantuzzo et al., in press]. Additionally, the parent version of the PIPPS was validated by the teacher version of the PIPPS. Multivariate analyses demonstrated congruence between the three PIPPS parent and teacher constructs. These analyses indicated a one-to-one correspondence between the parent and teacher factors of the PIPPS. This cross-validation documents the capability of the PIPPS assessment to obtain information about the same constructs of interactive peer play for preschool children across home and school environments. This study is also the first demonstration of congruence between parent and teacher reports of social competence constructs for preschool children within the context of play.

## Classroom-based Social Competency Intervention

**Partnership.** The PIPPS research process facilitated dialogue among the research partners regarding children's needs and strengths related to peer social competency. This sharing served as the basis for the development of the Resilient Peer Training (RPT) intervention to promote positive peer interactions in Head Start for children with poor peer play skills. The PIPPS assessment provided the research partnership team with the capacity to study the complete range of peer social competency for a population of Head Start children across home and school settings. Children with social competency needs were children who evidenced the lowest levels of Play Interaction and highest levels of either Play Disruption or Play Disconnection (or both). Resilient children, on the other hand, were children who came from the same stressful environments but showed very high levels of Play Interaction and low levels of Play Disruption and Play Disconnection. The research team constructed the RPT intervention to enhance the development of social competencies for the most needy children by capitalizing on the strengths of resilient peers and the natural support provided by teachers and parent volunteers in the classroom environment [Fantuzzo, Childs, et al. 1997].

*Development.* The development phase of the RPT intervention involved three major tasks: (a) selecting a resilient peer (Play Buddy) to pair with a child manifesting peer problems (Play Partner), (b) working with teachers to establish Play Corners in the natural classrooms for dyads to play, and (c) identifying and training parent volunteers (Play Supporter) from local Head Start sites to support positive play interactions between Play Buddies and Play Partners. At first the PIPPS rating system was used to identify resilient peers who were in Head Start centers with the children detected as having the greatest needs. The research team observed these children in play and noted how the resilient peers related to these less socially effective children. Children were selected as Play Buddies if they demonstrated play tactics that were effective in promoting play interactions with these more disconnected or disruptive children. Next, the team partnered with classroom teachers to design Play Corners where the RPT play sessions could occur. The principal aim of this partnership was to make sure that the RPT intervention was respectful of the teachers' classroom rules and routines and did not disrupt classroom ecology.

These participating teachers were resilient teachers. In the midst of their challenging teaching assignments, they volunteered to work with the research team to develop new strategies. These teachers were supportive and freely shared their ideas and concerns. They had two major concerns related to the supervision of the dyad's play in the play corner. First, they wanted the play supervised so that other children did not interrupt and distract the play of the dyad. Second, they wanted to be certain that the Play Buddies would receive support and encouragement for their contributions to the intervention. To address these concerns, we created a specific role in the RPT intervention for a parent volunteer, the Play Supporter. Play Supporters were resilient parents. By definition, they were authorative parents who were warm and nurturing and able to set firm limits with children. They were parents who volunteered regularly to work in Head Start classrooms and who enjoyed classroom contact with children. The Play Supporter's role in the RPT intervention consisted of initiating and supervising the daily dyadic play sessions in the classroom. This role was designed to provide a job to a resilient Head Start parent, who would receive training to reinforce and support the RPT intervention activity. Our Head Start partners soundly endorsed creating this job (paid position) for parents because of the dual benefits to the participating children and parents. Both the resilient parents and the resilient children were given special roles to help needy children, and they were affirmed and supported for their strengths. Therefore, RPT was designed to effect a twofold intervention purpose: (a) recognize and empower resilient teachers, parents, and children; and (b) use their competencies to promote the social competency of children who were having difficulty making beneficial connection with peers in play.

Daily RPT intervention sessions included the following sequence of activities. First, the Play Supporter entered the classroom and set up the Play Corner. The Play Corner was an area of the classroom, out of the main flow of traffic, that was designated for the Play Buddy and Play Partner to use as their special place to play. Next, the Play Supporter spent a few minutes one-on-one with the Play Buddy. The purpose of this time was to prepare the Play Buddy for the 20-minute play session with the Play Partner. During this time the Play Supporter concretely identified the play activities that the Play Buddy engaged in with the play partner that resulted positive play interactions. During the play sessions, the Play Supporter observed the play interactions from outside the Play Corner. At the end of the play session, the Play Supporter made supportive comments to the Play Partner and the Play Buddy about their interactive play. The intervention involved on average 20 play sessions spread over an 8-week period.

*Research Findings.* The research team conducted two studies to evaluate the effectiveness of the RPT intervention for socially isolated, African American children in Head Start. The studies involved 46 and 82 socially withdrawn children, respectively [Fantuzzo, Childs, et al. 1997]. The children were randomly assigned to either the RPT or control condition. The control condition was designed to control for the extra attention of being paired with a peer and spending time with this peer in a special play corner under the supervision of a parent volunteer. Children in the control condition met in the same play corners with the same set of toys for the same number of dyadic play sessions. Their play conditions were identical to the children in the RPT condition except that they were not paired with a Play Buddy, and the Play Supporter only supervised their play and did not prompt or encourage interactive peer play between dyad members. Pre- and Posttreatment data were collected. These data included observations of play behavior and standardized teacher-rating scales of social competencies.

Results from both studies supported the effectiveness of the RPT intervention. Socially withdrawn children showed a significant increase in positive interactive peer play behavior and a decrease in solitary play behavior as a result of the RPT Intervention. Treatment gains in observed social interactions were validated by teacher and parent ratings of social functioning. Children who received RPT were found to exhibit significantly higher self-control and interpersonal skills and interactive play. Treatment children also showed significantly less incidences of behavior problems than children in the control condition. Additionally, data indicated that the RPT interventions across Head Start centers and across studies were implemented with integrity (i.e., treatment carried out as planned at a 90% level or greater) and the research team received a 100% rate of cooperation from participating Head Start staff.

## System-wide Parent and Teacher Training to Promote Supportive Classroom Interactions

*Partnership.* The utility of the PIPPS and the effectiveness of the RPT intervention highlight the value of achieving a dynamic collaboration between teachers and parents to enhance children's social competency. Although parent involvement is a major emphasis in Head Start, the partnership activity evidenced by the previously described RPDA research represents a qualitatively different approach to parent involvement than typically implemented. Whereas previous ideas of parent involvement emphasized service and participation of parents, the RPDA partnership efforts seeks to establish equality and mutuality between parents, staff, and researchers. In this approach, partnership means shared decision making, rather than mere participation in decision making. It requires mutual respect between parents and staff relative to their respective roles, rather than a hierarchical relationship in which parents are subordinate to teachers and researchers. It also suggests a high level of mutuality in communication, whereby partners strive to establish common goals for children, work toward obtaining agreement on the method to reach those goals, and commit to building on strengths and resolving differences.

The fruits of this partnership activity captured the attention of the leadership in this large urban Head Start program with 3,000 families and over 300 staff [Fantuzzo, Childs, et al. 1997]. The leaders wanted to revise their system-wide teacher and parent training programs to generate dynamic teacher and parent partnerships. The Director of the Head Start program commissioned a steering committee to develop, implement, and evaluate a training approach to build community among Head Start staff and parents and to enhance collaborative learning. This committee was comprised of the Director and the Assistant Director, executive members of the Parent Policy Council, the coordinators of each of the component services in the program (Education, Health, Parent Involvement, and Social Services), and members of the research partnership from the University of Pennsylvania.

*Development.* The steering committee met for a number of intensive working sessions to establish guiding principles for this new training approach based on the prior research efforts. Three core elements were identified by the steering committee to serve as the basis for the development of the Collaborative Training Intervention:

*Conjoint Training.* Teachers and parents share in (a) identifying needs, (b) shaping the training, and (c) training experiences as colearners and coeducators of Head Start children.

*Exemplar-based Training.* Effective practices of exemplary teachers and parents are modeled for trainees.

*Field-based Training.* Exemplars and staff help trainees make the translation from structured learning sessions to their everyday functioning at the local Head Start site. This is accomplished by incorporating into the training sessions field-based activities designed to fit the realities of the local site.

An essential feature of the Collaborative Training intervention was conjoint teacher-parent training supported by exemplars. Parents were treated as cotrainees, not passive observers of teacher training. Head Start parent leaders made suggestions for both the content of training and how training should be conducted. As a result, the conjoint training included a recognition of (a) the unique set of resources that parents bring to home-school collaboration (e.g., knowledge about their child, sources of motivation, cultural values, and a capacity to carry classroom learning into the home) and (b) the need to actively encourage parents to use these resources to enhance learning. Teacher-parent exemplar teams were used to facilitate parental involvement by modeling active and respectful teacher-parent exchanges related to promoting developmentally appropriate adult-child classroom interactions.

The final Collaborative Training intervention emerged from nearly a year of piloting efforts to formulate the concrete methods of this approach. Nearly all of the training time was spent with parents and teachers participating in training together. This provided both groups with an opportunity to learn about the unique perspectives of the other group and experience each other as persons apart from the roles of teacher and parent. Training methods were experiential and included observing exemplary practices and receiving coaching from exemplars. Exemplars demonstrated practices of developmentally appropriate ways to support children's classroom learning experiences. Exemplars were staff and parents recruited from within Head Start based on criteria developed by a broad-based group of Head Start staff and parent leaders. Exemplars were videotaped working with children and parents in their classrooms during daily activities including breakfast time, circle time, small group activities, and transition time. During training, participants viewed these tapes and, in conjunction with the exemplars, identified guidelines for practices involving developmentally appropriate adult-child interactions and teacher-parent collaboration in the classroom. Trainees identified exemplary practices that they wanted to adopt and practiced the new methods they learned from exemplars and peers. Trainees were videotaped in their own classroom settings. They examined their own practices and received feedback on performance from coparticipants and exemplars. The training occurred in six training sessions over a 12-week period. Five of the sessions were half-days, while one session involved a full day of training. Training sessions were augmented by field-based activities that were designed to enhance participants' application of what they learned in the more structured training sessions to their classrooms. Classroom teams from the same center attended training together to encourage collaboration within teams as well as between teams.

*Research Findings.* The research team conducted two studies to evaluate the effectiveness of the Collaborative Training intervention for teachers and parents. The studies involved 24 and 70 classrooms respectively, with two teachers and two parent volunteers from each classroom as participants [Fantuzzo, Childs, et al. 1997]. The classrooms were randomly assigned to either the Collaborative Training intervention or control condition. The control condition consisted of the existing in-service training program that was operating separately for parents and teachers. This approach involved parents and teachers participating in workshops conducted by outside experts, who presented information that typically included demonstrations. The research team set the parameters for the Collaborative training to match the resources that were used for the comparison workshop training condition to control for staff time and program expenditures across training conditions. Posttreatment data were collected on reports of satisfaction and involvement in the training, reports of teacher-parent collaboration, and observational measures of adult-adult and adult-child supportive classroom interactions.

The results of the evaluation were favorable in many respects. First, in addition to reporting significantly higher levels of satisfaction with training, the Collaborative Training participants reported higher levels of adult-adult collaboration in the classroom than Workshop trainees. Both teachers and parents in this Collaborative Training group reported greater levels of teacher-parent collaboration than their workshop counterparts, and teachers in the Collaborative Training group reported greater levels of teacher-teacher collaboration as well. Moreover, compared to Workshop trainees, Collaborative Training parents reported significantly greater levels of involvement posttraining (as reflected in classroom volunteer hours and participation in center activities), and Collaborative Training teachers and parents were observed to make significantly more positive classroom initiations to other adults.

Collaborative Training was also associated with higher levels of adult-child classroom interactions than Workshop Training. Compared to Workshop trainees, both teachers and parents in the Collaborative Training group displayed significantly more positive interactions with children in the form of instruction, praise and encouragement, and supportive physical contact. Collaborative Training parents also engaged in more positive verbal exchanges with children and responded appropriately to children's initiations more often than Workshop Training parents.

The success of this program resulted in the Head Start leadership adopting the Collaborative Training intervention as the standard training. Additionally, new staff positions were created to implement this training model program-wide. One type of new position that was created was the Parent Educator Mentor position. This is a paid position for exemplary parents to help implement the Collaborative Training Intervention.

## Conclusion

As Kohler states [as cited in Viney & King 1998, p. 353], "A method is good if it is adapted to the given subject matter; and it is bad if it lacks regard for this material and misdirects research." The traditional illness model of mental health lacks regard for the realities of low-income minority children and families. With assessment systems based on sufficient manifestations of individual illness and treatment regimens consisting of formalized techniques administered by experts in hospitals or clinics, this model is not child centered. It is disconnected from children's competencies. Moreover, it is disconnected from the network of real and potential healthy relationships in children's lives that provide the only enduring framework of hope for healthy development. This model is antithetical to Head Start's mission and mandates. Head Start strives to restore lost hope by regarding the whole child and family and the benevolent influences that contribute to adaptive functioning. RPDA is a better fit for Head Start. This approach defines the *what* of mental health as child, family, and system competencies, and the *how* of mental health as the creation of authentic partnerships. This approach understands human well-being in terms of establishing and maintaining vital connectedness. In other words, mental health for children is associated with enhancing positive transactions between the children and their families, between children and children, and between home and school. Programmatically it involves making connections between assessment, intervention, and training that converge on promoting competencies for all participants and produce smarter and healthier systems.

The purpose of this chapter was to contrast illness and wellness orientations and demonstrate how the RDPA could be applied to Head Start. The above applications of the RPDA represent the initiation of an important learning process that is central to pursue wellness. This process consists of a partnership in which teachers, parents, and researchers come together to develop and validate competency-based methods for vulnerable Head Start children. The partnership involves gathering and sharing information regarding children's needs and competencies and using this knowledge and the competencies of natural helpers to promote supportive and nurturing environments for children.

To Head Start leadership: "Beware of desperate steps!" At the juncture of two ways to address the growing mental health concerns for vulnerable Head Start children, choose the least traveled path and pursue competency and community. Much work is needed to make this course a major thoroughfare for Head Start, but long and worthwhile journeys start with small steps in the right direction—Head Start leadership, choose the greatest good for the greatest number.

# References

American Psychiatric Association (1994). *Diagnostic and Statistical Manual of Mental Disorders.* Washington, DC: Author.

Boyd-Franklin, N. (1989). *Black families in therapy: A multisystems approach,* New York: Guilford.

Burns, B. (1991). Mental health service use by adolescents in the 1970s and 1980s. *Journal of the American Academy of Child and Adolescent Psychiatry, 30,* 144–150.

Campbell, S. B. (1997). Behavior problems in preschool children: Developmental and family issues. *Advances in Clinical Child Psychology, 19,* 1–26.

Cicchetti, D. & Lynch M. (1993). Toward an ecological/transactional model of community violence and child maltreatment: Consequences for children's development. Special Issue: Children and violence. *Psychiatry: Interpersonal and Biological Processes, 56:* 96–118.

Coolahan, K. C., Fantuzzo, J., McDermott, P., & Mendez, J. L. (1998). *Interactive peer play and school readiness: The relationship between play competencies and learning behaviors and classroom conduct.* Manuscript submitted for publication.

Costello, E., Burns, B., Angold, A., & Leaf, P. (1993). How can epidemiology improve mental health services for children and adolescents? *Journal of the America Academy of Child and Adolescent Psychiatry, 32*(6), 1106–1117.

Cowen, E. L. (1991). In pursuit of wellness. *American Psychologist, 46*(4), 404–408.

Fantuzzo, J., Childs, S., Hampton, V., Ginsburg-Block, M., Coolahan, K., & Debnam, D. (1997). Enhancing the quality of early childhood education: A follow-up evaluation of an experiential, collaborative training model for Head Start. *Early Childhood Research Quarterly, 12,* 425–437.

Fantuzzo, J., Coolahan, K., Mendez, J., McDermott, P., & Sutton-Smith, B. (1998). Contextually-relevant validation of peer play constructs with African American Head Start children: Penn Interactive Peer Play Scale. *Early Childhood Research Quarterly, 13,* 411–431.

Fantuzzo, J., Coolahan, K., & Weiss, A. (1997). Resiliency partnership-directed intervention: Enhancing the social competencies of preschool victims of physical abuse by developing peer resources and community strengths. In D. Cicchetti & S. L. Toth (Eds.), *Rochester Symposium on Developmental Psychopathology, Vols. 8 & 9: The effects of trauma on the developmental process* (pp. 463–490). Rochester, NY: University of Rochester Press.

Fantuzzo, J., Sutton-Smith, B., Coolahan, K. C., Manz, P. M., Canning, S., & Debnam, D. (1995). Assessment of preschool play interaction behaviors in young low-income children: Penn Interactive Peer Play Scale. *Early Childhood Research Quarterly, 10,* 105–120.

Fisher, E. P. (1992). The impact of play on development: A meta-analysis. *Play & Culture, 5,* 159–181.

Garbarino, J. (1995). The American war zone: What children can tell us about living with violence. *Journal of Developmental & Behavioral Pediatrics, 16*(6), 431–435.

Jensen, P. S., & Hoagwood, K. (1997). The book of names: DSM-IV in context. *Development and Psychopathology, 9*(2), 231–249.

Ladd, G. W., & Profilet, S. M. (1996). The Child Behavior Scale: A teacher-report measure of young children's aggressive, withdrawn, and prosocial behaviors. *Developmental Psychology, 36,* 1008–1024.

Mallory, B. L. & Kerns, G. M. (1988). Consequences of categorical labeling of preschool children. *Topics in Early Childhood Special Education, 8,* 39–50.

Messick, S. (1995). Validity of psychological assessment: Validation of inferences from persons' responses and performances as scientific inquiry into score meaning. *American Psychologist, 50* (9), 741–749.

National Association for the Education of Young Children. (1994). NAEYC position statement: A conceptual framework for early childhood professional development. *Young Children, 49,*(3), 68–77.

Pelligrini, A. (1992). Ethological studies of the categorization of children's social behavior in preschool: A review. *Early Education and Development, 3,* 284–297.

Piotrowski, C. S., Collins, R. C., Knitzer, J., & Robinson, R. (1994). Strengthening mental health services in Head Start. *American Psychologist, 49,* 133–139.

Raver, C. C. & Zigler, E. F. (1997). Social competence: An untapped dimension in evaluating Head Start's success. *Early Childhood Research Quarterly, 12,* 363–385.

Richters, J. E. & Cicchetti, D. (1993). Mark Twain meets DSM-III (R): Conduct disorder, development, and the concept of harmful dysfunction. *Development and Psychopathology, 5* (1/2), 5–31.

Sroufe, L. A. (1997). Psychopathology as an outcome of development. *Development and Psychopathology, 9*(2), 251–269.

Sutton-Smith, B. (1997). *The ambiguity of play*. Cambridge, MA: Harvard University Press.

U.S. Department of Health and Human Services. (1993). *Creating a 21st century Head Start: Final report of the advisory committee on Head Start quality and expansion*. Washington, DC: U.S. Government Printing Office.

U.S. Department of Health and Human Services, Administration on Children, Youth, and Families (1997). *Final rule—Head Start program performance standards*, 45 CFR Part 1304, Federal Register, 61, 57186-57227. Washington, DC: U.S. Government Printing Office.

U.S. Department of Health and Human Services (1999). *Mental health: A report of the surgeon general*. (Publication #017-024-01653-5). Washington, DC: Author.

Viney, W. & King, D. B. (1998). *A history of psychology* (2nd ed.). New York: Allyn & Bacon.

Yoshikawa, H. & Knitzer, J. (1997). *Lessons from the field: Head Start mental health strategies to meet the changing needs*. New York: National Center for Children in Poverty.

Zigler, E. & Styfco, S. J. (1994). Head Start: Criticisms in a constructive context. *American Psychologist, 49*(2), 127–132.

## Acknowledgments

Preparation of this chapter was supported in part by grants received from the U.S. Department of Health and Human Services' Head Start Bureau. A special thanks goes to our collaborators at Head Start: Director Jennifer Plumer Davis, Dr. Stephanie Childs, Office of Early Childhood, School District of Philadelphia, and Sam Mosca and David Silbermann of Head Start for their leadership and support.

# 12

## Interventions with Diverse Children and Adolescents: Contextualizing a Wellness Orientation

*Edison J. Trickett and Dina Birman*

Emory Cowen's commitment to a wellness orientation toward preventive interventions provides a welcome antidote to the increasing tendency of prevention science to focus on narrow and pathology-based prevention goals [see Mrazek & Haggerty 1994]. As outlined in his earlier work [Cowen 1991, 1994], Cowen's commitment to wellness opens up a range of possibilities for both generative research and intervention efforts. In those papers, Cowen nominates a sweeping array of potential paths to wellness, which cuts across levels of analysis ranging from attachment research and intervention to interpersonal problem solving to creating health-producing social environments and empowering conditions.

This vision of intervention to promote the development of strengths across multiple levels of the ecological context reconnects the prevention agenda with the origins and hopes of the field of community psychology [Bennett et al. 1966; Kelly 1970; Rappaport 1977]. It reminds us of the importance of personal and social resources in individuals and communities, which can enhance individual and community development [Trickett et al. 1972; Hobfoll 1988, 1989; Trickett & Birman 1989]. Further, the focus on wellness places issues of interventions intending to enhance well-being in a sociocultural context, not only because the very conception of wellness and adaptive functioning differs across cultures [Cowen 1994; Jenkins & Csordis 1997], but because interventions which venture beyond the individual level of analysis and outcome must devote conceptual

energy to understanding what the larger ecological context is like
[Rappaport 1994; Kelly 1971, 1986; Trickett 1996].

The purpose of this chapter is to discuss one particular aspect of
this larger wellness agenda: its implications for creating, conducting,
and assessing interventions designed to promote wellness in culturally diverse groups of children and adolescents. Many individually
based interventions have been conducted to improve the well-being of
children, ranging from programs designed to increase interpersonal
problem-solving capabilities [e.g., Weissberg & Elias 1993] to interventions intended to promote the positive adaptation to stressful life
transitions such as parental divorce [Wolchik et al. 1993]. In addition,
varied projects, such as Comer's school intervention program [Comer
& Haynes 1991] and Felner's School Transition Environmental Project
[Felner & Adan 1988] have been instigated to strengthen community
institutions and, in so doing, affect the well-being of children and
adolescents.

However, while conducted with diverse groups of children and
adolescents, few of the projects have conceptualized diversity as
central to the theoretical framework of the project and the definition
of wellness as represented in the selection of variables. Further, few
studies provide adequate sample description in terms of such potentially relevant constructs as ethnic identity or, when appropriate,
acculturative status of participating children and parents to allow an
examination of how self-defined diversity relates to program impacts
[see, however, Gonzales & Kim 1997].

## Cowen's Wellness Vision and Intervention with Diverse Children and Adolescents

While Cowen's devotion to empirical data is legendary, he has, in his
discussions of the wellness agenda, outlined a series of bold and
potentially revolutionary propositions that focus on the conceptual
frameworks underlying wellness interventions. These frameworks
have not been adequately reflected in published research, even those
studies cited by Cowen as exemplars of current wellness interventions
[Cowen 1991, 1994]. To set the stage for a discussion of the promotion

of well-being in diverse children and adolescents, we have selected three quotes from Cowen's 1994 paper that illustrate conceptual issues. We focus on the implications of these quotes for interventions with diverse children and adolescents, though their potential heuristic value extends far beyond our treatment of them. In so doing, we interpret Cowen's words as they inform the conduct of wellness interventions with diverse groups in diverse contexts. The three quotes are as follows:

> Built into any definition of wellness (or, for that matter, sickness) are overt and covert expressions of values. Because values differ across cultures as well as among subgroups (and indeed individuals) within a culture, the ideal of a uniformly acceptable definition of the construct is illusory. [p. 152]

> Pathways (to wellness) are differentially important (i.e. in regression language, have different beta weights) in different situations and at different points in the life span. Whereas beta weights for attachment are crucial in infancy, and attachment and competence strands are crucial in childhood, empowerment may be more relevant cross-sectionally for an inner-city minority youth than for a two-year-old in the suburbs. [p. 158]

> A key point to highlight in considering these complex wellness strands is that they are mutually enhancing elements in an elaborate system, not elements in competition with each other. Thus, competence without empowerment may restrict wellness just as much as empowerment without competence ... an exclusive emphasis on any one pathway would work against such a (synergistic) solution. [p. 159]

These three quotes express the cornerstones of developing wellness interventions relevant for children and adolescents from and in diverse cultures, contexts, and communities. They speak to the importance of attending to the cultural and local context in defining the *goals* and designing the *process* of interventions. The first quote stresses the necessity of defining wellness in the context of local cultures and community norms. The second quote highlights the importance of having interventions emerge from the specific conditions, populations, and ages of those for whom they are intended. The third quote speaks to the value of developing multiple additive or sequenced interventions where one builds on another over time, with the goal of affecting both individuals and context. This overall image is not business as usual in the area of interventions conducted by psychologists. Indeed, such a vision raises a number of questions about interventions with diverse children and adolescents in diverse cultural contexts. To some of these we now turn.

## Diversity and the Cowen Wellness Agenda

The concept of diversity has had a variety of meanings over time [Trickett, Watts, & Birman 1993] and includes a number of related but distinct constructs often used in the literature, such as culture, race, ethnicity, social class, and religion. When we speak of diversity, we draw attention both to the positive cultural values and practices of all people in context, including whites, as well as to issues of disenfranchisement and oppression for various groups.

Like diversity, culture has been defined in multiple ways [Lonner 1994]. We use it to refer broadly to folkways, customs, norms, and traditions shared by individuals who, in differing degrees, identify with groups and transmit aspects of this history and sets of traditions to succeeding generations. Culture shapes the meanings of wellness and pathology. For example, Triandis [1994] and other cross-cultural psychologists have suggested that individualism and collectivism is one dimension on which cultures differ, with Western countries such as the U.S. promoting individualism, independence, and responsibility for oneself, and other countries such as Japan promoting collectivism, interdependence, and responsibility to others. From this perspective, what is seen as appropriate behavior in a collectivistic context may be seen as dependency and inability to separate when viewed through an individualistic lens, whereas a collectivistic society might view rampant individualism as culturally inappropriate.

With respect to sociopolitical issues, a history of discrimination and truncated opportunities shapes meanings and can create differing adaptive issues for minority and majority children and adolescents. For example, Ogbu [1991] presents a compelling portrait of a subgroup of African American adolescents who can succeed academically in majority institutions only at the cost of having their peers view them as "acting white." In contrast to the norms for many white students, succeeding academically for this group may come at the price of losing the connection to peers and community. Such a situation complicates the definition of "wellness," and, in turn, the development of achievement-enhancing interventions for these students.

While attention to diversity surely includes a consideration of broad cultural and sociopolitical issues, children and adolescents within any given sociocultural group differ in terms of their response to these overarching factors. They differ in terms of identification with the group, their affect about group membership, and their interest in behaving in ways consistent with group norms and traditions. Pursuing the wellness agenda with diverse groups thus means understanding both broad sociopolitical and cultural contours and the diversity of response to them within such groups. For example, sample descriptions need to extend beyond the genetically questionable construct of race or the implicit monolith of ethnicity and attend to the degree to which individuals purported to represent diverse groups identify with those groups. When children are from other countries the construct of acculturation arises as both a conceptual and measurement issue as it relates to wellness [Birman 1994].

In addition, while cultural variation and sociopolitical dynamics with diverse children and adolescents are central aspects of interventions, cultural values and racial attitudes are always filtered through the circumstances of specific communities and institutions. Even for children from the same cultural group, the definition of wellness and the effectiveness of interventions will differ depending on a variety of local conditions.

For example, refugees from Somalia have resettled in the U.S. in communities as diverse as a predominantly white rural area of Maine and a predominantly African American urban community in Maryland. While those few Somali refugee adolescents enrolled in a high school in Maine share some experiences and world-views with the larger and more visible group of Somali refugee students in a suburban, predominantly African American high school in Maryland [Ford 1997], the adaptive requirements and resources in those contrasting communities presumably yield important differences in their experiences. Such differences may be linked to contrasting attitudes and assumptions about them made by the surrounding community, peers and school personnel; the relative strength and resourcefulness of the ethnic communities; and the existence of local resources.

For example, in suburban Maryland the existence of an ethnic community of Somalis provides social support, acculturative advice, and role models. Such a context can enhance a sense of cultural continuity and serve as a buffer from externally imposed acculturative stressors. In the more isolated, rural context in Maine, the few adolescents experience less of the stresses of urban life but have fewer ethnic supports to aid the transition to this country. Further, they are more likely to experience acculturation as a "sink or swim" situation of immersion in the dominant culture.

While the urban context may seem to provide more resources and options for adolescents, there are indeed potential costs to the adolescents in the ethnic enclave and potential benefits to the more isolated Maine adolescents. The presence of a visible Somali enclave in suburban Maryland, by creating a new group, may inadvertently create intergroup tensions with differing groups of American students. Ford [1997], for example, reports on a high school where African American students had expectations that these African refugees would assimilate into the African American community and resented what they perceived as separatism of the refugees. Here, a "critical mass" engendered intergroup issues around acculturation styles.

On the other hand, in Maine, the fact that there are too few refugees to form a visible group makes them seem more approachable to the white Americans. Ironically, this can create a welcoming context devoid of intergroup tensions. Further, because there are too few refugees of any one group to form an ethnic enclave, refugees of different ethnic backgrounds may reach out to one another to form a multicultural support network.

Such contextual differences in the communities of resettlement of these adolescents create dramatically different experiences of adjustment to American high school, each with its own advantages and disadvantages. In the suburban context, the acculturative task for the Somali adolescents is to develop the kind of bicultural style which allows an integration of Somali culture with the African American and white cultures that surround them. The intervention goal is to create an environment that both reinforces a positive sense of identity while simultaneously providing safe avenues of social integration with the broader culture(s).

In Maine the acculturative tasks for the adolescents are enacted without the benefit of a supportive cultural surround or knowledge of the cultural background of the new arrivals, but with much good will and less suspicion on the part of the larger community. Here the adaptive options are more likely to be based on individual preferences about acculturative style in the face of ever-present assimilationist demands of the more homogeneous culture. In this context, the intervention goal is to work with critical settings in the dominant culture, such as the school, to minimize the potential isolation a refugee might feel, and to help build connections with other persons or groups to create an environment that can appreciate the validity of Somali culture in the face of an overwhelming assimilationist environmental press.

These same contextual conditions may be linked to differential definitions of successful outcomes. One may hypothesize that, for a small ethnic enclave within an urban community, successful adaptation would involve making difficult choices about whether to assimilate and reap the benefits of success within the dominant culture, or remain ethnically identified and maintain one's emotional ties to the supportive ethnic community. Because such choices may carry political overtones in some ethnic communities, it is particularly difficult in such contexts to develop a bicultural or acculturative style. Such a situation is consistent with our work with adolescents from the former Soviet Union living in an engulfing American Jewish community [Birman et al. in preparation].

In the rural community, however, successful adaptation may be more clearly linked to an assimilationist style and is more likely to be construed a matter of survival rather than a political act. In such communities, joining with the larger culture may provide the only opportunity for friendships with other peers and support from school personnel.

The implications of such complexity are that creating interventions for wellness for diverse children and adolescents requires exploration of both the larger sociocultural contexts, as well as understanding of the specific local context. It is critical to understand the cultural values and explore the "ethnic validity" [Tyler 1993] of the wellness construct within a population. It is also important, however, to attend to the ecological validity of interventions as they fit or do not fit with the particular characteristics of the community, such as ethnic density, the policies and norms of the institutions such as schools and community agencies, and, more generally, the "culture" of the particular local environment.

The need to attend to local ecology requires a very different way of doing business for psychologists intending to design wellness interventions. The notion that ecological conditions vary means that designing manualized, packaged interventions that can work across contexts, albeit with modifications, is not the preferred strategy. Rather, it becomes important to develop a process that can allow interventions to emerge from collaboration and involvement with the local community, so that definitions of wellness and the mechanics of how the intervention will take place can have both ethnic and ecological validity. Such an approach calls attention to the centrality of the research relationship in community intervention [e.g., Kelly & Hess 1987; Trickett et al. 1985], a topic which has been relatively neglected in the reporting of intervention studies [see Durlak & Wells 1997].

In sum, Cowen's earlier cited comments when applied to diverse children and adolescents challenge not only the narrowness of the pathology-premised prevention agenda, but also the normative practice of intervention research as reflected in current scholarly literature. These practices, as discussed elsewhere [Trickett 1997], focus on the acontextual assessment of individual outcomes, a lack of reporting about potential cultural issues in any aspect of the intervention, and a relative neglect of how interventions are modified when applied in differing sociocultural communities.

The remainder of the paper focuses on some of the many implications of Cowen's conceptual agenda as reflected in the previously cited quotes. The intent is to provide illustrative data-based examples of projects that focus on wellness and diverse groups of children and adolescents. These studies also clarify the kinds of questions that arise when diversity itself is a central rather than peripheral concern.

## Cultural Variation in the Wellness Construct

Cowen's first quote focuses on the folly of assuming that well-being assumes the same form across cultural groups and subgroups. While he focuses on the notion of values, indeed important in understanding cultural differences in the concept of wellness, values themselves reflect an underlying sociocultural framework embedded in definable historical and contextual circumstances. Thus, where values come from and how they are expressed locally becomes an area of inquiry on which wellness interventions and their evaluation may be built.

For example, the ethnographic research of Burton and colleagues [e.g. Burton et al. 1995; Burton et al. 1996] on intergenerational patterns of childrearing among African American inner-city teenagers suggests that for these economically disadvantaged teens, "adolescence may not be clearly defined as a distinctive life-course stage that occurs between childhood and adulthood" [p. 398]. Burton's work clarifies how the residual of truncated life options related to oppression and poverty, limited resources, and the "accelerated life course" resulting from a foreshortened life expectancy intersect to shape the time perspectives, coping strategies, and locally defined successful adaptations of these adolescents. For example, physical survival, pure and simple, becomes a bottom line indicator, "making it on the streets" a sign of success, and having the ability to get out of one's community of origin another.

Burton's work further suggests that the definition of adaptive coping flows from these contextual circumstances. Thus, in the community of scarce physical and social resources she studied, caring about one's neighbors and community becomes a particularly prized quality. Quoting a community leader's description of a young man [cited in Burton et al. 1996]: "Anthony may not have finished high school, and he may not have a job, but he is a treasure to our community. He helps the young mothers around the neighborhood with their kids. He does the grocery shopping for some of the old folks here who can't get out. And he keeps the peace between rival street gangs in the community" [p. 402].

Such qualities of local relevance may not fit easily into commonly used notions of wellness for adolescents. From the cross-cultural perspective, Burton et al.'s finding suggests that a more collectivist orientation is implicit in the value system of the community they studied. As Oyserman and Harrison [1998] note, "The social roles and membership associated with ethnic and racial groups involve common fate and interdependence, aspects of collectivism [p. 283]". These observations suggest that when diversity is taken into account, outcomes of interest must include locally defined achievements, and that such traditional markers as dropping out of school are at best inadequate in capturing the lives of those for whom intervention is intended.

A related perspective on how cultural context may affect valued outcomes is found in the work on rites of passage interventions with African American youth. Watts [1993], for example, cites the outcome of "giving back to the community" as one prized by activists who worked in manhood development organizations. In like manner, Brookins [1996] suggests that such programs should socialize youth to "be prepared to commit themselves to identification of innovative ways of changing the existing value system of the society" [p. 408]. Thus, one implication of Cowen's assertion about the varied expressions of wellness across cultural contexts involves the discovery of new kinds of outcome variables that link individuals more closely to cultural context than the kinds of outcomes that dominate psychological research at present.

In addition to outcomes, the concepts of risk and resilience take on new meanings when cultural or subcultural differences are central. Jarrett [1997], for example, has applied the more general perspective of Rutter [1987] and Garmezy and Rutter [1983] to low-income African-American youth. She offers a variety of ethnographic insights into the kinds of coping strategies families use to reduce the impact of risk for their adolescent children, including the close monitoring of youth activities and associations, demonstrating high academic expectations, inculcating religious and humanistic values, and linking their children with resource-rich individuals and institutions in the community. Such coping strategies increase the resilience of adolescents in these communities to withstand the varied risks.

In addition, attention to such locally defined strategies draws attention to potential avenues for intervention with these adolescents.

Research such as this highlights the importance of Cowen's caveat about the cultural influences on wellness by adopting a coping and adaptation perspective on the meaning of behavior rather than attempting to medicalize it through attributing it to internal dysfunction. This issue, implicit in Cowen's quote, is beautifully articulated in Richter and Cicchetti's [1993] paper "Mark Twain meets DSM-III: Conduct disorder, development, and the concept of harmful dysfunction." Here the authors contrast antisocial behavior due to dysfunctions in natural mechanisms with antisocial behavior attributable to adaptive coping in deviant environments. In so doing, they provide several examples where behavior that would yield a DSM-III diagnosis of conduct disorder represents a rational adaptation to living in dangerous and disenfranchised environments. Both Huckelberry Finn and Tom Sawyer represent examples of diagnosable individuals whose behavior suggests that a coping and adaptation perspective may be more useful as a tool for understanding both their circumstances and their coping strategies.

Cowen's comments, and the examples noted here serve as reminders that the concept of positive outcomes may be contextual rather than universal. If outcomes and wellness are be understood as individual efforts to cope and adapt to the demands of the surrounding culture, community, and institutions, then the definition of what is positive will be different across situations, and even among individuals in similar circumstances.

## The Differential Importance of Alternative Pathways to Wellness

Cowen's second quote draws attention to the importance of understanding the sociocultural context before deciding on or designing interventions, since "pathways (to wellness) are differentially important (i.e., in regression language, have different beta weights) in different situations and at different points in the life span." This deceptively simple assertion carries quite dramatic implications for interventions with diverse children and adolescents. If, as Cowen suggests, "empowerment may be more relevant cross-sectionally for an inner-city minority youth than for a two-year-old in the suburbs" [Cowen 1994, p. 158], then the orienting intervention question centers on what kinds of interventions are appropriate in diverse cultural contexts. If pathways themselves vary across developmental level and context, then interventions to promote wellness should evolve from a knowledge of local context. Such a stance argues that we make secondary the popular concept of attempting to disseminate "proven" or "manualized" interventions, which preordain a specified problem and solution across varied communities, and focus instead on the relevance or fit between the developmental level(s) of the population, context, and content of the intervention.

This perspective is not one readily found in the intervention literature in general, much less as applied to diverse children and adolescents. More often the issue of diversity is limited to a discussion of the cultural relevance or appropriateness of preordained interventions. Here, attention to issues of diversity among children and adolescence is indeed discussed. For example, Rotheram-Borus and Tsemberis [1989] examined the cultural assumptions of social competency training programs (SCT) and their congruence with diverse communities that differ in sociocultural norms and values, suggesting that "SCT programs have implicit values that may be compatible or conflicting with the values of the teachers, children, and parents of a culturally diverse community" [p. 298]. Van Hasslelt et al. [1993] provide an example of a model program of a broad-based intervention with African American families and adolescents that addresses the issue of cultural relevance and includes a social competency component. Petosky et al. [1998] integrate an American Indian spiritual and cultural perspective into their multilevel intervention with elementary school Ojibwe children. Gonzales and Kim [1997] provide additional examples of interventions involving diverse children and adolescents that focus on "providing parents with childrearing and family management skills and facilitating strong parent-child bonds" [p. 503].

However, Cowen's vision seems far more grand and calls for a rethinking of how interventions may be linked to context. Among the many implications of this notion is the importance for intervention-ists to develop local knowledge as a prelude to intervention design. This, in turn, promotes the potential of collaborative relationships with those in local settings who can inform both the process and content of the intervention [Kelly 1986]. Such a strategy is emerging as a movement among health educators [e.g., Robertson & Minkler 1994; Airhihenbuwa 1994] who focus on the multiple implications of such concepts as empowerment and community participation as pathways to improving community health. For example, Stark [1992] describes the emergence of a coalition of self-help groups and non-profit organizations involved with children and youth as an empower-ment effort in the Healthy Cities Project in Munich, and Sonty [1992] outlines the evolution of a multimodal approach to prevention in India that involves members of the target population in program development and whose ideology is acceptable to those for whom it is intended. Good et al. [1997] provide an enlightening case study of the evolution of a series of interventions designed to enhance parent-school relations. In this instance, an environmental assessment of the school and community was followed by the building of family partici-pation structures to bridge the gap between family and school.

Such examples provide both experiential and empirical food for thought about working with community organizations to affect the well-being of diverse groups of children and youth. However, their longitudinal nature and improvisational quality make the evaluation of the collaborative process complex. By its very nature, it does not fit neatly into the "clinical trial" perspective, which currently holds sway as the "gold standard" in the evaluation of preventive interventions.

*Interdependence of Differing Paths to Wellness*

Cowen's third quote draws attention to the notion that complex wellness strands represent "mutually enhancing elements in an elaborate system." Consequently, interventions with "an exclusive emphasis on any one pathway would work against" a synergistic solution which takes multiple pathways into account. The conceptual and action implications of this comment are profound and once again complex. Conceptually, it places both the rationale for and effects of any specific intervention in the context of the varying levels and kinds of influences present in any specific context. It suggests that outcomes of interventions be assessed broadly and across multiple spheres, since influences outside the scope of any discrete intervention *per se* can either facilitate or undermine its effects. Thus, it is less fruitful to dedicate one's intervention energy to a single wellness strand or intervention option than to develop what McGuire [1983], in the context of conducting research *per se*, calls a research strategy rather than research tactics.

In elaborating on the implications of a contextualist theory of knowledge for the conduct of research, McGuire states:

> Tactics deal with specific methodological issues that arise within the conduct of a single study, whereas strategy involves the broader issues that arise in designing a multistudy program of research, including choice of topic, planning an integrated series of studies, and deciding where to start. ... The contextualist view of knowledge stresses that an adequate understanding of either a phenomenon or a theory requires that it be investigated through a program of research planned to reveal the wide range of circumstances that affect the phenomenon and the rich set of implicit assumptions that limit the theory, thus making explicit the contexts in which one or another relationship obtains. [p. 22]

Such a research strategy is equally valid as a metaphor for interventions with diverse children and adolescents. It suggests that before discrete interventions are planned, a larger intervention program based on an assessment of diverse potential pathways and their local relevance be developed. Doing so, as in McGuire's approach, necessitates considerable reconnaissance of the intervention context to see where to begin, how to develop plans for future intervention plans or options, and where to expect synergy of interventions as well as where not to. Altman [1995], in an overview of a public health perspective on community intervention, provides four elements of intervention consistent with Cowen's comments: "(1) integrate interventions into a community infrastructure, (2) use comprehensive, multilevel intervention approaches, (3) facilitate community participation and promote community capacity building, and (4) conduct thorough needs assessment/environmental reconnaissance in order to tailor interventions to the community context" [p. 229].

Interventions have been reported involving varied diverse groups of children and adolescents that illustrate the spirit of Cowen's notion and the elements suggested by Altman. The Stanford Three Communities Project to increase health-promoting behaviors [Maccoby 1990] and Kegeles, Hays, and Coates' [1996] description of a multiple component community-level intervention to reduce risk behaviors related to AIDS both involve community collaboration and multilevel intervention efforts. Other projects have focused on the empowerment concept as it relates to the well-being of children, such as the earlier described family-school intervention [Good et al. 1997].

More often, however, interventions do not involve a wellness or community development orientation per se, but a both/and perspective on the prevention of some adverse outcomes and the promotion of settings, community development, and community resources more generally. The earlier described intervention by Pekosky, Van Stelle, and De Jong [1998] included not only a culturally-based school curriculum designed to affect substance abuse in adolescents, but also a variety of empowerment activities for teachers and community leaders in the American Indian community in which they worked. In addition, Delgado [1996] describes a natural support system intervention to prevent use of alcohol and other drugs among African American, Latino, and Asian American youth. However, one central goal of the intervention was to strengthen indigenous networks for community problem solving. Other empowerment projects with similar both/and goals in Hispanic and Native American communities are outlined by McFarlane and Fehr [1994], Aguirre-Molina and Gorman [1995], and Rowe [1997].

However, the deep implications of Cowen's idea on the interdependence of interventions based on multiple pathways has not taken hold in the scholarly literature on prevention or wellness. The development of an intervention program for diverse children and adolescents, which accounts for multiple intersecting pathways and interventions, that prepare the way for subsequent interventions has not been central to intervention efforts in the field. Blending this vision with issues of diversity as outlined above constitutes a wide-ranging, intellectually challenging, and long-range agenda for wellness interventions.

## Conclusion

Drawing on Cowen's perspective on the development of a wellness agenda, the present paper has pursued three related aspects of Cowen's vision as inferred from quotations in his 1994 paper on the topic. Taken together they suggest an intervention agenda with children and adolescents which explicitly acknowledges potential sociocultural differences as well as similarities in values across diverse groups in diverse social contexts. They further include the notion of differentiated and coordinated interventions which are tailored to the local situation and developmental level. These suggestions, stated by Cowen in a matter of fact and almost self-evident way, carry quite revolutionary implications for the conduct of intervention research and for theory building in the field. They include the study of culture in childhood and adolescence as central rather than peripheral, the importance of environmental assessment as a prelude to the development of interventions in contrasting sociocultural communities, and the value of a long-range developmental time perspective on the individual and community-level effects of interventions.

While many of the interventions mentioned above involve some of these notions, such as cultural analysis, environmental assessment, and multiple intervention activities, the broader picture that emerges suggests three areas where inquiry might usefully be directed in the future in pursuing the wellness agenda with diverse children and adolescents. First, while occurring in diverse sociocultural contexts, most intervention studies do not, as a rule, clarify whether and in what ways cultural diversity is implicated in the definition of positive outcomes or wellness, the design of interventions, or the evaluation of impact beyond the individual level of analysis. Thus, they only begin to provide answers to the kinds of culturally central intervention questions outlined by Pasick, D'Onofrio, and Otero-Sabogal [1996] in their elegant discussion of third-generation health promotion research: "(1) What is the meaning of culture in health promotion? (2) What is the role of culture in understanding health behavior? (3) What is the role of culture in the design of interventions? (4) What do the relationships of culture to behavior and intervention mean for cultural tailoring (of interventions to diverse groups)?" [p. S142]. These authors' description of the similarities and differences in conducting a cancer detection intervention in Hispanic, Vietnamese, and Chinese communities, while not directed at children and adolescents, is a useful heuristic model for furthering knowledge linking diversity to wellness.

Second, most of the reported interventions which focus on children and adolescents in diverse communities and include multiple intervention components are stronger on the description of process issues than on the development of the kind of "meat and potatoes" outcome data so highly valued in the field. While process data are particularly instructive with respect to conducting interventions in varied sociocultural contexts [Kelly 1986; Trickett 1996], they need to be integrated with and linked to outcome data in a clearer manner.

Third, neither the traditions of the field nor the vicissitudes of external funding agencies promote one of the most intriguing aspects of Cowen's perspective; namely, that interventions can be sequenced over time and across levels of analysis, with one building on what was learned in a preceding intervention effort. For example, in the description of a school-level intervention, Trickett and Birman [1989] found that in assessing the high school experience of international students' influences at varied levels of the ecological environment, from school system policy to school culture to teacher understanding of the lives of culturally diverse students, each contributed to the school experience of these students. Such a multilevel perspective allowed the development of sequenced interventions aimed at differing levels of the school and school system. Placing such issues in the context of cultural variation in the meaning of wellness provides a considerable challenge for the field.

The spirit of Cowen's call for a wellness agenda for children and adolescents is particularly timely in the context of the changing demography of the United States. Werner [1993] stated it well: "Due to the vagaries of contemporary wars and changing immigration laws, the United States sees today a virtual explosion of young people who seek refuge and a chance for better opportunities. In California, each year some 1 million young immigrants arrive from Latin America, Southeast Asia, and the Middle East, whose resilience has been severely tested by civil wars in El Salvador, Guatemala, and Honduras and by political persecution in Southeast Asia and the Middle East. Among them are the children of the Vietnamese boat people who survived pillage and rape at sea, the Highland Hmong, and Cambodian teenagers who witnessed the holocaust of the Pol Pot regime when they were young children. There is a lot we can learn from these resilient survivors!" [p. 514]. While California is somewhat unusual in the number and variety of cultural groups who reside there, the diversity of many communities across the nation is rapidly increasing as descendants of white Europeans constitute an increasingly smaller proportion of the population. This requires much greater attention to diversity of world-views, histories, experiences, and notions of success and wellness on the part of social scientists who must adapt their enterprise to these changes.

Through a tenacious insistence on the importance of wellness, Emory Cowen has provided a set of ideas that can be useful not only for the study of wellness *per se*; they can also focus attention on how culture, support structures, and professional commitments can be crafted to appreciate both what's healthy in diverse children and adolescents as well as what protects us when our genes, peers, families, schools, or communities do not.

# References

Aguirre-Molina, M. & Gorman. D. M. (1995). The Perth Amboy community partnership for youth: Assessing its effects at the environmental and individual levels of analysis. *International Quarterly of Community Health Education, 15*(4), 363–378.

Airhihenbuwa, C. O. (1994). Health promotion and the discourse on culture: Implications for empowerment. *Health Education Quarterly, 21*(3), 345–353.

Altman, D. G. (1995). Strategies for community health intervention: Promises, paradoxes, pitfalls. *Psychosomatic Medicine, 57*, 226–233.

Bennett, C. C., Anderson, L. S., Cooper, S., Hassol, L., Klein, D. C., & Rosenblum, G. (Eds.). (1966). *Community psychology: A report of the Boston Conference on the Education of Psychologists for Community Mental Health*. Boston: Boston University Press.

Birman, D. (1994). Acculturation and human diversity in a multicultural society. In E. J. Trickett, R. J. Watts, & D. Birman (Eds.), *Human diversity: Perspectives on people in context* (pp. 261–284). San Francisco: Jossey-Bass.

Birman, D., Trickett, E. J., & Vinokurov, A. (in preparation). Acculturation across contexts and over time: The distinctive patterns of Jews from the former Soviet Union.

Brookins, C. C. (1996). Promoting ethnic identity development in African American youth: The role of rites of passage. *Journal of Black Psychology, 22*(3), 388–417.

Burton, L. M., Allison, K., & Obeidallah, D. (1995). Social context and adolescence: Perspectives on development among inner-city African-American teens. In L. Crockett & A. C. Crouter (Eds.), *Pathways through adolescence: Individual development in relation to social context* (pp.119–138). Hillsdale, N. J.: Erlbaum.

Burton, L. M., Obeidallah, D., & Allison, K. (1996). Ethnographic insights on social context and adolescent development among inner-city African-American teens. In R. Jessor, A. Colby, & R. A. Shweder (Eds.), *Essays on ethnography and human development* (pp. 397–418). Chicago: University of Chicago Press.

Comer, J. P. & Haynes, N. M. (1991). Parent involvement in schools: An ecological approach. *Elementary School Journal, 91*, 271–277.

Cowen, E. L. (1991). In pursuit of wellness. *American Psychologist, 46*, 404–408.

Cowen, E. L. (1994). The enhancement of psychological wellness: Challenges and opportunities. *American Journal of Community Psychology, 22*(2), 149–180.

Delgado, M. (1996). Implementing a natural support system AOD project: Administrative considerations and recommendations. *Alcoholism Treatment Quarterly, 14*(2), 1–14.

Durlak, J. A. & Wells, A. M. (1997). Primary prevention mental health programs for children and adolescents: A meta-analytic review. *American Journal of Community Psychology, 25*(2), 115–152.

Felner, R. D. & Adan, A. M. (1988). The School Transitional Environmental Project: An ecological intervention and evaluation. In R. H. Price, E. L. Cowen, R. P. Lorion, & J. Ramos-McKay (Eds.), *14 ounces of prevention* (pp. 111–122). Washington, DC: American Psychological Association.

Ford, M. (1997). *Enhancing communication between newcomer and native-born youth.* Unpublished manuscript. Baltimore, MD: Maryland Office for New Americans.

Garmezy, N. & Rutter, M. (Eds.). (1983). *Stress, coping, and development in children.* New York: McGraw-Hill.

Gonzales, N. A. & Kim, L. S. (1997). Stress and coping in an ethnic minority context. In S. A. Wolchik & I. N. Sandler (Eds.), *Handbook of children's coping: Linking theory and intervention* (pp. 481–511). New York: Plenum Press.

Good, T. L., Wiley, A. R., Thomas, R. E., Stewart, E., McCoy, J., Kloos, B., Hunt, G. D., Moore, T., & Rappaport, J. (1997). Bridging the gap between schools and community: Organizing for family involvement in a low-income neighborhood. *Journal of Education and Psychological Consultation, 8*(3), 277–296.

Hobfoll, S. E. (1988). *The ecology of stress.* New York: Hemisphere.

Hobfoll, S. E. (1989). Conservation of resources: A new attempt at conceptualizing stress. *American Psychologist, 44,* 513–524.

Jarrett, R. L. (1997). Resilience among low-income African American youth: An ethnographic perspective. *Ethos, 25*(2), 219–229.

Jenkins, J. H. & Csordas, T. J. (Eds.) (1997). Ethnography and sociocultural processes: A symposium. *Ethos, 25*(1).

Kegeles, S. M., Hays, R. B., & Coates, T. J. (1996). The Mpowerment project: A community-level HIV prevention intervention for young gay men. *American Journal of Public Health, 86*(8), 1129–1136.

Kelly, J. G. (1970). Antidotes for arrogance: Training for a community psychology. *American Psychologist, 25,* 524–531.

Kelly, J. G. (1971). The quest for valid preventive interventions. In G. Rosenblum (Ed.), *Issues in community psychology and community mental health* (pp. 109–140). New York: Behavioral Publications.

Kelly, J. G. (1986). Context and process: An ecological view of the interdependence of practice and research. *American Journal of Community Psychology, 14,* 581–589.

Kelly. J. G. & Hess, R. E. (Eds.). (1987). *The ecology of prevention: Illustrating mental health consultation.* New York: Haworth Press.

Lonner, W. J. (1994). Culture and human diversity. In E. J. Trickett, R. J. Watts, & D. Birman (Eds.), *Human diversity: Perspectives on people in context* (pp. 230–243). San Francisco: Jossey-Bass.

Maccoby, N. (1990). Communication and health education research: Potential sources for education for prevention of drug use. *National Institute on Drug Abuse: Research Monograph Series, 93*, 1–23.

McFarlane, J. & Fehr, J. (1994). De Madres a Madres: A community primary health care program based on empowerment. *Health Education Quarterly, 21*(3), 381–394.

McGuire, W. J. (1983). A contextualist theory of knowledge: Its implications for innovation and reform in psychological research. In L. Berkowitz (Ed.), *Advances in Experimental Social Psychology* (Vol. 16) (pp. 1–47). New York: Academic Press.

Mrazek, P. J. & Haggerty, R. J. (Eds.). (1994). *Reducing risks for mental disorders: Frontiers for preventive intervention research.* Washington, DC: National Academy Press.

Ogbu, J. (1991). Minority coping responses and the school experience. *Journal of Psychohistory, 18*(4), 433–456.

Oyserman, D. & Harrison, K. (1998). Implications of cultural context: African American identity and possible selves. In J. Swim & C. Stangor (Eds.), *Prejudice from the target's perspective* (pp. 291–300). New York: Academic Press.

Pasick, R. J., D'Onofrio, C. N., & Otero-Sabogal, R. (1996). Similarities and differences across cultures: Questions to inform a third generation for health promotion research. *Health Education Quarterly, 23* (Supplement), S142–S161.

Petosky, E. L., Van Stelle, K. R., & De Jong, J. A. (1998). Prevention through empowerment in a Native American community. *Drugs and Society, 12*(1/2), 147–162.

Rappaport, J. (1977). *Community psychology: Values, research, and action.* New York: Holt, Rinehart & Winston.

Rappaport, J. (1994). Empowerment as a guide to doing research: Diversity as a positive value. In E. J. Trickett, R. J. Watts, & D. Birman (Eds.), *Human diversity: Perspectives on people in context* (pp. 359–382). San Francisco: Jossey-Bass.

Richter J. E. & Cicchetti, D. (1993). Mark Twain meets DSM-III-R: Conduct disorder, development, and the concept of harmful dysfunction. *Development and Pychopathology, 5*, 5–29.

Robertson, A. & Minkler, M. (1994). New health promotion movement: A critical examination. *Health Education Quarterly, 21*(3), 295–312.

Rotheram-Borus, M. J. & Tsemberis, S. J. (1989). Social competency training programs in ethnically diverse communities. In L. A. Bond & B. E. Compas (Eds.), *Primary prevention and promotion in the schools* (pp. 297–318). Newbury Park, CA: Sage Publications.

Rowe, W. E. (1997). Changing ATOD norms and behaviors: A Native American community commitment to wellness. *Evaluation and Program Planning, 20*(3), 223–233.

Rutter, M. (1987). Psychosocial resilience and protective mechanisms. *American Journal of Orthopsychiatry, 57,* 316–331.

Sonty, N. (1992). A multimodal approach to prevention: A review of India's Integrated Child Development Scheme. In G. W. Albee, L. A. Bond, & T. V. C. Monsey (Eds.), *Improving children's lives: Global perspectives on prevention* (pp. 177–190). Newbury Park, CA: Sage Publications.

Stark, W. (1992). Empowerment and social change: Health promotion within the Healthy Cities Project of WHO—Steps toward a participative prevention program. In G. W. Albee, L. A. Bond, & T. V. C. Monsey (Eds.), *Improving children's lives: Global perspectives on prevention* (pp. 167–176). Newbury Park, CA: Sage Publications.

Szapocznik, J. & Kurtines, W. (1980). Acculturation, biculturalism, and adjustment among Cuban Americans. In A. M. Padilla (Ed.), *Acculturation: Theory, models, and some new findings* (pp. 139–159). Boulder, CO: Westview Press.

Triandis, H. (1994). *Culture and social psychology.* New York: McGraw-Hill.

Trickett, E. J. (1996). A future for community psychology: The contexts of diversity and the diversity of contexts. *American Journal of Community Psychology, 24,* 209–229.

Trickett, E. J. (1997). Ecology and primary prevention: Reflections on a meta-analysis. *American Journal of Community Psychology, 25*(2), 207–214.

Trickett, E. J. & Birman, D. (1989). Taking ecology seriously: A community development approach to individually based preventive interventions. In L. A. Bond & B. E. Compas (Eds.), *Primary prevention and promotion in the schools* (pp. 361–390). Newbury Park, CA: Sage.

Trickett, E. J., Kelly, J. G., & Todd, D. M. (1972). The social environment of the high school: Guidelines for individual change and organizational development. In S. Golann & C. Eisdorfer (Eds.), *Handbook of community mental health* (pp. 331–406). New York: Appleton Century Crofts.

Trickett, E. J., Kelly, J. G., & Vincent, T. A. (1985). The spirit of ecological inquiry in community research. In E. Susskind & D. Klein (Eds.), *Community research: Methods, paradigms, and applications* (pp. 5–38). New York: Praeger.

Trickett, E. J., Watts, R. W., & Birman, D. (1993). Human diversity and community psychology: Still hazy after all these years. *Journal of Community Psychology, 21,* 264–279.

Tyler, F. B. (1993). Ethnic validity: A model for families in uncharted seas. *Journal of Social Distress and the Homeless, 1*(3), 203–222.

Van Hasslelt, V. B., Hersen, M., Null, J. A., Ammerman, R. T., Bukstein, O. G., McGillivray, J., & Hunter, A. (1993). Drug abuse prevention for high-risk African American children and their families: A review and model program. *Addictive Behaviors, 18,* 213–234.

Watts, R. J. (1993). Community action through manhood development: A look at concepts and concerns from the frontline. *American Journal of Community Psychology, 21*(3), 333–360.

Weissberg, R. P. & Elias, M. J. (1993). Enhancing young children's social competence and health behavior: An important challenge for educators, scientists, policymakers, and funders. *Applied and Preventive Psychology, 2,* 179–190.

Werner, E. E. (1993). Risk, resilience, and recovery: Perspectives from the Kauai Longitudinal Study. *Development and Psychopathology, 5,* 503–515.

Wolchik, S. A., West, S. G., Westover, S., Sandler, I. N., Martin, A., Lustig, J., Tien, J-Y, & Fisher, J. (1993). The Children of Divorce Parenting Intervention: Outcome evaluation of an empirically based program. *American Journal of Community Psychology, 21*(3), 293–332.

# 13

## The Development of Psychological Wellness in Maltreated Children

*Dante Cicchetti, Sheree L. Toth, and Fred A. Rogosch*

## Introduction

Throughout a significant period of his influential career as an academic psychologist, Emory Cowen has been a staunch advocate for the importance of allocating much of the field's energies and resources toward promoting and building the development of positive mental health [Cowen 1980, 1985; Cowen et al. 1996]. Given the vast economic expense of treating mental disorders in children, adolescents, and adults [Institute of Medicine (OM) 1985, 1989, 1994], as well as the waste and erosion of potential that human disorder, misery, and dysfunction entail, Cowen [1991, 1994] has argued that a social strategy focused on the promotion and implementation of wellness-enhancement as early as possible in the developmental course is likely to be a more effective approach than are strategies designed to repair existing deficits and mental disorders.

Wellness constitutes what goes right in psychological development and adjustment. It is conceived as a dynamic condition. In the words of Cowen [1994], wellness "is not an etched in granite, immutable state" [p. 152]. Rather, states of wellness can be eroded under conditions of adversity and be enhanced or brought about by favorable circumstances or protective processes. Cowen stated that the challenge that lies ahead is the identification of the factors that advance or restrict wellness, so that once identified, they can be utilized to develop preventive interventions that enable individuals who have experienced great adversity to develop wellness.

Child maltreatment may represent one of the greatest failures of the environment to offer opportunities for fostering psychological wellness. Child maltreatment, according to the stringent operational criteria utilized in the third National Incidence Study [USDHHS 1996], involves moderate harm from physical or sexual abuse and serious harm resulting from neglect. The NIS-3 estimated that 1,555,800 American children were abused or neglected according to the harm standard in 1993. Maltreating families do not provide many of the expectable experiences that extant theories of normal development postulate are necessary for the acquisition of competent adaptation [Cicchetti & Lynch 1995]. Consequently, the maltreating environment is likely to exert a substantially negative impact on children's capacity to negotiate the progression of developmental tasks and challenges in an optimal fashion. Thus, maltreated children's ability to achieve psychological wellness should be greatly constrained, especially because maltreating parents are, at best, an aberration of the supportive, nurturant adults expected by the child in the evolutionary context of species-typical development [Rogosch et al. 1995]. Moreover, numerous studies reveal that maltreating families characteristically provide fewer opportunities for achieving psychological wellness outside the family than are expected from an environment that is "good enough" [Winnicott 1958, 1965] to foster positive development.

Child maltreatment exemplifies a pathogenic relational environment that poses substantial risk for undermining psychological wellness across a broad spectrum of domains of adaptation. Both the proximal environment of the immediate family context and more distal factors associated with the community conspire to undermine the attainment of psychological wellness in maltreated children. In this chapter, we utilize the ecological-transactional model of child maltreatment and the organizational perspective on development to guide our review and analysis of the literature on pathways through which maltreated children may achieve psychological wellness.

## An Ecological-Transactional Model of Maltreatment

Cicchetti and Lynch [1993] have proposed an ecological-transactional model that can be used to examine the manner in which serious disturbances in caregiving environments, such as child maltreatment, impact individual development, thereby impeding the achievement of psychological wellness. Cicchetti and Lynch's [1993] model is useful in illustrating how forces from each level of the social ecology, as well as characteristics of the individual parent and child, can exert reciprocal influences on each other and shape the course of adaptation and the development of psychological wellness. Thus, the multilevel ecology of child maltreatment can be conceived as demonstrating broad-based environmental failure and indicating a significant deviation from the average expectable environment. In combination with characteristics of the individual parent and child, these disturbances affect the probabilistic course of maltreated children's development.

According to Cicchetti and Lynch [1993], potentiating and compensatory risk factors associated with maltreatment are present at each level of the ecology. Risk factors within a given level of the ecology can influence outcomes and processes in surrounding levels of the environment. These ongoing transactions determine the amount of risk, both biological and psychological, that the child faces. At higher, more distal levels of the ecology, such as the macrosystem (e.g., culture, society) and the exosystem (e.g., community) [cf. Bronfenbrenner 1977], potentiating factors increase the likelihood of conditions that support maltreatment being present. For example, cultural acceptance of corporal punishment and restricted availability of affordable day care are features of the macrosystem and exosystem, respectively, that may increase the risk for maltreatment. In contrast, compensatory factors decrease the potential of maltreatment eventuating [Coulton et al. 1995; Korbin et al. 1998]. For example, at the macrosystem level, a prosperous economy and low unemployment rate may decrease the risk for neglect; at the exosystem level, active community and neighborhood programs may reduce isolation, thereby decreasing the potential for maltreatment. Risk factors within the microsystem (i.e., the family) also contribute to the adaptiveness of family functioning, as well as to the presence or absence of maltreatment. Characteristics of the microsystem exert the most direct effects on children's development because it is the level of the ecology most proximal to the child.

The manner in which children handle the challenges presented to them by family, community, and societal dysfunction is seen in their own ontogenic (i.e., individual) development. It is the particular pathway that individual development takes that ultimately results in adaptation (i.e., wellness) or maladaptation. An increased presence at all ecological levels of the enduring vulnerability factors and transient challengers associated with different forms of violence and maltreatment represents a deviation from the average expectable environment, making the successful resolution of stage-salient developmental issues problematic for maltreated children. The result is a greater likelihood of negative developmental outcomes, low levels or an absence of psychological wellness, and increased psychopathology.

Within the organizational perspective, development is conceived as consisting of a series of stage-salient developmental tasks that must be successfully resolved and, although decreasing in their relative importance as development proceeds, nonetheless continue to affect adaptation over the life span [Cicchetti & Schneider-Rosen 1986; Waters & Sroufe 1983]. A hierarchical picture of adaptation emerges in which the successful resolution of an early stage-salient issue increases the probability of subsequent successful adjustment, whereas early difficulties in competent adaptation challenge subsequent strivings toward successful adjustment and psychological wellness and may potentiate the emergence of dysfunction and psychopathology.

Although more distal early developmental factors and current influences are both viewed as important to the process of development, theorists who adhere to the organizational perspective do not consider the child to be a passive recipient of environmental input [Cicchetti & Tucker 1994]. Rather, active individual choice and self-organization are thought to exert critical influences on development. Early experience and prior levels of adaptation neither destine the child to continued maladaptive functioning nor inoculate the child from future problems in functioning. Moreover, because it has been demonstrated that not only can biological factors impact on psychological processes, but also that psychological experiences can modify biological processes [Cicchetti & Tucker 1994; Eisenberg 1995], developmental plasticity across the life course may take place through self-organization.

# The Impact of Maltreatment Experiences on the Development of Psychological Wellness in Children

In order to examine the effects of maltreatment on the probability of maltreated children achieving psychological wellness, we next review research on maltreatment for each of the pathways to wellness articulated by Cowen [1994]. The five major pathways leading to psychological wellness proposed by Cowen [1994] include: 1) forming wholesome (i.e., secure) early attachments; 2) acquiring age-appropriate competencies; 3) exposure to settings that favor wellness outcomes (e.g., family, schools, church, community and social agencies, work sites); 4) the ability to control one's own destiny (i.e., empowerment); and 5) coping effectively with stress, an ability that individuals who function resiliently possess, even in the face of serious adversity. Further, Cowen [1994] has stated that these elements differ in a number of ways, including when they are most temporally relevant, their malleability, and the particular operations needed to bring about constructive modifications. Likewise, these pathways are conceptualized as interdependent, such that early failures to move toward wellness may restrict a person's ultimate wellness potential. We utilize Cowen's [1994] proposed framework to examine the development of psychological wellness in maltreated children. Although maltreatment poses a severe risk to child adaptation and, relatedly, to the attainment of psychological wellness, it is important to note that information included in this section is derived from group data. Not all maltreated children are similarly affected by maltreatment, and some succeed despite extreme adversity. The fact that maltreatment may impede the attainment of wellness provides critical information that can be used to inform prevention and intervention strategies, thereby ensuring that even greater numbers of maltreated children will succeed in avoiding the negative sequelae of maltreatment.

## 1. The Formation of Secure Early Attachments

Research has demonstrated that experiences with the caregiver in infancy contribute to the quality of the attachment relationship that infants develop with their mothers. Achieving security in the attachment relationship provides the infant with a secure base from which the infant begins to explore the environment more actively. As development proceeds, the character of the attachment relationship is represented internally. Internal working models of the caregiver and of the self that are consistent with experiences in the attachment relationship are developed, and these models are later used as a basis for interpreting and organizing other subsequent relationships.

Not surprisingly, the attachment relationships of maltreated infants consistently have been shown to be predominantly insecure [Cicchetti 1989], with 70% to nearly 100% of maltreated infants exhibiting insecure attachment organizations. Not only are the attachment organizations of maltreated infants insecure, but also research has demonstrated that maltreated infants frequently evidence atypical patterns of insecure attachment. Specifically, during interactions with their caregivers, maltreated infants have been observed to inconsistently employ avoidant and resistant attachment strategies (Type A/C) [see Crittenden 1988]. Disorganization and disorientation in the attachment behaviors of maltreated infants also have been found [Carlson et al. 1989]. Bizarre behaviors, including interrupted movements and expressions, freezing, stilling, and apprehension, have been observed during interactions between maltreated infants and their caregivers. The disorganized/disoriented pattern (Type D) has been shown to be quite prevalent in maltreated infants, ranging as high as 80% [Carlson et al. 1989; Lyons-Ruth et al. 1991]. Frightened and frightening behavior by the caregiver has been linked to these unusual insecure attachment patterns [Main & Hesse 1990].

Examination of the ongoing development of attachment patterns in maltreated children reveals that these children continue to exhibit insecure attachments, although the atypical patterns become less prevalent [Cicchetti & Barnett 1991]. The stability of attachment classifications among maltreated children also indicates that those maltreated children classified as secure in infancy and the preschool period later shift to insecure classifications, whereas those classified as insecure in infancy are likely to remain insecure during the preschool years [Cicchetti & Toth 1995]. In older, school-age maltreated children, evidence for continued insecurity in the internal working models of attachment figures has been demonstrated [Lynch & Cicchetti 1991].

Thus, early difficulties for maltreated children in attaining a secure attachment relationship with the primary caregiver are likely to potentiate continued disturbances in interpersonal relationships as development proceeds. The existing evidence suggests that interventions to alter the internal working models of maltreated children are essential in order to redirect maltreated children on a trajectory toward psychological wellness.

## 2. The Acquisition of Age-Appropriate Competencies

Maltreated children do not fare better as they negotiate the successful resolution of the subsequent stage-salient developmental issues delimited by organizational theorists: the development of an autonomous self, the formation of effective peer relationships, and adaptation to school [Cicchetti & Lynch 1995]. Specifically, maltreated children have been shown to: 1) reveal disturbances in the development of the self [Cicchetti 1991; Toth et al. 1997]; 2) form ineffective peer relationships [Rogosch & Cicchetti 1994; Shields et al. 1994]; and 3) manifest difficulties in adapting successfully to the school environment [Cicchetti et al. 1993; Eckenrode et al. 1993; Toth & Cicchetti 1996b]. Moreover, histories of child maltreatment are associated with increased rates of behavior problems and psychopathology. A number of investigations have revealed that school-aged maltreated children manifest increased depression, higher levels of depressive symptomatology, and behavior problems at home and at school, when compared to nonmaltreated children [Cicchetti & Toth 1995].

In general, problems seem to become more severe and differences between maltreated and nonmaltreated children seem to become more pronounced as children get older. Thus, interventions to promote successful adaptation to school, facilitate academic success, and develop rewarding relationships with peers are critical for maltreated children in order to encourage subsequent age-appropriate competencies that will place them on a positive trajectory toward the development of psychological wellness [Weissberg & Greenberg 1998].

## 3. Exposure to Settings That Favor Wellness

Bronfenbrenner [1977] described the exosystem as the formal and informal social structures that create the context in which individuals and families function. These social structures include neighborhoods, informal social networks, and formal support groups. The exosystem also encompasses characteristics of these extrafamilial social systems such as the availability of services, the presence of employment, and the pervasive socioeconomic climate. This conceptualization of the exosystem also draws from Bronfenbrenner's [1977] notion of a "mesosystem" that incorporates the interconnections among settings such as school, peer group, church, and workplace [cf. Cowen 1994].

Several aspects of the exosystem have been associated with maltreatment. Poverty conditions, for example, place families under great stress. Although maltreatment occurs across the socioeconomic spectrum, it is disproportionately present among impoverished families. In the most recent National Incidence Study of Child Abuse and Neglect, it was discovered that children from families whose incomes were below $15,000 annually were 22 times more likely to experience some form of abuse and/or neglect than were children from families whose annual incomes exceeded $30,000 [USDHHS 1996].

Unemployment is another aspect of the exosystem that has been associated with child maltreatment. Steinberg, Catalano, and Dooley [1981] demonstrated that increases in child abuse are preceded by periods of high job loss. The relationship between unemployment and violent behaviors toward children appears to be strongest among fathers [Wolfner & Gelles 1993].

The neighborhoods in which families reside also may play a role in the incidence of maltreatment. A particular area of interest in this vein is the burgeoning literature on community violence. Neighborhoods with the high rates of violence undoubtedly are stressful environments for family functioning. For example, Lynch and Cicchetti [1998] found that, in general, rates of maltreatment were higher among children who reported higher levels of violence in their community. This finding provides corroborative evidence for the prediction from an ecological-transactional approach that aspects of the exosystem can create increased risk for problems in the microsystem. Specifically, community violence was associated with the rate of physical abuse and the severity of neglect. Children who reported higher exposure to violence in their neighborhoods were more likely than those from low reported-violence neighborhoods to have been physically abused. Although the severity of the physical abuse experiences of children from high- versus low-violence neighborhoods did not differ, the severity of neglect experiences did. Children who reported more violence in their community were also more severely neglected than children from communities where there was less reported violence.

Evidence was also obtained demonstrating how factors from different levels of the ecological context mutually shape individual development. Both child maltreatment and exposure to community violence were related to multiple indicators of children's adaptation. Maltreated children, in particular, manifested higher levels of externalizing and internalizing behavior problems. The negative impact of maltreatment on children's behavior was evident even when the effects of children's prior functioning were accounted for. A history of sexual abuse was associated with an increased probability of having clinically significant levels of externalizing behavior problems. Moreover, regression analyses revealed that the severity of children's neglect experiences was related positively to their internalizing behaviors, traumatic stress reactions, and depressive symptomatology, and negatively to self-esteem. These findings suggest that in a context where children may be exposed to violence in the community, severe parental neglect may further contribute to behavioral and emotional maladaptation. Having parents fail to recognize and meet one's basic needs and/or deprive one of consistent access to external supports, as is frequently the case for neglected children, may be especially problematic for children growing up in stressful, violent communities.

In investigating the prevalence of maltreatment in particular neighborhoods, Garbarino and colleagues [Garbarino & Crouter 1978; Garbarino & Sherman 1980] found that some neighborhoods have higher rates of maltreatment than would be expected, and that some neighborhoods have lower rates of maltreatment than would be expected based on socioeconomic conditions alone. Child abuse rates have been found to be higher in poor neighborhoods with fewer social resources than in equally disadvantaged neighborhoods where social resources are perceived to be more plentiful. Parents in these high-abuse-rate neighborhoods do not use resources preventively, they do not engage informal supports such as scouting or youth groups, and they usually rely on formal public agencies only when intervention is necessary. On the other hand, parents in neighborhoods with lower than expected abuse rates make more constructive use of resources and experience greater satisfaction with their neighborhoods as a context for child and family development. In fact, parents who are most successful in coping with these challenges from the exosystem appear to make active attempts to protect their children physically and psychologically from the dangers of their environment while employing more achievement-oriented socialization practices with their children [Dubrow & Garbarino 1989]. Community programs that foster informal and formal bonds among neighbors may be beneficial for strengthening the social fabric of communities, thereby reducing the alienating contexts in which maltreatment occurs. Improving the cohesion and safety of neighborhoods also promotes contexts where psychological wellness will be more likely.

Social isolation from neighborhood networks, support groups, and extended family also are associated with maltreatment [Thompson 1995]. The possible cause of social isolation among maltreating families involves some interaction between characteristics of individual families and characteristics of the environment [Crittenden 1985; Garbarino 1977]. Even if resources are available, maltreating families often fail to make use of social supports. As a result, maltreating families are likely to lack the support and resources that could ameliorate negative family functioning [Thompson 1995]. Moreover, these additional supports are especially necessary in light of the many ecological risk factors that typically occur in families that maltreat their children [Cicchetti & Lynch 1993].

In addition to the difficulties that maltreated children have in succeeding in school which were noted earlier, given the impoverished, high-risk neighborhoods and communities in which maltreating families reside, the schools that many maltreated children attend are likely to be of poor quality and not to provide any extrafamilial support for the children. Despite the fact that the harmful effects of emotional maltreatment also have been well documented [Hart & Brassard 1991; Rosenberg 1987], several leading scholars in the field have expressed concern over the occurrence of emotional abuse in the schools. As Broadhurst [1986] poignantly stated, "Educators ... also include those who use verbal abuse ... as a means of behavior control. Administrators, who see only the result—subdued, fearful children (which they may interpret as a quiet classroom)—without examining the causes, in effect become accomplices to the emotional abuse" [p. 20]. Similarly, Garbarino and Gilliam [1980] posed the chilling question ..."Where else may we find the legally and socially sanctioned abuse of children? We point to that social institution which, after the family, is the most important socializing agent in America, namely the school" [p. 97].

The insecure working models of attachment figures and of the self in relation to others that characterize the relationships of maltreated children also adversely affect their potential to derive support from school personnel, even when staff are emotionally available. Moreover, because maltreating families move often and their children may change schools several times in one year, maltreated children often have little opportunity to establish long-term, intimate relationships with their teachers. Rather, transitory residences and school placements may add to the experience of loss and unavailability of significant adults that become incorporated into maltreated children's internal working models.

Identification of children who frequently change schools and altering school policies to allow for continuity of school placements could enhance the opportunity for maltreated children to benefit from school. Further, the structure of school systems can make it difficult for children with self and interpersonal deficits to form intimate relationships with teachers. During the elementary school years, children change teachers every year, and once they advance to secondary school, children no longer have one primary teacher with whom to relate. Although children with secure internal working models are likely to be able to form positive relationships with teachers, children whose working models of others are organized around fear and mistrust may have difficulty getting close to a novel adult during the course of a single school year. Thus, changes in the organization of schools allowing maltreated children to have multiyear contact with the same teacher could be an important environmental intervention that could contribute to the promotion of wellness in maltreated children.

Given the mounting evidence for these environments' independent and interactive effects on maltreated children's functioning, community level interventions are important for altering these contexts in order to foster the development of psychological wellness.

*4. The Promotion of Empowering Conditions That Contribute to a Sense of Playing an Active Role in Creating One's Own Destiny*

Maltreating parents' prior developmental histories may be the first contributor to their sense of feeling disempowered to exert control over their outcomes in life. Many maltreating parents were maltreated during their own childhoods, thereby contributing to the development of negative internal working models of the self and the self in relation to others, parental psychopathology, and difficulties in coping with stressful life events and in handling the tasks of parenting successfully [Cicchetti & Lynch 1993].

Likewise, once identified as maltreating, the social service system may, in many ways, parallel the dynamics of the maltreating family by fostering dependency as opposed to competence, autonomy, and a sense of perceived control and responsibility for one's destiny. When social service agencies provide for the minimal necessities of food and shelter while also restricting families from having savings accounts or taking other steps to manage their own financial affairs, or deducting benefits when low-paying, part-time work is obtained, a dynamic of dependency is fostered that works against the development of feelings of empowerment for maltreating parents [Howes & Cicchetti 1993]. This reality is demonstrated by studies that have found differences in outcome for children from families who were multigenerational recipients of welfare, versus children in families who accessed such supports on a more short-term basis [cf. Bolger et al. 1995;

Kaufman & Cicchetti 1989]. Welfare systems need to provide the scaffolding to empower impoverished families to become more self-sufficient. Education programs, job training, provision of day care, and maintenance of health care benefits are examples of ways that the social service system can foster more effective transitions to economic independence. In contrast, a paternalistic approach with threats of abrupt termination of benefits seems designed to punish parents. Inadvertently, added resulting financial stress may increase the risk for child maltreatment in these families.

Similar to their parents, maltreated children's sense of control over their own destiny is compromised by the parenting they receive [Rogosch et al. 1995]. Specifically, abusive parents often employ punishment, threats, coercion, and power assertion, and use reasoning and affection less often in disciplining their children [Trickett & Susman 1988]. Even with infants, abusive parents are more controlling, interfering, and hostile [Crittenden 1981]. These parenting strategies do not promote independent functioning in the child and thwart striving and attainment of autonomy. Aversive behavior in abusive families is more likely to be reciprocated, with escalating negative exchanges of longer duration, than those found in nonabusive families [Lorber et al. 1984]. Additionally, maltreated children are often exposed to domestic violence, and they reside in stress-laden and unsupportive settings [Thompson 1995; Wolfe & Jaffe 1991].

Finally, the intrusion of state intervention into maltreating families lives further exacerbates feelings of uncontrollability for both children and parents. In cases of extreme abuse or neglect, children may be suddenly removed from their homes and placed into foster care. Once in the foster care system, neither children nor families can predict subsequent events or time sequences that ensue. Children may be moved from foster home to foster home, or between biological and foster parents in unexpected and sudden ways. School changes often frequently accompany these shifts in living arrangements, thereby further disrupting any sense of stability that a child may have developed. Most significantly, minimal preparation or explanation is provided to help children understand the turmoil that they are experiencing, further undermining any sense of control that they may have. Consequently, both maltreating parents and maltreated children are highly likely to feel a compromised sense of control in their lives. Such life conditions are not conducive to fostering empowerment. Therefore, the alteration of practices by Child Protective Services and foster care systems to incorporate strategies to promote empowerment for families are important for furthering psychological wellness for maltreated youngsters.

## 5. The Ability to Cope and Adapt in a Resilient Fashion in the Face of Major Life Stress and Adversity

For over a decade, Cowen and his colleagues have embarked on a series of cross-sectional and longitudinal investigations of young, highly stressed, urban inner-city children with stress-resilient (SR) and stress-affected (SA) outcomes [Cowen et al. 1997]. As Cowen, Wyman, Work, and Parker [1990] suggested, the investigation of pathways to resilience is an important aspect of developing an enhanced understanding of psychological wellness. These thoughts are in keeping with those of Masten [1989], who stated that "to understand and prevent maladaptation, we will do well to understand resilience in development; they are different parts of the same story" [p. 289]. There is no doubt that the occurrence of child maltreatment, whether through physical abuse, sexual abuse, emotional abuse, and/ or neglect, represents an extremely stressful, frequently protracted experience.

However, despite the fact that maltreatment exerts a deleterious impact on the developmental process, not all children are equally affected by the experience of maltreatment. Indeed, it would be surprising if all maltreated children displayed the same developmental profile, given their diverse environments, maltreatment experiences, and personal resources. Clearly, the contributions of maltreatment and other contextual variables, as well as the interactions among these stressors must be examined over time in order to understand the dynamic systems processes that influence how the various aspects of children's ecologies eventuate in diversity in child developmental outcome, adaptive or maladaptive.

Unfortunately, to date there have been few studies that have focused on elucidating the processes that lead to resilient functioning in maltreated children. Resilience has been conceptualized as the individual's capacity for adapting successfully and functioning competently, despite experiencing chronic stress or adversity or following exposure to prolonged or severe trauma [Masten & Coatsworth 1998]. Within the context of this operationalization, it is important that resilient functioning not be conceived as a static or trait-like condition, but as a state in dynamic transition with intra- and extra-organismic forces [Cicchetti & Schneider-Rosen 1986; Egeland et al. 1993]. Thus, discovering the processes whereby individuals initiate their self-righting tendencies [cf. Cicchetti & Rizley 1981; Waddington 1957] when confronted with acute and chronic adversity will shed light on how dynamic and active self-organizing strivings exert a critical role in determining whether an adaptive or a maladaptive pathway will be traversed [Cicchetti & Tucker 1994].

Because resilience is the product of an ongoing, dynamic developmental process, the presence of resilience, at least up to the point in the life span that children have been investigated, is best revealed through longitudinal studies. Unfortunately, not only have there been a paucity of studies on the correlates of resilience in maltreated children, but also there have been even fewer longitudinal studies on the later adaptation of maltreated children who are functioning adaptively. In order to emphasize aspects of resilience specific to maltreatment above and beyond the influences of poverty and other psychosocial risks, we limit our review to those studies of maltreated children that employed a comparison group of nonmaltreated children.

Egeland and Farber [1987] conducted a longitudinal follow-up investigation of a sample of maltreated and nonmaltreated disadvantaged young children. Children were assessed as infants, toddlers, and preschoolers, with competence defined as the successful resolution of the stage-salient developmental issue of each period. The findings of Egeland and Farber [1987] are disconcerting, as there was not even one maltreated child who consistently functioned competently across each age period assessed.

Herrenkohl, Herrenkohl, and Egolf [1994] conducted a longitudinal investigation of a large group of maltreated and nonmaltreated children who were assessed at three time periods ranging from when the participants were between 18 months and 6 years of age, of elementary school age, and in late adolescence. Twenty-five of 191 school-age children who had been maltreated prior to age 6 were identified as resilient. Twenty-three of these resilient children were reassessed during adolescence. Their data attest to the dynamic nature of resilience, as only 14 (i.e., 61%) of the 23 children who were high-functioning in elementary school had graduated from high school or were still enrolled in high school. Moreover, only six of the group of 14 adolescents had maintained a B or better grade point average. Strikingly, two had C averages, and six had D averages. In addition, Herrenkohl et al. [1994] identified a number of personal and contextual factors that contributed to the ongoing competent functioning of the 14 adolescents. These protective factors included average or above-average intellectual performance, absence of physical abuse, the presence of at least one stable caregiver, and positive parental expectations regarding their child's academic performance.

In an investigation of maltreated and nonmaltreated adolescent females, Moran and Eckenrode [1992] found that the personality characteristics of internal locus of control for good events and higher self-esteem served as protective factors for maltreated adolescents, mitigating their risk for depression. More specifically, child maltreatment before the age of 11, in concert with lower self-esteem and more external locus of control for good events, were related to an increased risk for depression. Moran and Eckenrode [1992] proffered the interesting speculation that internality for good, but not bad events buffered the effects of maltreatment because the presence of such a personality characteristic in maltreated adolescents suggests that they may believe in their ability to make good things happen for themselves, a major asset if one lives in a world that is basically hostile and hopeless.

Cicchetti and Rogosch [1997] examined the longitudinal adaptation of a group of over 200 school-age children drawn from low socioeconomic backgrounds. Approximately 60% of the children were indicated as maltreated by Child Protective Services personnel. The children in this study experienced a variety of risks to their development, including single parenting, relationship instability, limited maternal education, family unemployment, persistent poverty, dependency on the state for subsistence as reflected in the receipt of Aid to Families with Dependent Children, racism as a consequence of their minority status, and parental psychopathology. The presence of these cumulative risk factors has been demonstrated to be related to numerous difficulties in childhood, such as compromised socioemotional and cognitive development, psychiatric disorder, and engaging in criminal behavior [Loeber & Stouthammer-Loeber 1986; Rutter 1979; Sameroff et al. 1987; Seifer et al. 1992]. In contrast to many studies in the area of resilience, wherein some individuals have undergone more stressful experiences than others, with most participants experiencing minimal risks [Downey & Coyne 1990; Richters & Weintraub 1990], all of the children in this investigation encountered substantial and chronic psychosocial adversity. Additionally, the children who had been maltreated also had experienced severe dysfunction in the parent-child relationship.

Not surprisingly, given the extant literature on the cumulative risks that maltreatment experiences add to the experience of poverty on developmental processes, a higher percentage of nonmaltreated than of maltreated children were found to be resilient according to clearly operationalized indicators (e.g., high prosocial skills, low aggression, low withdrawal, low behavior problems, low depressive symptoms, no academic risk). Moreover, a higher percentage of maltreated (40.6%) than nonmaltreated (20%) children were shown to exhibit functioning in the lowest range of adaptive functioning across the three years of the investigation. Strikingly, 9.8% of the maltreated children compared to only 1.3% of the nonmaltreated children displayed zero competence indicators—that is, an absence of resilient strivings across the three-year assessment period. The not-insignificant percentage of maltreated children who exhibited no resilient strivings over the course of the longitudinal investigation is cause for great concern. Because self-righting tendencies are characteristics inherent to all living organisms, the consistent absence of such strivings over time in nearly 10% of the maltreated children examined is extremely aberrant and alarming.

However, resilient maltreated children were identified. Twelve percent of the maltreated children evidenced either a high number of resilience indicators over three years or a pattern of increasing improvement over time. Differential predictors of resilience were found for maltreated and nonmaltreated children. Specifically, for maltreated children, positive self-esteem, ego resilience, and ego overcontrol (i.e., the ability to adopt a more reserved, controlled, and rational way of interacting and relating) predicted resilient functioning, whereas relationship features and ego resilience were more influential for the development of resilience in nonmaltreated children.

When one considers the disturbed parent-child relationship that exists between maltreated children and their caregivers [Cicchetti & Toth 1997], these results possess considerable intuitive appeal. Specifically, given the poor quality attachment relationships that are characteristic of maltreated children and their mothers, it is not surprising that maltreated children might not emphasize relationships as they embark upon pathways to resilient functioning. For example, Toth and Cicchetti [1996b] found that for maltreated children who reported optimal/adequate (i.e. secure) relationships with their mothers, higher competence in their overall school functioning was not attained. In fact, for teacher-rated externalizing symptomatology and social acceptance, maltreated children with nonoptimal (i.e., insecure) patterns of relatedness to mother evidenced more positive adaptation than did maltreated children with optimal/adequate patterns of relatedness.

The findings of Toth and Cicchetti [1996b], and of Cicchetti and Rogosch [1997], in conjunction with those of Moran and Eckenrode [1992], coalesce to suggest that self-reliance and self-confidence, in concert with interpersonal reserve, may bode well for the development of resilient adaptation in maltreated children. The power of personal conviction in maintaining resilient self-organizing strivings, even against the backdrop of severe and chronic adversity, is congruent with the finding that positive future expectations for the self are a predictor of resilient functioning in highly stressed, disadvantaged youngsters [Wyman et al. 1993]. Moreover, these findings attest to the importance of reliance upon the self, confidence in the self, and interpersonal reserve and highlight the role that children play in actively constructing their outcomes and in influencing their ultimate adaptation.

In summary, some small percentage of maltreated children are capable of coping and adapting resiliently. Given our focus on pathways to psychological wellness, it is instructive to inquire as to how maltreated children were able to develop ego-control, ego-resiliency, and positive self-esteem while experiencing adverse circumstances. Discovering the processes by which maltreated children develop adaptive personality organizations and self-esteem despite their adverse community and family experiences is a central challenge for understanding resilience in development. It also will be critical to examine whether employing less commonly utilized pathways to achieving competent adaptation is successful in contributing to children remaining competent over time or makes children more vulnerable to manifesting later deviations or delays in development [Cicchetti & Schneider-Rosen 1986; Luthar 1991]. Although far too few children with histories of maltreatment evidence resilience, the challenge for us in promoting wellness in maltreated youngsters is not only to intervene so as to promote resilience, but also to determine how best to foster the utilization of the other possible pathways to wellness described by Cowen [1994].

## The Promotion of Psychological Wellness in Maltreated Children

Now that researchers possess an appreciable amount of knowledge about the factors that may erode the development of psychological wellness in maltreated children, as well as have some insight into those processes that contribute to resilient adaptation, we offer several prescriptions that we believe hold promise for promoting wellness in children who so often fail to have the benefits offered by the pathways to wellness articulated by Cowen [1994].

*The primary prevention of maltreatment must be a priority.* Given the adverse effects associated with child maltreatment and the high likelihood that children who have been maltreated will not achieve psychological wellness, it is critical that concerted efforts be made to prevent the occurrence of maltreatment. In recent years, some promising interventions directed at the prevention of child abuse and neglect have been developed. Specifically, David Olds, Harriet Kitzman, and their colleagues [Kitzman et al. 1997; Olds et al. 1997], have demonstrated that a psychoeducational home-based outreach model of intervention is effective in preventing child abuse and neglect. In view of the demonstrated utility of this intervention, it is clear that resources should be directed toward implementing programs such as this on a widespread basis. Although this would represent a significant commitment of financial resources, the savings with respect to human suffering, lost productivity, and social costs associated with addressing the aftermath of maltreatment (e.g., foster care, special education services, residential treatment, incarceration, etc.), far outweigh the necessary expenditures.

*In view of the burgeoning rates of child abuse and neglect, interventions also must be directed toward the prevention of the sequelae associated with maltreatment.* Although there is no doubt that resources must be directed toward stopping the occurrence of child maltreatment, it is equally critical that efforts to prevent the adverse consequences of maltreatment in children who have been abused or neglected be intensified. It is clear that child maltreatment in the United States has reached epidemic proportions. In fact, the most recent National Incidence Study [USDHHS 1996] found that the rate of abuse and neglect in 1993 (23.1 per 1000 children) evidenced an increase of 67% compared to 1986 and a 149% increase since 1980. The rate of children seriously injured due to maltreatment increased 299% between 1986 and 1993. Clearly then, until our efforts to prevent maltreatment become more widely used and effective, we cannot ignore the effects on victims of maltreatment. Unfortunately, overwhelmed child protection agencies often intervene with only the most severe cases. Because statistics show that a large number of children suffer severe maltreatment prior to the age of 5, it is especially important that the provision of services to young children be increased. Moreover, because early insults to development may exert much more severe and cumulative consequences over time [Cicchetti 1989; Cowen 1994], young maltreated children are at extreme risk for future maladaptation and mental disorders.

*Intervention must be provided in close proximity to the occurrence of maltreatment.* Related to the above point, it is important that intervention services be provided as soon as possible after an act of maltreatment has been identified. In some cases of maltreatment, a child may appear to be asymptomatic immediately following the abuse, but may exhibit clinically significant symptoms years later. We believe that all children who have been maltreated require immediate support to help them avert future maladaptive trajectories. Rather than being psychopathology based, such interventions can strive to enhance those competencies that have been shown to be operative in children who develop resilience in the context of significant environmental stress.

*In providing both preventive and psychotherapeutic interventions, various levels of the ecology must be considered and addressed.* As discussed in this chapter, it is clear that the functioning of maltreated children is compromised via various levels of their social ecologies, from proximal to more distal. Additionally, it is apparent that unless interventions are directed toward these different ecological levels, opportunities to attain psychological wellness will be severely restricted. Findings on the additive effects of community violence in contributing to maladaptive outcome in maltreated children are emerging, and the clear increases in violence in our communities jeopardize not only maltreated, but all children [Lynch & Cicchetti 1998]. As a society, we must gain a better understanding of those factors that are contributing to increases in community violence, and we must be prepared to take action to stem this pernicious influence on our youth. Although historically focused on promoting educational competencies in children, the potential value of the schools in helping to promote psychological wellness in maltreated and high-risk children cannot be minimized. In this regard, the work of Cowen and his colleagues [1996] serves as an exemplary model.

*Interventions need to be developed that foster self-determination in school-age maltreated children.* In view of findings that elucidate different pathways to resilience in maltreated and nonmaltreated children, efforts to develop interventions directed toward facilitating self-determination in maltreated children should be a priority [cf. Ryan et al. 1995]. Many current psychotherapeutic interventions emphasize relationship-building as a strategy to minimize the negative sequelae of abuse and neglect. Although such an approach possesses considerable merit in the early years of life, when children's working models of relationships may be less entrenched and more amenable to modification [Toth & Cicchetti 1996a], as children mature, it may be more effective to help them develop a sense of self-efficacy, self-reliance, and a belief in their ability to affect their own destinies. Strategies such as these flow from Cowen's delimitation of the importance of empowering experiences as one pathway to psychological wellness [see also, Rappaport 1981, 1987]. Community-based programs that provide success and achievement would be beneficial for challenging negative self-views and fostering improved self-perceptions.

Although self-determination has been found to be one pathway to resilience in maltreated children, it is important to note that we must continue to examine additional pathways that may be present as a function of the period of development that is being addressed or the context in which resilience is being assessed. Part of the problem in providing maltreated children with timed, guided interventions is identification of the specific vulnerabilities and competencies these children exhibit in order to formulate individual and community-based interventions focused on the amelioration and remediation of deficits or the promotion of wellness. Utilizing these children's *strengths* can facilitate the change process [Masten et al. 1990; Toth & Cicchetti 1993]. Additionally, it is important to recognize that resilience has been shown to evidence developmentally-related changes, such that what fosters resilience at one point in time may not do so at an earlier or later period. Therefore, a developmental perspective must be incorporated into interventions.

*Social Service agencies need to become increasingly sensitive to the importance of empowerment for children and families, and to modify their intervention strategies accordingly.* As discussed earlier in this chapter, involvement with social service agencies following the occurrence of maltreatment may further erode the capacity of children and parents to experience any sense of being in control of their own destinies. Although well-intended, interventions initiated by such agencies may be perceived as punitive and coercive by families. If parents seek services not through any desire to change or recognition of a need for assistance, but rather as a function of the threat that unless they attend therapy they will lose their children, then it is unlikely that they will derive much benefit from services. Similarly, when children are placed in foster care, they frequently become pawns in a complex game involving court personnel, therapists, and case-workers. Often neither parents nor children understand the processes in which they are involved and consequently may develop anger and, eventually, apathy and helplessness. A thorough review of current approaches to addressing maltreatment-related concerns should be undertaken by legislative bodies and social service agencies to deter-mine how best to intervene effectively on behalf of maltreated chil-dren without eliminating feelings of empowerment in children and families.

*Mechanisms must be developed that allow for the early provision and subsequent continuity of services for maltreated children.* With the ascendance of managed care in this country, insurance limits are being placed on mental health services that affect the development and provision of both prevention and intervention services. Although this reality is of concern in all areas of mental health, it may be particularly damaging with respect to the prevention efforts and service provision directed toward the area of child maltreatment. With respect to prevention, the majority of mental health funding streams are disorder-based. Rather than taking a proactive approach similar to that utilized by preventive medicine, insurers are reluctant to pay for mental health services unless a diagnoseable mental disorder has been identified. Clearly, such a stance works against the promotion of psychological wellness and is the antithesis of preven-tion, as it is only after a disability has emerged that the service system is mobilized. Additionally, because psychological wellness is not a static condition, even maltreated children who demonstrate wellness at one point in time may subsequently experience difficulties. There-fore, efforts should be directed toward helping those children who are functioning well to maintain their psychological wellness. Unless pathology-based methods of allocating funding are modified, we will no doubt continue to see an escalation in the occurrence and negative aftermath of child abuse and neglect.

With respect to the treatment needs of children who have been maltreated, funding constraints are equally likely to be detrimental. Because the effects of maltreatment may be insidious, developmentally-related sequelae of maltreatment may emerge over time. Moreover, symptomatology may not immediately consolidate into a diagnoseable mental disorder, despite the detrimental effects being exerted on the course of development. If services are withheld pending a clear diagnoseable condition, then it is probable that the needs of very young children will be overlooked. Additionally, time limits imposed by insurers may impede the course of therapy due to the likelihood that a maltreated child will require more time to trust and become involved in a therapeutic process. Children with histories of maltreatment may experience new difficulties over time as a function of changing developmental capacities and challenges related to developmental transitions or changing life circumstances. Therefore, periodic booster interventions may be required to help maltreated children attain cumulative protection from these potentially disruptive influences. Toward this end, funding mechanisms that provide for repeated access to and continuity of treatment will be critical for maltreated children.

## Summary

In this chapter we have examined the effects of child maltreatment in relation to the five pathways to psychological wellness proposed by Cowen [1994]. Our review has shown that maltreated children are at high risk for failing to attain wellness via these routes. Society must grapple with the reality of increasing rates of child maltreatment and must evaluate how best to triumph over this insidious social problem. Cowen's pathways to wellness suggest a number of possible avenues to averting the occurrence and negative effects of child maltreatment. Additionally, it is possible that by better understanding how some maltreated children develop in a competent fashion, further insights on alternate pathways to wellness will be gained. It is clear that broad-based, community initiatives must be directed toward the problems of child abuse and neglect. By moving toward the promotion of wellness as opposed to the prevention of disorder, it is likely that many more children and families will benefit. To date, our efforts to eliminate child abuse and neglect have been far from successful, as reflected in the escalating rates of child maltreatment. The concept of psychological wellness offers some new perspectives on this ancient problem and may help guide the development and implementation of innovative and effective strategies.

## Acknowledgments

Our work on this chapter was supported, in part, by grants from the William T. Grant Foundation, the National Institute of Mental Health, the Office of Child Abuse and Neglect, and the Spunk Fund, Inc.

## References

Bolger, K., Patterson, C., Thompson, W., & Kupersmidt, J. (1995). Psychosocial adjustment among children experiencing persistent poverty and intermittent family economic hardship. *Child Development, 66,* 1107–1129.

Broadhurst, D. (1986). *Educators, schools, and child abuse.* Chicago: National Committee for the Prevention of Child Abuse.

Bronfenbrenner, U. (1977). Toward an experimental ecology of human development. *American Psychologist, 32,* 513–531.

Carlson, V., Cicchetti, D., Barnett, D. & Braunwald, K. (1989). Disorganized/disoriented attachment relationships in maltreated infants. *Developmental Psychology, 25,* 525–531.

Cicchetti, D. (1989). How research on child maltreatment has informed the study of child development: Perspectives from developmental psychopathology. In D. Cicchetti & V. Carlson (Eds.), *Child maltreatment: Theory and research on the causes and consequences of child abuse and neglect* (377–431). New York: Cambridge University Press.

Cicchetti, D. (1991). Fractures in the crystal: Developmental psychopathology and the emergence of the self. *Developmental Review, 11,* 271–287.

Cicchetti, D. & Barnett, D. (1991). Attachment organization in pre-school aged maltreated children. *Development and Psychopathology, 3,* 397–411.

Cicchetti, D. & Lynch, M. (1993). Toward an ecological/transactional model of community violence and child maltreatment: Consequences for children's development. *Psychiatry, 56*, 96–118.

Cicchetti, D. & Lynch, M. (1995). Failures in the expectable environment and their impact on individual development: The case of child maltreatment. In D. Cicchetti & D. Cohen (Eds.), *Developmental psychopathology, Vol. 2: Risk, disorder, and adaptation* (pp. 32–71). New York: Wiley.

Cicchetti, D. & Rizley, R. (1981). Developmental perspectives on the etiology, intergenerational transmission and sequelae of child maltreatment. *New Directions for Child Development, 11*, 32–59.

Cicchetti, D. & Rogosch, F.A. (1997). The role of self-organization in the promotion of resilience in maltreated children. *Development and Psychopathology, 9*(4), 799–817.

Cicchetti, D. & Schneider-Rosen, K. (1986). An organizational approach to childhood depression. In M. Rutter, C. Izard, & P. Read (Eds.), *Depression in young people: Clinical and developmental perspectives.* (pp. 71–134). New York: Guilford.

Cicchetti, D. & Toth, S. L. (1995). A developmental psychopathology perspective on child abuse and neglect. *Journal of the American Academy of Child and Adolescent Psychiatry, 34,* 541–565.

Cicchetti, D. & Toth, S. L. (1997). Transactional Ecological Systems in Developmental Psychopathology. In S. S. Luthar, J. Burack, D. Cicchetti, and J. Weisz (Eds.), *Developmental psychopathology: Perspectives on risk and disorder* (pp. 317–349). New York: Cambridge University Press.

Cicchetti, D., Toth, S. L., & Hennessy, K. (1993). Child maltreatment and school adaptation: Problems and promises. In D. Cicchetti and S. L. Toth (Eds.), *Child abuse, child development and social policy* (pp. 301–330). Norwood, NJ: Ablex.

Cicchetti, D. & Tucker, D. (1994). Development and self-regulatory structures of the mind. *Development and Psychopathology, 6,* 533–549.

Coulton, C., Korbin, J., Su, M., & Chow, J. (1995). Community level factors and child maltreatment rates. *Child Development, 66,* 1262–1276.

Cowen, E. L. (1980). The wooing of primary prevention. *American Journal of Community Psychology, 8,* 258–284.

Cowen, E. L. (1985). Person-centered approaches to primary prevention in mental health: Situation-focused and competence enhancement. *American Journal of Community Psychology, 13,* 31–48.

Cowen, E. L. (1991). In pursuit of wellness. *American Psychologist, 46,* 404–408.

Cowen, E. L. (1994). The enhancement of psychological wellness: Challenges and opportunities. *American Journal of Community Psychology, 22,* 149–179.

Cowen, E. L., Hightower, A. D., Pedro-Carroll, J. L., Work, W. C., Wyman, P. A., & Haffey, W. G. (1996). *School-based prevention for children at risk: The Primary Mental Health Project.* Washington, DC: American Psychological Association.

Cowen, E. L., Work, W. C., & Wyman, P.A. (1997). The Rochester Child Resilience Project (RCRP): Facts found, lessons learned, future directions divined. In S. S. Luthar, J. A. Burack, D. Cicchetti, & J. R. Weisz (Eds.), *Developmental psychopathology: Perspectives on adjustment, risk, and disorder* (pp. 527–547). New York: Cambridge University Press.

Cowen, E., Wyman, P., Work, W., & Parker, G. (1990). The Rochester Child Resilience Project: Overview and summary of first year findings. *Development and Psychopathology, 2,* 193–212.

Crittenden, P. M. (1981). Abusing, neglecting, problematic, and adequate dyads: Differentiating by patterns of interaction. *Merrill-Palmer Quarterly, 27,* 201–208.

Crittenden, P. M. (1985). Maltreated infants: Vulnerability and resilience. *Journal of Child Psychology and Psychiatry and Allied Disciplines, 26,* 85–96.

Crittenden, P. M. (1988). Relationships at risk. In J. Belsky & T. Nezworski (Eds.), *Clinical implications of attachment theory* (pp. 136–174). Hillsdale, NJ: Lawrence Erlbaum Associates.

Downey, G. & Coyne, J. C. (1990). Children of depressed parents: An integrative review. *Psychological Bulletin, 108,* 50–76.

Dubrow, N. F. & Garbarino, J. (1989). Living in a war zone: Mothers and young children in a public housing project. *Child Welfare, 68,* 3–20.

Eckenrode, J., Laird, M., & Doris, J. (1993). School performance and disciplinary problems among abused and neglected children. *Developmental Psychology, 29,* 53–62.

Egeland, B., Carlson, E., & Sroufe, L. A. (1993). Resilience as process. *Development and Psychopathology, 5,* 517–528.

Egeland, B. & Farber, E. (1987). Invulnerability among abused and neglected children. In E. J. Anthony & B. Cohler (Eds.), *The invulnerable child* (pp. 253–288). New York: Guilford.

Eisenberg, L. (1995). The social construction of the human brain. *American Journal of Psychiatry, 152,* 1563–1575.

Garbarino, J. (1977). The human ecology of child maltreatment: A conceptual model for research. *Journal of Marriage and the Family, 39,* 721–732.

Garbarino, J. & Crouter, A. (1978). Defining the community context for parent-child relations: The correlates of child maltreatment. *Child Development, 49,* 604–616.

Garbarino, J. & Gilliam, G. (1980). *Understanding abusive families.* Lexington, MA: Lexington Press.

Garbarino, J. & Sherman, D. (1980). High-risk neighborhoods and high-risk families: The human ecology of child maltreatment. *Child Development, 51,* 188–198.

Hart, S. & Brassard, M. (1991). Psychological maltreatment: Progress achieved. *Development and Psychopathology, 3,* 61–70.

Herrenkohl, E. C., Herrenkohl, R., & Egolf, M. (1994). Resilient early school-age children from maltreating homes: Outcomes in late adolescence. *American Journal of Orthopsychiatry, 64,* 301–309.

Howes, P. & Cicchetti, D. (1993). A family/relational perspective on maltreating families. Parallel processes across systems and social policy implications. In D. Cicchetti & S. L. Toth (Eds.), *Child abuse, child development and social policy* (pp. 249–300). Norwood, NJ: Ablex.

Institute of Medicine (1985). Research on mental illness and addictive disorders: Progress and prospects. *American Journal of Psychiatry, 1142*(Supplement), 1–41.

Institute of Medicine (1989). *Research on children and adolescents with mental, behavioral, and developmental disorders.* Washington, DC: National Academy Press.

Institute of Medicine (1994). *Reducing risks for mental disorders: Frontiers for preventive intervention research.* Washington, DC: National Academy Press.

Kaufman, J. & Cicchetti, D. (1989). The effects of maltreatment on school-aged children's socioemotional development: Assessments in a day camp setting. *Developmental Psychology, 25,* 516–524

Kitzman, H., Olds, D., Henderson, C., Hanks, C., Cole, R., Tatelbaum, R., McConnochie, K., Sidora, K., Luckey, D., Shaver, D., Engelhardt, K., James, D., & Barnard, K. (1997). Effect of prenatal and infancy home visitation by nurses for pregnancy outcomes, childhood inquiries, and repeated childbearing: A randomized controlled trial. *Journal of the American Medical Association, 278,* 644–652.

Korbin, J. E., Coulton, C. J., Chard, S., Platt-Houston, C., & Su, M. (1998). Impoverishment and child maltreatment in African-American and European-American neighborhoods. *Development and Psychopathology, 10*, 215–233.

Loeber, R. & Stouthamer-Loeber, M. (1986). Family factors as correlates and predictors of juvenile conduct problems and delinquency. In M. Tonry & N. Morris (Eds.), *Crime and justice.* (Vol. 7) (pp. 29–149). Chicago: University of Chicago Press.

Lorber, R., Felton, D. K., & Reid, J. B. (1984). A social learning approach to the reduction of coercive processes in child abusive families: A molecular analysis. *Advances in Behavior Research and Therapy, 6,* 29–45.

Luthar, S. S. (1991). Vulnerability and resilience: A study of high-risk adolescents. *Child Development, 62*(3), 600–616.

Lynch, M. & Cicchetti, D. (1991). Patterns of relatedness in maltreated and nonmaltreated children: Connections among multiple representational models. *Development and Psychopathology, 3,* 207–226.

Lynch, M. & Cicchetti, D. (1998). An ecological-transactional analysis of children and contexts: The longitudinal interplay among child maltreatment, community violence, and children's symptomatology. *Development and Psychopathology, 10,* 235–257.

Lyons-Ruth, K., Repacholi, B., McLeod, S., & Silva, E. (1991). Disorganized attachment behavior in infancy: Short-term stability, maternal and infant correlates, and risk-related subtypes. *Development and Psychopathology, 3,* 377–396.

Main, M. & Hesse, E. (1990). Parents' unresolved traumatic experiences are related to infant disorganized attachment status: Is frightened and/or frightening parent behavior the linking mechanism? In M. Greenberg, & D. Cicchetti, & E. M. Cummings (Eds.), *Attachment in the preschool years* (pp. 161–182). Chicago: University of Chicago Press.

Masten, A. (1989). Resilience in development: Implications of the study of successful adaptation for developmental psychopathology. In D. Cicchetti (Ed.), *Rochester symposium on developmental psychopathology, Vol. 1: The emergence of a discipline* (pp. 261–294). Hillsdale, NJ: Lawrence Erlbaum Associates.

Masten, A., Best, K., & Garmezy, N. (1990). Resilience and development: Contributions from the study of children who overcome adversity. *Development and Psychopathology, 2,* 425–444.

Masten, A. S. & Coatsworth, J. D. (1998). The development of competence in favorable and unfavorable environments: Lessons from research on successful children. *American Psychologist, 53*, 205–220.

Moran, P. B. & Eckenrode, J. (1992). Protective personality characteristics among adolescent victims of maltreatment. *Child Abuse and Neglect, 16*, 743–754.

Olds, D., Eckenrode, J., Henderson, C., Kitzman, H., Powers, J., Cole, R., Sidora, K., Morris, P., Pettitt, L., & Luckey, D. (1997). Long-term effects of home visitation on maternal life course and child abuse and neglect: Fifteen-year follow-up of a randomized trial. *Journal of the American Medical Association, 278*, 637–643.

Rappaport, J. (1981). In praise of paradox: A social policy of empowerment over prevention. *American Journal of Community Psychology, 9*, 1–25.

Rappaport, J. (1987). Terms of empowerment/exemplars of prevention: Toward a theory of community psychology. *American Journal of Community Psychology, 15*, 121–148.

Richters, J. E. & Weintraub, S. (1990). Beyond diathesis: Toward an understanding of high-risk environments. In J. Rolf, A. S. Masten, D. Cicchetti, K. G. Nuechterlein, & S. Weintraub (Eds.), *Risk and protective factors in the development of psychopathology* (pp. 67–96). New York: Cambridge University Press.

Rogosch, F. & Cicchetti, D. (1994). Illustrating the interface of family and peer relations through the study of child maltreatment. *Social Development, 3*, 291–308.

Rogosch, F., Cicchetti, D., Shields, A., & Toth, S. L. (1995). Parenting dysfunction in child maltreatment. In M. H. Bornstein (Ed.), *Handbook of parenting* (Vol. 4) (pp. 127–159). Hillsdale, NJ: Lawrence Erlbaum Associates.

Rosenberg, M. S. (1987). New directions for research on the psychological maltreatment of children. *American Psychologist, 42*, 166–171.

Rutter, M. (1979). Protective factors in children's responses to stress and disadvantage. In M. W. Kent and J. E. Rolf (Eds.), *Primary prevention in psychopathology: Social competence in children* (Vol. 8) (pp. 49–74). Hanover, NH: University Press of New England.

Ryan, R., Deci, E., & Grolnick, W. (1995). Autonomy, relatedness, and the self: Their relation to development and psychopathology. In D. Cicchetti & D. Cohen (Eds.), *Developmental psychopathology, Vol. 1: Theory and methods* (pp. 618-655). New York: Wiley.

Sameroff, A. J., Seifer, R., Barocas, R., Zax, M., & Greenspan, S. (1987). Intelligence quotient scores of 4-year-old children: Social-environmental risk factors. *Pediatrics, 79*, 343–350.

Seifer, R., Sameroff, A., Baldwin, C., & Baldwin, C. (1992). Child and family factors that ameliorate risk between 4 and 13 years of age. *Journal of the American Academy of Child and Adolescent Psychiatry, 31*, 893–903.

Shields, A., Cicchetti, D., & Ryan, R. (1994). The development of emotional and behavioral self regulation and social competence among maltreated school-age children. *Development and Psychopathology, 6*, 57–75.

Steinberg, L., Catalano, R., & Dooley, D. (1981). Economic antecedents of child abuse and neglect. *Child Development, 52*, 975–985.

Thompson, R. A. (1995). *Preventing child maltreatment through social support: A critical analysis*. Thousand Oaks, CA: Sage Publications.

Toth, S. L. & Cicchetti, D. (1993). Child maltreatment: Where do we go from here in our treatment of victims? In D. Cicchetti & S. L. Toth (Eds.), *Child abuse, child development and social policy* (pp. 399–4389). Norwood NJ: Ablex.

Toth, S. L. & Cicchetti, D. (1996a). Patterns of relatedness and depressive symptomatology in maltreated children. *Journal of Consulting and Clinical Psychology, 64*, 32–41.

Toth, S. L. & Cicchetti, D. (1996b). The impact of relatedness with mother on school functioning in maltreated youngsters. *Journal of School Psychology, 3*, 247–266.

Toth, S. L., Cicchetti, D., Macfie, J., & Emde, R. N. (1997). Representations of self and other in the narratives of neglected, physically abused, and sexually abused preschoolers. *Developmental Psychology, 24*, 270–276.

Trickett, P. K. & Susman, E. J. (1988). Parental perceptions of childrearing practices in physically abusive and nonabusive families. *Developmental Psychology, 24*, 270–276.

U. S. Department of Health and Human Services, National Center on Child Abuse and Neglect. (1996). *Child abuse and neglect case-level data 1993: Working paper 1*. Washington, DC: U.S. Government Printing Office.

Waddington, C. H. (1957). *The strategy of genes*. London: Allen and Unwin.

Waters, E. & Sroufe, L. A. (1983). Competence as a developmental construct. *Development Review, 3*, 79–97.

Weissberg, R. P. & Greenberg, M. T. (1998). School and community competence-enhancement and prevention programs. In W. Damon (Series

Ed.), *Handbook of Child Psychology* (5th ed., Vol. 4) (pp. 877-954). New York: Wiley.

Winnicott, D. W. (1958). *Through pediatrics to psycho-analysis: Collected papers.* New York: International Universities Press.

Wolfe, D. A. & Jaffe, P. (1991). Child abuse and family violence as determinants of child psychopathology. *Canadian Journal of Behavioural Science, 23,* 282–299.

Wolfner, G. D. & Gelles, R. J. (1993). A profile of violence toward children: A national study. *Child Abuse and Neglect, 17,* 197–212.

Wyman, P. A., Cowen, E. L., Work, W. C., & Kerley, J. H. (1993). The role of children's future expectations in self-system functioning and adjustment to life stress: A prospective study of urban at-risk youth. Milestones in the development of resilience. *Development and Psychopathology, 5,* 649–661.

# 14

## *Porgy and Bess* and the Concept of Wellness

*Seymour B. Sarason*

**Prologue**. Years ago I was asked to present a paper at the dedication of the new psychology building at the University of Rochester. The paper was "Psychology To the Finland Station in The Heavenly City of the Eighteen Century Philosophers." A week before the dedication, it became apparent that my father would die in a few days. I sent the paper to Emory, who read it at the dedication. He was intrigued by the title and agreed with the content of the paper. So, when I was asked to contribute to this festschrift, I wanted another strange title with, I hoped, appropriate contents. I gave up, reluctantly. But then I read a book on the history of Gershwin's *Porgy and Bess* at the same time I was agonizing about what I could write about wellness that would not embarrass me or cause Emory to worry about my state of wellness. I hope I have not failed on both counts, although the likelihood of the former is far greater than the latter.

The premiere performance of George Gershwin's *Porgy and Bess* in the mid-1930s engendered mixed reactions. Was it a Broadway musical or an opera? Should it be considered a serious effort to elevate the level and quality of American music or pretentious, overambitious, and flawed? Did it depict a realistic picture of a black culture of a particular time and place or one that was derogatory, misleading, and unacceptable? Was it or would it be a footnote in the history of American music or one that history would have to acknowledge as a major work of music, American or otherwise? When a work of art (of any kind) elicits such a range of contrasting, passionate reactions, how do we explain it? That question, of course, takes force by virtue of the fact that more than 60 years after it first opened, *Porgy and Bess* had become the most frequently performed and acclaimed American "musical-opera" outside of the United States. Within the United States, it is regarded as a work of art transcending time and place. It is in the repertory of the Metropolitan Opera Company.

The act of classifying is an obvious feature of human behavior from our earliest days. Is this person friend or foe? Like or unlike me? Is this person gay or straight? Radical or conservative? Is this a healthy or unhealthy thing to eat? Is this action legal or illegal, moral or immoral? There are several reasons we "naturally" categorize, but two are most relevant to my purposes; one is obvious and the other less so, but the two are interrelated. The more obvious reason is that classifying serves the function of a guide to what we should think, feel, and do. Far more often than not, our act of classification is automatic and nonreflective (i.e., we do not "decide" to classify, it just happens). But there are times when we feel we need to classify because something in the external context is strange or problematic, and when we say we want or have to decide, it is because we assume that the way we classify (define our options) is in some ways important to us.

The less obvious reason, especially in regards to matters cultural, is that classifying is associated with values. The act of classifying never takes place in a social, value-free vacuum. Values precede and are reinforced by the act of classifying. So, when musical critics saw *Porgy and Bess* and had to decide whether it was an opera or musical, "serious" or "light," those categories reflected values. If it was an opera, it had more worth than if it was a Broadway musical. Granted that a particular musical may be more worthy than other musicals— it may in fact be deemed to be in the pantheon of great musicals—it is not as worthy as an opera similarly judged in that genre. What are the criteria of worthiness? The musical critic will say that opera deals with the most important human feelings and situations: passionate love, jealousy, hate, shame, guilt, fear, revenge, war, murder, etc. It does so by capitalizing on the capacity of the human voice to express those features with a range and force appropriate to them. For example, despite the scores of times I have listened to *Rigoletto*, I am still more than moved when I hear the "tremendous revenge" duet, expressing, as it does, rage and revenge so compellingly. If we accept the critic's criteria, we have to ask how come the operatic canon contains operas that are basically comedic (e.g., *Barber of Seville, Marriage of Figaro*) or lack the most passionate emotions (e.g., *The Bartered Bride, Falstaff, Oberon, Fledermaus*)? The critic would probably respond by saying that, however worthy these operas may be, they are not as worthy as those that deal with life's tragedies, but they are nevertheless worthy enough to be regarded as deserving of canon status—i.e., they may not be great opera but to classify them as a Broadway musical would be ridiculous. It is hard to avoid the conclusion that the critic believes criteria for classifying a work as an opera, as well as judging its worthiness, are objective or impersonal, validated by time.

Why, then, were some critics ambivalent about how to classify *Porgy and Bess*? If the criteria are impersonal and clear, why the ambivalence? One reason is that the *range* of feeling-emotion in *Porgy and Bess* is comparable to that of what is called opera; it is clearly not the June-moon Broadway musical. The second reason is its dramatic themes or substance are, directly and indirectly, about America's tragedy: race. When critics of the time thought of opera, it did not need to be said that they meant European opera. There were, of course, some American operas but they proved, to most critics, that quality opera by American composers was not on the musical horizon, and when they came to see *Porgy and Bess*, their set and expectation were not neutral. That reason was associated with the third reason: the music was composed by someone who came out of the jazz-blues-popular music tradition. That was a kind of red flag to critics who classified music as either serious or popular, and who valued the former infinitely more than the latter. I am not hell-diving into the minds of the critics when I say that none of them came to *Porgy and Bess* with the expectation that the likes of George Gershwin could compose music they would regard as operatic. They had already classified American music in ways that expressed values about worthiness.

They came to *Porgy and Bess* with a "show me" attitude: "Prove to me that my classification and associated value assignment are wrong." They were defending strongly held personal and professional beliefs, which, it needs to be emphasized, were not unrelated to the fact that they were Americans. They would not agree that their reactions were personal, professional, and cultural.

Why did (and do) audiences flock to see *Porgy and Bess* here and abroad? Unlike critics, members of an audience (at least most of them) did not come to see *Porgy and Bess* with a clear classification scheme and its explicit or implicit values. The so-called average person came with questions. Will it move me? Will it stimulate my thinking? Will it instruct me? Will I like it? Will I want to see it again? Will I tell others to see it? They did not ask if it was an opera or a musical and were not prepared to say that if it was the former, it had greater value than if it was the latter. What was crucial for many of them was that they knew that it was composed by the person who wrote "Rhapsody in Blue," "An American in Paris," and scores of popular songs they had listened to and sung countless times. Unlike the critics, they came with high hopes and expectations, uncluttered with issues of musical classifications and traditions. And it is important for what I shall say later (I will get to wellness!) to note that what I have said about audiences did not hold for the American South. It was assumed that it would be many decades (if not more) before *Porgy and Bess* could be performed in the South. Five years after its premiere, World War II started, the world changed, and that assumption went by the boards, as did the evaluation of *Porgy and Bess*—whether it was an opera or a musical seemed beside the point.

What I have said is not novel: classification in the realm of human affairs serves (among other things) personal, professional, and cultural purposes. Classification becomes mischievous in its consequences when those purposes are not recognized. Let me (very briefly) illustrate that point by calling attention to an article by Garner (1972). Garner discusses the classification of research into two categories: basic and applied. Although he restricts his focus to psychology, the general import of what he says goes far beyond psychology. In a nutshell, here are his major points:

- There is an unnecessary, historically invalid, distinction between basic and applied research.

- That way of classifying research is associated with a value judgement that basic research is superior to, more worthy than, applied research. (That is a theme I discussed in my paper for the dedication of the new psychology building at the University of Rochester).

- Employing examples from World War II, Garner describes how the applied problems psychologists studied influenced basic research in psychology in the post-World War II era.

- Basic research is not "superior" to applied research. Each seeks to answer *different* questions. Each depends on and is influenced by the other.

Garner (a dear friend and colleague who was mightily disappointed when Emory declined to came to Yale) is regarded as the quintessential basic researcher. He has received every award such a researcher can be given. What most psychologists do not know is that, for a good part of his long career, he was an applied researcher, i.e., working on very practical problems requiring practical answers. He did not and does not value that research as inherently less worthy than his basic research, as if it had less of a Platonic essence of value. Different questions lead to different answers. A practical question can influence the substance and direction of basic research, and vice versa. The crucial question is how well their intended purposes are achieved, and calling one basic and the other applied, and implying differences in social value says more about snobbishness than it does about research. There is lousy basic research just as there is lousy applied research, just as there are lousy operas and lousy Broadway musicals. The word lousy is pejorative. I employed it in order to indicate that in both science and the arts there are examples where over time what had been devalued became highly valued, what had been deemed appropriately classified at one time is differently classified at another time.

What is wellness? However you define it, wellness is a category in a classification that contains the category nonwellness. You could argue that wellness should not be seen in terms of classification but rather as a continuum anchored on one end by exemplary wellness and on the other end by obvious nonwellness. For my purposes here, the concept of continuum still leaves you with the question of what wellness is—as a state, process, or both. If you cannot get agreement on a provisional, semi-clear definition of wellness, we will—inevitably I would say—continue to classify on egregiously oversimplified grounds that insure that we will some day have a DSM-100 psychiatric diagnostic manual. Is wellness the absence of pathology? The concept of wellness has gained currency as a reaction to the limitations of the view that the goal of prevention is to prevent this or that psychological pathology. Without in any way "putting down" efforts at preventing this or that pathology—unlike how critics put down *Porgy and Bess*—wellness advocates sought to determine those characteristics and capacities that enable people to confront and overcome obstacles to achieving their goals and fulfilling their social responsibilities.

There are two problems inherent in the concept of wellness. The first is that the word wellness implies a value judgment. Take, for example, parents who are appalled by who attends and what is taught and how in public schools. They decide that they will exercise their right to educate their child at home. How do we judge the wellness of these parents? To the several hundred thousand parents who are exercising their legal rights, that is an insulting, demeaning question. Just what you would expect, they would say, from psychologists who, if they were honest, would admit that they believe the capacity of parents to screw up the development of their children is near bottomless? To these parents their wellness is a given, not something to be understood and judged. The psychologists could reply by saying that he or she is not questioning the parental right to provide home instruction. But just as not all physicians should be physicians, and all teachers should not be teaching, not all parents are "fit" to be solely responsible for home instruction. Besides, the psychologist might add, not all young children will flourish in the social context of home instruction; by virtue of temperament and more, some children, far from flourishing, will not become psychologically well people. The conversation, of course, will be nonproductive of agreement. Each of the parties has a different and strongly held conception of what makes for wellness, although the psychologist, I would hope, would admit (at least to him or herself) that his or her concept of wellness is fuzzy and leaves much to be desired in regard to clarity and empirical grounding.

Let us imagine the following:

1.  In order for parents to be allowed to provide home instruction, they and their child must be evaluated from a wellness perspective. That evaluation will be confidential—not available to the state or parents—and in no way will jeopardize the legal rights of the parents. The evaluation will contain conclusions, judgments, predictions, and the grounds for making them.

2.  Similar evaluations will be conducted at what would be the end of elementary, middle, and high schools.

3.  Similar evaluations will be made of children's wellness.

It would take a group of wellness psychologists several months, meeting daily, to reach a conscionable degree of agreement about (a) their conception of wellness and the investigative methods appropriate to it, (b) what would be confirming and disconfirming evidence for their conception of wellness, (c) how to justify the "should and ought" in their perspective in contrast to the shoulds and oughts undergirding competing conceptions of wellness.

Assume the data are in and analyzed. What will be said in the event that there is no or little agreement between the conclusions-predictions and the level and quality of the ability of parents and child to cope effectively with problems that have come their way? What will we say if the "real life" performance of the children are remarkably above that of comparable children who did not have home instruction? I need not list other outcome scenarios. The point here is how to remain committed to a conception at the same time we are open to its correction, not only because of very shaky empirical data, but also because the very conception of wellness obviously contains the imprint of value judgments about what makes for the good life. A rose is a rose is a rose. An opera is an opera is an opera. Wellness is wellness is wellness. Words are not the things to which they refer. In the realm of human affairs, our words and labels bear the imprint of what we have come to believe is good or bad, right or wrong, productive or unproductive. It is an imprint of which we are hardly aware. It is an imprint we do not explore or want to explore. We treasure and defend our categories, just as the critics defended theirs in the case of *Porgy and Bess.* But to those of us whose stock-in-trade is understanding human behavior, flushing out that imprint is not or should not be a matter of choice or preference. If at best we can do that only partially, we are obliged to do the best we can. To proceed as if we have no such obligation—as if that imprint does not exist or, if it does, it contains no features about which we need worry—serves only the purpose of maintaining our personal and professional self-esteem.

I am reminded here of something Freud wrote near the end of his life. It was addressed to the psychoanalytic community, too many of which Freud came to believe were convinced of two things. The first was that by virtue of their psychoanalytic training, they understood and could control tendencies interfering with their obligations to help others. The second was that psychoanalytic theory and therapy were the only and best way to alleviate individual misery and dysfunction and, in the case of theory, ultimately to change society and prevent (or mammothly reduce) the incidence of such misery and dysfunction. Although he does not say it explicitly, those are two beliefs Freud held earlier in his life. Those beliefs, especially the first, Freud asserted, are illusory, dangerous, and self-defeating. The psychoanalytic relationship, he says, is inherently corrupting. On the one hand, the analyst is the object of a patient's hostility and hatred, arousing in the analyst feelings hard to control. On the other hand, the analyst is seen by the patient as all-knowing, all-powerful, an object deserving of love, devotion, gratitude, and willing subordination. Those contrasting, conflicting reactions inevitably corrupt, in small and large ways, the analyst and analytic relationship, which is why Freud went on to recommend that analysts be reanalyzed every five years, a suggestion that no one heeded or *discussed* then or since. At least some of the critics of *Porgy and Bess* were ambivalent. They were certain about how they classified and regarded themselves. It was in that paper that Freud asks the analysts what conclusions they would draw if he told them that one of his female patients went into a deep depression several years after an apparently successful analysis. Would they say the analysis had been incomplete, that it had left untouched or unexplored a psychological vein of pathology? Would their conclusion in any way be altered if he told them that the depression followed the burial of her young child? Did they really believe that analytic therapy inoculates them to any or all catastrophies life may bring?

I found what Freud said instructive in two ways—one obvious, one less so. The obvious one is that however critical you may be of Freud, you have to admire how, over the course of his lifetime, he had the courage to change his mind about a lot of things. If he had his own rigid classifications in regard to who and what were supportive of or enemies of his theorizing, he restlessly sought to improve and enlarge his theory, albeit within the category of orthodoxy (the truth). The second way in which what Freud said was instructive, to me, was his use of a depressed woman to make his point. The Freudian part of me prevents me from saying that the example he uses for illustrative purposes was, so to speak, random. One of the most upsetting experiences earlier in Freud's life was the death of a young grandson much beloved by him, a loss that caused sustained grief, and it is not unwarranted to say that he was depressed. Not a "severe" depression, of course, but something that was more than sadness. As we know, Freud had a jaundiced, unflattering, querulous view of women. Men were to women as opera was to *Porgy and Bess*. The resilience of men was greater than that of women, and that is implied in his use of a woman to illustrate his point. However, Freud was using the example as a way of asking: What is wellness and what is pathology? Are extreme reactions to *all* traumas in life to be labeled pathological? Freud provided no answer. If he was not asking those questions and, therefore, not providing answers, I have to say that there are many people today who wrestle with those questions in trying to explain reactions in the Nazi concentration camps.

Freud and his case example brings me to the second problem in a conception of wellness. Wellness is not a feature in or of an individual. It refers to interpersonal phenomena suffused with the imprint of time and era, i.e., culture and cultural change (of which the critics of *Porgy and Bess* could not conceive). My book *Barometers of Social Change* was my attempt to understand the vast post-World War II social-cultural change. Although I tried to be as dispassionate as possible, there are times in that book when it is clear that I view *some* of those changes as an ill wind that blows no good. And one of those winds concerns a conception of wellness that puts a premium on self-expression, a lineal descendant of catharsis as the crucial ingredient in wellness. Am I an aged fogie unable to comprehend that the world has changed? Was I, like the critics of *Porgy and Bess*, a prisoner of criteria for classifying and judging human behavior, which said more about my past than the nature of "real" wellness? I will not be around when the issue gets decided *provisionally*. Maybe that is just as well.

**Epilogue**. After I sent Emory a copy of *Caring and Compassion in Clinical Practice*, he sent me a 15-page, single-spaced critique. It was clear, incisive, telling, laced with Cowanesque humor. The guts of his critique was that my concepts of caring and compassion were, to say the least, fuzzy, incomplete, and ultimately misleading and confusing. He was, I had to admit, annoyingly and largely correct. When, in the past decade, he directed his focus to the nature and study of wellness, I wondered whether he would make the mistakes he said I made about the concepts of caring and compassion. He has not. Emory is a far more conservative (in the best sense of that word) psychologist than I am. No less a thinker than I am, he is more reflective than I am. He mulls and remulls, he needs to feel more certain than I do about the validity of what he writes, although what he writes is the tip of an iceberg I call creative imagination. I confess to the fantasy that derived from the time that Emory talked at the Yale Psycho-Educational Clinic in the mid-1960s. The fantasy was that he and I would spend our teaching careers in the same department and "rear" several generations of graduate students (having the same personal and intellectual qualities our Rochester and Yale graduate students had, of course). How different and better (of course) psychology in general and our field in particular would be! That is not arrogance, because fantasy is intended to give expression to our arrogances. I assume that a conception of wellness does not rule out such arrogant fantasies.

I wrote this paper because I know how Emory is struggling with the concept of wellness. This paper will not be all that helpful to him in his struggle. I request that he not respond to it with the critique I know that mind of his will come up with. I make that request to protect the fragility of my state of wellness. This paper, Emory, is my way of hearing again Gershwin's "Of Thee I Sing."

## References

Garner, W. (1972). The Acquisition and Application of Knowledge. *American Psychologist, 27,* 941–946.

# 15

## The Importance of Being Emory: Issues in Training for the Enhancement of Psychological Wellness

*Stanley F. Schneider*

## Change and Continuity as Overarching Issues in Training for Psychological Wellness

*The Importance of Being Emory* is the title I used for a small appreciation of Emory Cowen presented during a tribute to him in 1996 [Schneider, 1996]. Its inclusion in the title of this chapter is deliberate because of the continuity and further elaboration of certain ideas presented earlier. I began the 1996 appreciation by noting that I honored Cowen "especially because he has changed, and in his clearly argued, meticulously researched, and articulately differentiated and defined fashion he has taken a giant step beyond his beloved playground of primary prevention and led all of us to the much more comprehensive arena of the enhancement and promotion of wellness" [p.1]. Of course, Cowen [1994] has long included the promotion of psychological health and well-being in his notion of primary prevention, but the historical inattention to those aspects of prevention is largely responsible for his recent work and for the creation of this volume. Note also that the title of this chapter specifies the enhancement of psychological wellness, although there are other forms of wellness that bear upon and are affected by psychological wellness (e.g., physical, spiritual, economic). The inclusion of the title of the earlier appreciation is deliberate also because the first issue to concern us in training for psychological wellness is that of *change and continuity*. In his seminal article on

psychological wellness, Cowen [1994] indicates clearly that he considers psychological wellness to be a paradigm shift, a radical depar-
ture from current thinking and practice. This is no overstatement. At
the same time, he thinks of wellness-illness as a continuum, rejecting
the binary conception based on risk so common in mental health, and
considers wellness to be more than the absence of disease, something
with "positive marker characteristics," and that the ideal of wellness
and the goal of its enhancement apply to all people, including those
who are ill [p. 153]. I shall use Cowen's 1994 paper, which I consider
to be the most cogently argued and thoughtful work on psychological
wellness, and some others as springboards for many of the questions
and issues in this chapter.

My original thoughts about this article took the form of a
dialogue with myself, or rather between my contextual self—so long
identified with mental health training—and my current self, trying to
envision a new field. By asking several questions, I hope to explore
some issues and suggest a substantive agenda for psychological
wellness training. I have been able to find very little written about
issues of training for psychological wellness, but even more important, it seemed necessary to approach this topic *de nouveau* since the
concept and the activities associated with psychological wellness
require a fresh look at almost everything we've been about. Consider
this chapter, then, to be a work in progress, an attempt to abandon
preconceptions, an exercise in undoing ourselves or whatever term
seems to you to capture the need for a new frame of reference. This is
not an effort to deny the past or to abandon the contexts of psychology, prevention, mental health, community, or other identifiers of our
cumulative preoccupations, or to neglect the relationships that exist
between psychological wellness and these domains. It would not be
possible to do that. Rather, it is a concern that if we do not wrench
ourselves sufficiently from our comfortable conceptual cocoons, we
shall find it too easy to slip back into them and leap less than we
should.

I admit to a restless uneasiness about the requirements of this
change. Although I had been coming around slowly to an increased
concern with the promotion of well-being, Cowen's 1994 article had

a profound effect on me. I recommended it highly in some valedictory remarks [Kent, 1995] on the occasion of my retirement from the National Institute of Mental Health (NIMH), emphasizing the importance of his ideas for the future and the almost inescapable necessity of enhancing wellness as a matter of health economics. We need to focus on change, on psychological wellness, while at the same time we borrow from our roots in prevention, psychology, and mental health, all of them transcended by the notion of psychological wellness, but each of them accommodated congenially by it [Cowen, 1994]. This is more easily said than done, since those roots are deep and pervasive.

## The Socioeconomic Context of Psychological Wellness Training

What is the social and economic context in which this change must occur, and why would the change required by this paradigm shift be more difficult than others experienced by psychologists (e.g., from classical learning theory to cognitive psychology, or from a predominant nature-nurture emphasis to a recognition of biology-environment reciprocity)? In these earlier paradigm shifts, the social structure is not aligned against the change. However, the entire health macrosystem rewards an emphasis on the understanding, treatment, and cure of illness and disease. *That is what is paid for* It is one important reason why the NIMH prevention mission is so bonded to a risk-based conception of illness. There are indications of greater attention to prevention, still very disease oriented, at the National Institutes of Health (NIH). The great paradox is that there is no lack of interest in maintaining and improving health among the general public. Indeed, we are surfeited with recommendations regarding diet, exercise, alcohol consumption, tobacco use, and various other facets of lifestyle that aim to improve health. This interest does not yet extend to psychological wellness with the intensity shown in physical health, but the trend may work to our advantage in the future. There is little indication that health-oriented funds would be used to promote or enhance psychological wellness. There have been earlier indications of possible support of prevention and health promotion.

Several years ago I was able to report [Schneider, 1993] that the then-Assistant Secretary of Health, Philip Lee, stated that the administration's health plan called for paying to keep people healthy, a phenomenal change in the system of incentives. Of course, we know what happened to the Clinton health plan, but the fact that this kind of thinking had permeated to Lee's level suggests that it may resurface at some point. We should do everything to encourage that.

Why are the issues of the socioeconomic context and constraints on expenditures for psychological wellness important? Because that context defines some of the activities that graduates of psychological wellness training programs will need to be prepared for, and it is relevant to jobs they need to do. It suggests that they require preparation for expertise and involvement in social and economic health policy, to the point of affecting legislation, to a much greater extent than others we have historically trained. These are some thoughts regarding the significance and urgency of change, and resistance against it in the socioeconomic context. The importance of continuity becomes apparent with the next major issues for discussion. Since almost nothing is written about training for psychological wellness, reliance on training material for prevention and some other areas was mandatory. It seemed necessary and appropriate to borrow from prevention at least two major characteristics of training: (a) the conceptual framework of an ecologically based, contextual life course development perspective; and (b) the importance of multidisciplinary programs containing academic and field experience covering a wide substantive bandwidth. The importance of these features, which are actually trajectories in constant transactional relationship, cannot be overemphasized.

## The Conceptual Basis of Training for Psychological Wellness

There seems to be little question about the value of a life course developmental and ecological orientation [see Weissberg & Greenberg 1998, Cowen 1994, Lerner & Miller 1993] as the conceptual framework for training in psychological wellness. This orientation is valuable also in training for prevention [Mrazek & Haggerty 1994], developmental psychopathology [Cicchetti & Toth 1991], and applied developmental psychology [Fisher et al. 1993]. The developmental life course contextual research agenda is described cogently in Lerner & Miller [1993, see especially pp. 354-358]. In the following material, it should be understood that pathways to psychological wellness over the life course must be reflected in appropriate academic work accompanied by intensive field-based research and experience. Students must not only know the literature of attachment; cognitive, social, and emotional competence; empowerment, sense of self, self-efficacy; stress and resilience; families, schools, peer groups, workplaces; relationships, intimacy, loss—the stuff that shapes our lives—but they need firsthand experience with as much of this as possible, working closely and in a diversity-sensitive fashion with individuals, families, other relational networks, settings, organizations, communities, and systems. This should not be called an internship—a term now in very general use, but still too medical in its aura. Psychological wellness students will not be *practicing or experimenting on* as much as *joining and participating with*. The following sections deal with suggested pathways to psychological wellness during four periods in the life course. The issue of field experience elucidating these pathways is discussed in a section on experiential training below.

## *Pathways to Psychological Wellness Before and During Childhood*

When do we begin to consider the life course for an individual, and what are some of its contexts? We might start with a couple's decision to have a child, the relationship of the couple at the time, and the family setting in which these factors are embedded, including biological, sociocultural, and economic information. The point in time can, of course, yield vastly different individual circumstances. There may be no decision in an entirely unplanned pregnancy, or no family as such for one or both prospective parents. Any available information should be provided on the course of the pregnancy, keeping in mind the contextual factors already mentioned, and including the availability, access to, and quality of medical or nursing care during the pre- and postnatal periods. Consideration and understanding of these important periods and transitions can provide necessary material to appreciate the "givens" and early stress experiences of a child.

During early childhood we can use Cowen's [1994] pathways to psychological wellness as examples, vivifying and appreciating attachment (and, I would add, temperament of the child) not only from the vast literature on the subject, but by examples of the range of attachments from those that are secure and warm to instances where there appears to be no connection at all between caregiver and infant or child. A similar script is possible for the development of age-related competencies. The body of family process research is one aspect pertinent for these pathways and for others, as the child grows older. The creation of settings that favor psychological wellness presents a somewhat different problem. The family, which is the major actor together with the developing child in matters of attachment and early competencies, must share control increasingly with the child's peers and with others in settings that begin to affect the life of the child (e.g., day care centers, preschools, and schools), all of which may vary in the degree to which they enhance psychological wellness. One of the questions prompted by the pathway of coping effectively with stress is that of the relationship between physical health and psychological wellness. Some knowledge of this relationship should be required as part of psychological wellness training. It is an area that is pertinent throughout the life course. Illnesses beyond those usually expected in childhood, such as diabetes and asthma, may provide sufficient stress to affect psychological wellness, as may any severe or chronic condition. There are other compelling reasons to be interested in the physical health—psychological wellness relationship. The area of physical wellness is considered a significant pathway to general wellness in adolescence [Crockett and Petersen 1993, see below]. Moreover, one of the subdisciplines in psychology of particular relevance to psychological wellness is health psychology, which has not only a rich literature on the relationship of stress to health, but also a tradition of exploring the problems and potentialities of influencing a disease-oriented biomedical culture to consider behavioral and psychological factors in physical health and illness. Psychological wellness advocates can learn from health psychologists.

The complexity, age-relatedness, interdependence, complementarity, and developmental change in these pathways, along with others to be mentioned during development, call for methodological sophistication that is staggering. One problem, for example, is the necessity for better-defined outcomes for psychological wellness and measures for them. The diversity resulting from plasticity, growth, resilience, and adaptation during development, together with the possibilities for overcoming negative circumstances, far exceeds the diversity in psychopathology [see Cicchetti 1996, p. 35, for a similar view]. Yet we have a body of knowledge in the nosology of psychopathology that, despite its problems, can serve as a basis for outcome measures. No such refinement exists for psychological wellness, and the danger of substituting pollyannishness for substance in a wellness vocabulary is a real one unless further thought is given to this issue.

## Pathways to Psychological Wellness in Adolescence

What substantive and experiential content might be relevant to students of psychological wellness in later stages of development? Crockett and Petersen [1993] identify six goals for adolescent development, which can be considered as pathways to psychological wellness for this stage of the life course. They are:

> (1) to promote physical health and well-being through proper nutrition and exercise, development of a positive body image and healthy sexuality, and adoption of a healthy lifestyle; (2) to promote cognitive maturity, including the capacity for abstract, formal reasoning, social-cognitive skills, and autonomous decision making; (3) to promote self-esteem and a positive sense of personal identity, including positive future goals and a sense of self-efficacy and social responsibility; (4) to promote supportive relationships with family, peers, and other important adults; (5) to provide opportunities for educational and occupational success; and (6) to avoid pitfalls that would interfere with the positive developmental outcomes outlined above. [p. 31]

The authors state that these goals "reflect a dual emphasis on promoting health-enhancing behaviors and simultaneously weakening health-compromising behaviors" [p. 31], an important contribution put forth by Perry and Jessor [1985]. Compas [1993] describes a multiaxial framework of positive adolescent mental health, defined as:

> [A] process characterized by development toward optimal current and future functioning in the capacity and motivation to cope with stress and to involve the self in personally meaningful instrumental activities and/or interpersonal relationships. Optimal functioning is relative and depends on the goals and values of the interested parties, appropriate developmental norms, and one's sociocultural group. [pp. 166-167]

Positive adolescent mental health "cannot be characterized by a single profile or developmental trajectory" [p. 167], and multiple different developmental paths during adolescence may be considered adaptive. Elliott [1993] provides evidence that health-compromising behaviors in early adolescence (ages 11-14) have consequences that are much more significant for future difficulty than similar behaviors in later adolescence (ages 18-20).

This material adds some important dimensions to the remarks previously made regarding paths to wellness during childhood. Crockett and Petersen's goals of adolescence show some continuity with Cowen's [1994] pathways. The promotion of cognitive maturity and social-cognitive skills links directly with the earlier age-related competencies; the self-esteem and increase in autonomy are analogs of empowerment. The promotion of supportive relationships with family and other important adults can be seen as a ripening derivative of early attachment. The significance of peer relationships is especially critical in adolescent development. Nothing is said about settings that enhance psychological wellness as such, but the goal of providing opportunities for educational and occupational success is related to that pathway. The goal of promotion of physical health, well-being, positive body image, and healthy lifestyle incorporates some of the added factors suggested earlier in this chapter on physical health, as well as healthy sexuality, a factor particularly salient for adolescence, although it should also be included in preadolescence and what quaintly used to be called "latency period" children and in later stages of the life course. The last goal—avoidance of pitfalls that would interfere with positive development—can be generalized across the life course, growing with age as one achieves greater judgment and discretion. Elliott's findings are excellent reminders of how important it is to consider age clusters within more general developmental stages. Compas' work reflects, in its emphasis on multiple developmental paths, how important diversity is in any consideration of psychological wellness.

### Suggested Pathways to Psychological Wellness During Adulthood

Literature on psychological wellness in the adult years is scant. One of the ironies of psychology is how much attention is directed toward reparative therapies during adulthood and how little attention is paid to adult development. A very large chunk of life is lived between the ages of 21 and 60 or 65, and there are certainly age-related differences bearing on psychological wellness during this period. Freud's views about the significance of loving and working direct attention to two salient areas during adult development, and Sarason's essay [1996] about the changing nature of these aspects of life should dispel any question about the continually developing and evolving aspects of the pathways to psychological wellness. Sarason's point, briefly, is that ideals of a single loving relationship or a single career have been powerfully undermined in recent times. Yet it is possible to look at relationships with other people and comment on their scope and character, which change over time, but which have qualities like intimacy, sharing, depth, and commitment that are adult and that contribute to psychological wellness. It is during these years that relationships with one's own parents undergo significant changes and, if there are children, relationships with them will be among the most important new ones formed. Think of attachment now from the view of the parent of an infant or young child. The ability to love, care for, and engage a child—to facilitate attachment from the parent's side—will enhance psychological wellness in the parent. So will the understanding of and respect for the aging of the parents' parents. The capacity to develop and sustain a loving and healthy sexual relationship with a significant other, to share the tapestry of small intimacies, to grow and change in ways that enrich relationships, are features of a pathway to psychological wellness. It is possible that the scope of interpersonal relationships and social competence becomes wider as well as deeper during these years, that qualities like empathy and trust play greater roles in life. The maintenance and growth of competencies in work, the sense that work is productive, meaningful, enjoyable, and a source of pride and accomplishment are important factors in enhancing psychological wellness.

The issue of empowerment and its associated attributes in adult life is worth more exploration. It is important to feel in control of one's destiny, to feel a stake in the future, to feel capable, optimistic, and that one "can do," but this must be tempered by respect for others, by a sense of fairness and equity, by an always-judicious use of power. Adults can help create workplaces and other settings that enhance psychological wellness for themselves and for others; this is but one aspect of social responsibility and a sense of community, which are important in psychological wellness. The ability to cope with stress continues to be a significant element in psychological wellness throughout the life course. Maintaining a healthy lifestyle, avoiding situations that compromise health and psychological wellness, and capacities to deal maturely with things like the increasing autonomy of children, loss of loved ones, relocation, divorce, loss of job, and other potential stresses of the adult years are essential to psychological wellness. The ability to enjoy friends and be enriched by leisure time activities is another important element in enhancing psychological wellness; these activities may invigorate us physically and/or expand our cognitive and emotional lives.

### Suggested Pathways to Psychological Wellness in the Later Years

Older adults illustrate the effects of demographic change on empowerment, social policy, and even legislation. Increased longevity, and therefore increased numbers, has given this group clout it did not previously possess. How common were retirement communities, senior fares or rates, elder hostels, and the influence of AARP a generation ago? In the years beyond 60 or 65 (or, with some of these entities, increasingly before that time), some of the following things appear to be important in enhancing psychological wellness. (1) Interpersonal relationships may be less extensive than during the prior period, but it will enhance psychological wellness if those retained are riper, richer in nuance and caring, more trusting and less competitive, and particularly generous to the very young. Contact with and support of a spouse or significant other, of children and friends, are critical. (2) Despite the normal loss of certain memory functions, the ability to retain cognitive competence and interest in activities of the mind is of paramount importance. This includes the mastery of new technologies, such as the computer in the present generation, which will increase in number and the speed with which they become part of daily life. The attainment of wisdom in addition to cognitive competence (they are quite different) can be a real plus, since it brings a measure of respect and veneration to the bearer, sure to boost self-esteem. (3) The ability to deal constructively with the diminution of physical and sexual vigor, i.e., accepting the situation with grace and even humor while continuing as much as possible to engage in these activities in whatever ways are comfortable, will be valuable. At the same time, the maintenance of robust physical health is a great contributor to psychological wellness. (4) The ability to cope with illness or the loss of loved ones, such as a spouse, partner, or friends, will do much to preserve psychological wellness. The cumulative effect of such losses is not only greater at this time of life, but is a constant reminder of one's own mortality, and the acceptance of the inevitability of the latter is especially important. (5) Retirement is one of the most common changes during these years, and the creative uses of leisure time and/or continued work of some sort are vital to psychological wellness. So is the ability to relax. (6) Settings retain their importance in the enhancement of psychological wellness. Those that acknowledge some limitations and lessen stress while at the same time encouraging independence and social interaction are to be prized. (6) Finally, continued personal growth, the ability to feel good about oneself and that what one does is worthwhile, enhance psychological wellness during this period of marked change.

## Substantive Knowledge and Experience for Psychological Wellness Training

What substantive knowledge and experience are relevant and important for the domain of psychological wellness? Cowen [1994] has some suggestions. Beginning with a review of necessary collaborative efforts in risk-driven primary prevention programs mentioned by Coie [Coie et al. 1993], which "include sociology, epidemiology, econometrics, psychopathology, criminology, child development, education, and several areas of psychology," Cowen asserts the need for cross-discipline contributions to program development and research is even stronger in psychological wellness, calling "for major inputs from social policy makers, urban planners, political scientists, child development specialists, and educators, among others" [p. 174]. Elsewhere, Cowen [1997b] states, "Should a field's guiding objectives be recast, associated professional training must also change; that is, new roles and activities that vivify the shift must be articulated" [p. 97]. He goes on to describe the best known primary prevention or wellness enhancement programs as those that "(a) train children in skills and competencies that promote wellness outcomes; and (b) modify class and school environments with that same goal in mind," but acknowledges that proactive wellness promotion roles are still evolving and "not yet either widely perceived or meaningfully incorporated into the preparation of school mental health professionals" [p. 113]. These remarks are elaborations of Cowen's basic arguments and changes as they pertain to a particular setting (schools) and its professionals. They do not address explicitly graduate research training for psychological wellness.

In my earlier tribute [1996] to Cowen I asked if it was farfetched to suggest that the major interlinked pathways to wellness described by him [1994] and the research accomplishments that address them comprised much of the subject matter of basic behavioral and social science research. "The pathways reflect early attachment; cognitive, social, and emotional development; the relationships between persons and environments; matters of identity, self-efficacy, self-other relations, as well as empowerment and equity as social constructs; and they reflect the abilities and resilience to deal with stress" [p. 5]. Throughout the history of NIMH, it has been accepted as a maxim that it is essential to know about normal development in order to understand psychopathology. Support of the basic behavioral sciences rested on this maxim. From the time of the institute's first research grant in 1947 on the basic structure of the learning process until the present, that has been so. However, in recent years the case for basic behavioral science, unlike that for neuroscience, had to be made by demonstrating more clearly its relevance to mental illness. In this regard, the demands were not unlike those for prevention. Cowen [1996] notes that the concluding sentence of the recent NIMH report on behavioral science [NIH-NIMH 1995] recommends increased funding for this area as part of a general societal investment in research related to mental illness, and he asks, "Isn't the possibility worth considering, for a moment, that the sound initial promotion, and maintenance, of wellness may, in fact, be among the most promising of all strategies for preventing mental illness?" [pp. 243-244]. I would answer this question with a resounding "yes." The basic behavioral sciences play an important role in understanding, treating, and preventing mental illness, but in addition I suggest strongly that *behavioral and social sciences research be yoked to psychological wellness as part of a strategy to enhance their survival and growth.* Relevant and significant findings from the behavioral and social sciences across the life course will constitute a major portion of the substantive base of psychological wellness and of defining and demonstrating the outcomes vital to psychological wellness. The tasks of continuing to refine our knowledge about what leads to constructive lives and to convey it in meaningful language to the public, policymakers, and settings form a large kernel of psychological wellness education and training.

Additional and valuable suggestions regarding the substance of psychological wellness training come from the growing literature on prevention. Mrazek and Haggerty [1994] discuss core sciences for prevention research: neuroscience, genetics, epidemiology, and developmental psychopathology, but the sections of the volume on training are concerned primarily with support mechanisms, supply of researchers, and career-level considerations. The model provided [pp. 458-460] for training prevention researchers calls for knowledge of risk and protective factors (biological and psychosocial) for onset of mental disorders; ability to transform this knowledge into preventive interventions; the design, conducting, and analysis of such interventions in the real world, and the incorporation of sound decisions regarding clinical, ethical, and economic issues into the research.

Weissberg and Greenberg [1998] in their comprehensive review of school-based programs address training for competence enhancement and prevention research. Competence enhancement is one of the pathways to psychological wellness for children [Cowen 1994,

1996]. After reviewing the four roles for prevention researchers described by Price [1983], problem analyst, innovation designer, field researcher, and diffusion researcher, Weissberg and Greenberg indicate that to carry out these roles effectively, prevention researchers who specialize in programming for young people require training in several areas. These include:

> [D]evelopmental epidemiology and knowledge of social-environmental and behavioral trends; a life span developmental and ecological theoretical orientation with sensitivity to human diversity; knowledge of social, cognitive, and biological risk and protective factors for social, health, and mental/emotional problems; culturally appropriate assessment approaches with diverse populations; design and implementation of multicomponent prevention programs in natural settings—particularly with families, schools, and communities; multidisciplinary approaches to the prevention of problem behaviors such as substance use, unsafe sex, and delinquency; clinical field trial research designs and data-analytic techniques for longitudinal prospective interventions; methods to design, conduct, and evaluate collaborative, community action research; strategies to disseminate effective prevention practices; and principles of scientific integrity and ethics in conducting prevention research. [p. 924]

This is a full plate. Training for psychological wellness requires almost all of the above, with the possible exception of detailed exposure to clinical trials. The training must be geared to psychological wellness rather than to psychopathology. However, developmental psychopathology should be incorporated into the training of psychological wellness students. Is that paradoxical? I think not. If the maxim about knowing "normal" development to understand psychopathology is true, the reverse is also valid [see Cicchetti 1993, for a persuasive account of this issue). Since we are talking about a continuum (psychological wellness for all people) rather than a binary system, we will be concerned about wellness possibilities for those who are on the entire continuum. Indeed, I think that an increased understanding of psychological wellness will provide new insights into the understanding of psychological illness.

*Research and Methodology in Psychological Wellness Training*

Unquestionably, the methodological requirements of psychological wellness training will be formidable. A multiplicity of methods is dictated by the plethora of disciplines that may be participating in the research, and also by the fact that units and levels of analysis may range from the individual to large-scale systems, all of them changing during the course of their development and in their relationships with each other. A wise comment on this general problem has been provided by Cairns [1986]:

> There is an intimate relationship between the subject matter of an area and the research methods that are appropriate. On this basis, the methods of developmental study present special problems precisely because they are addressed to dynamic and changing phenomena. The most important stuff of development has multiple antecedents and it generates multiple consequences. Moreover, true novelties and new patterns of behavioral organization arise in the course of ontogeny. These distinctive features of development would seem to require a fresh view of the basic methods of science. [p. 109]

The final draft [Sandler et al. 1992] on training prepared for the NIMH reports on the Prevention of Mental Disorders [NIMH 1993] and A Plan for Prevention Research [NIH-NIMH 1996] is actually more pertinent to substantive training issues than the reports themselves, and its section on methodology is exceptionally strong. The draft states:

> Ideally, methodologists in prevention should have expertise in the following areas: Experimental and quasi-experimental design, and passive observational design with a focus on longitudinal studies; sampling; measurement; epidemiology; analysis of variance and regression; continuous and discrete multivariate analysis; longitudinal data analysis; survival—that is—event-history analysis; attrition analysis

and the treatment of missing data; and structural equation and latent growth-curve modeling. In reality, this list may be too demanding for any one individual; the exact set of skills required will depend upon the problem under investigation. Moreover, the list is not static, but will grow with the development of new methodologies. [pp. 8-9]

Sandler [personal communication, July 17, 1998] has added natural experiments, case studies of change, qualitative and ethnographic studies, and randomized trials to this list.

What kind of research strategies do psychological wellness programs require? Weissberg and Greenberg [1998] provide an excellent review of current prevention science randomized control trial (RCT) methods contrasted with collaborative community action research (CCAR). They conclude that both approaches are valuable in prevention research. RCT affords greater scientific control, whereas CCAR, a contextually based collaboration involving community participants and researchers, is better suited to the needs of diverse communities. There is little doubt about which strategy would impress scientific review committees, but CCAR may be more appropriate to enhancement of psychological wellness because its ecological perspective "(a) emphasizes how people, settings, and events can serve as resources for the positive development of communities; and (b) considers how these resources can be managed, coordinated, ... created, ... preserved and enhanced," looking at the "strengths, competencies, and potential" of settings rather than "weaknesses, deficits, and problems" [p. 932]. If multiple strategies are appropriate for prevention research, they are probably even more pertinent for psychological wellness research, as previous remarks about multidisciplinary participation and multiple units and levels of analysis suggested.

*Four Areas Requiring Additional Emphasis in Psychological Wellness Training*

There are four areas that need a bit more weight in the cursory descriptions of training relevant to psychological wellness. Cowen [1997a] mentions the "givens" and "early stress experiences" as largely laid down and uncontrollable elements in the child's very early years. In order not to minimize the importance of these factors, a basic understanding of developmental neurobiology and genetics should be part of psychological wellness training [see also Cicchetti 1993, 1996]. It would be valuable to comprehend the reciprocal relationships that exist, and continue to develop and change across the life span, between biological and environmental factors. Emde [1996] points out that "dynamic changes in genetic and environmental influences on behavior [occur] over time" and that "genetic change may come about as a result of changes in the environment." Cairns and Cairns [1994], suggest that it is an error to think of context only in terms of external events, pointing out that, "Each of us has an internal context that is at once dynamic and regulatory," and they go on to ask, "What ultimately calls the shots in behavioral regulation—one's internal state or one's environment?" Their answer:

> One advance of the modern developmental synthesis has been to unravel the apparent dualism between biology and environment. Over development, elements of the internal context can be brought into alignment with elements of the social ecology, and vice-versa. The upshot is that forces under the skin and forces outside become loosely correlated over time, creating a network of constraints and regulatory guides for living. Long-term changes in behavior occur when modifications are sufficiently potent to affect reorganization in both systems. [p. 268]

A second, and usually absent, area for added emphasis is that of emotional competence, that is, the development of age related and appropriate emotions. When we speak of the development of competencies as a critical pathway to psychological wellness in the young child, they tend to be seen predominantly as cognitive and social (interpersonal) in nature. Cicchetti and Toth [1991] are among the few authors to distinguish between socioemotional and social-cognitive development [p. 253]. Dunn [1994] points out that children who are two or three years old begin to express emotions not seen earlier, such as pride, shame, guilt, jealousy, and embarrassment. She then indicates that what develops with, or as a result of, emotional development includes understanding of other people, understanding the social world, understanding oneself; the development of intimacy and power in close relations; and also the development of membership in a particular culture. These observations link aspects of emotional development with features that are central to psychological wellness, and her comment regarding membership in a culture gives credence, from a different perspective, to Weisner's [1994] contention regarding the importance of a cultural place as the single most important influence in a child's development (see below). Another factor related to emotional development is that of self-regulation [Masten & Coatsworth, 1998], characterized by the authors as the gain of increasing control over attention, emotions, and behavior, which appears to "be linked with the development of competence in multiple domains from an early age" [p. 208].

A third area for additional emphasis is knowledge of, and experience in, socioeconomic and political matters. Practical understanding of health economics will be helpful in order to convince policymakers of the value of psychological wellness. Insuring that knowledge influences laws and social systems and that an informed public has the tools to help facilitate change are vital aspects of the promotion of psychological wellness. Think for a moment about Cowen's [1994] phrase "wellness for the many". Who makes up the many? Certainly an important segment of the many includes those who have poorer educational opportunities and health care and who may also suffer inequities in justice. Some portion of this group may be helped by extraordinary personal and/or community effort, but for many others ultimately political action and legislation will be necessary. These may also be required to create or modify settings and social environments that favor wellness. Green [1984], writing about these issues, considers the dilemma facing the health educator who is also committed to health promotion:

> The complexity of the behavioral change processes now presenting themselves for intervention … dwarfs and even trivializes health education as the singular intervention. The more sweeping organizational, economic, and environmental changes necessary to support these behaviors conducive to health call for a return to the principles of community

organization and community development, in which education is applied as much to the decision makers, opinion leaders, and gatekeepers as to the people whose behavior is in question. ... even this level of education is insufficient where there are powerful economic interests at stake, as with the tobacco industry... Aggressive political advocacy and action is required to dislodge these 'manufacturers of illness'... This does not require that the fundamental nature of health education should change from a science-based profession to a political party. ... Educated political action is a form of voluntary behavior conducive to health, so it qualifies as *one* of the goals of health education. [p. 190]

Green comments on health education and health promotion, pointing out that, "Just as health care is too large an enterprise to be left entirely to physicians, so is health promotion too large an enterprise to be left entirely to health educators" [p. 191]. It is noteworthy that 14 years after Green's comments, the tobacco industry is just now being called to account. I would submit that psychological wellness is a more complicated, subtle, and controversial arena than physical health, and that the multiple resistances to it will make it that much more difficult to achieve agreement on action. The general reluctance of many scientists to become involved in policy matters shows small signs of change. Lerner & Miller [1993] present a view that should inform psychological wellness training:

[P]olicy and program endeavors do *not* constitute secondary work, or derivative applications, conducted after research evidence has been compiled. Quite to the contrary, policy development and implementation, and program design and delivery, become integral components of developmental contextual research; the evaluation component of such policy and intervention work provides critical feedback about the adequacy of the conceptual frame from which this research agenda should derive. [p. 357]

A fourth area that deserves additional highlighting is the cultural context of wellness and illness, an area sufficiently complex to demand extraordinary knowledge and sensitivity. Among the collaborative disciplines essential to training in psychological wellness, cultural anthropology should be near the top. This suggestion has implications also for methodology. Weisner [1996] asks an intriguing question and provides answers that resonate to some extent with those of Cowen [1994]:

> If you could do one thing to influence a child's development, and could pick something that would be the single most important influence, what would it be? ... The responses are quite predictable: touch and hold the child close for attachment and bonding; provide it with nutrition, physical security, and good medical care; talk with it responsively and often; provide it with a quality education, both formal and informal; find playmates for it; give it a sense of self-esteem; make sure its parents are wealthy. What comes to mind are qualities of the dyadic interactional system in which a child develops, or the physical needs of the developing organism, or the need for stimulation to encourage cognitive and social competencies, or the importance of a kind of self. ... Although every one of these responses is undeniably important in the development of a child, in my view none of these is the most important—the most important is to give the child a specific culture in which to mature and develop. ... By a 'cultural place' I mean the cultural beliefs, practices, meaning, and ecological setting characteristic of members of that community (where the child is going to grow up). ... Ethnography is the most important method in the study of human development because it ensures that the cultural place will be incorporated into understanding development. [pp. 305-306]

Weisner's inclusion of the phrase "make sure its parents are wealthy" is frank and pertinent. Few authors have confronted this problem so directly and simply. The danger that wellness is a prerogative only, or mostly, of those who are affluent is a major issue in a nation where the gap between the wealthy and the poor is growing. Although there is recognition of the importance of sociocultural factors in wellness and in prevention, there are also signs that it is honored more in the breach than in the observance. Weissberg and Greenberg [1998] remark that a recent analysis of "primary prevention programs for children and adolescents provided disquieting data regarding the state-of-the-practice of most prevention intervention research. ... The race and ethnicity of participants were not reported in 48% of the studies—a problematic finding in a field where the sociocultural appropriateness of interventions is critical" [p. 926]. A recent Internet survey of prevention training [Eddy et al. 1998] reflected the opinions of members of the Early Career Prevention Network and other prevention researchers, slightly over half of them either now in training status, junior faculty, or research appointments. Areas of perceived competence and need/relevance were clustered into two content groups, a "core" cluster (e.g. trial design, program design, and evaluation) and an "auxiliary" cluster (I wish they had used different cluster descriptors), which included administration, ethics, community collaboration, gender and culture issues, developmental timing, and scientific collaboration, plus history, economics, and funding. Results show that the perceived competence and need/relevance of the "core" content group was rated higher than the "auxiliary" group. The authors call the finding "disturbing," since they feel that the future of prevention research and interventions is centered in the auxiliary content areas. "Most notably," they state, "gender and culture appear to be extremely important factors in the dissemination, use, and effectiveness of interventions...and sound economic analyses are becoming increasingly important in terms of bringing prevention into policy debates" [p. 15].

## Experiential Training in Psychological Wellness

I assume that the leaders of the training program would fashion an academic sequence that involved the best available expertise representing the multidisciplinary mix of faculty. Students in a comprehensive doctoral program would be exposed to the life course trajectory and to field experience relevant to each major period of the life course. Since collaboration among the participating disciplines is essential to the success of wellness training programs, team participation by a mix of students and faculty in academic and field work would represent the ideal model. In their field experience, students would be exposed to the range of people, relationships, settings, person-setting interactions, cross-cultural issues and policy issues for each period of the life course. Suggested pathways to psychological wellness over the life course have been presented in a previous section of this chapter. Although a research agenda based on a "normal" developmental perspective is recommended as a model for training programs, the degree of complexity, interdependence, age-relatedness, complementarity, and developmental change [Cowen, 1994] must be emphasized yet again. There is nothing simple or "pat" about the material suggested here; the range of human diversity and plasticity and the diversity of person-environment interactions should be sufficient warning against formulaic or cliched approaches to these issues. A few lines above, I used the word normal in quotes. Why? Because a comprehensive program would honor Cowen's [1994] thinking about the prospect of psychological wellness for all people, even for those who are ill. Therefore, might exposure to a psychiatric ward or a drug treatment setting be part of the experiential training for psychological wellness students? Absolutely, because the value of contrast as a teaching device can be extraordinarily powerful.

Two major requirements of psychological wellness training have been mentioned: (1) the conceptual underpinning of an ecological life course development; and (2) a substantive arc from developmental neurobiology and genetics to political science, cultural anthropology, and areas like econometrics, law, and urban planning. It seems to me that the first will be easier to implement, because the second depends so much upon the availability of expertise (and of cooperation) at a particular institution. We should not expect that political scientists or economists will be interested in life course development, but for a program to work well, they should have some idea of what that means, why it is important, and why their talents are needed for connections to social policy and legislation.

A third requirement for training in psychological wellness is an integration of academic and field experience wherever possible. This kind of articulation is not a new problem, and it has in fact plagued clinical psychology throughout its history. Cicchetti and Toth [1991] are clearly cognizant of the problem in their proposal for training developmental psychopathologists, and Fisher, Rau, and Colapietro [1993] go even further in their attempt to increase the constructive interaction between academic and field sites in their interesting program for applied developmental psychology. Fisher and her colleagues seek to ensure close and continuing relationships between faculty members and field supervisors and to see that field experiences are tailored to the skills and career goals of the students. My own views on the problem of integration of academic and internship training in clinical psychology have become more critical over time. In an address on the issue of accreditation, I described the Boulder model of training in clinical psychology to be stillborn for the most part, and added, "The internship represented the great structural fragmentation of clinical psychology. It provided many graduate departments with the opportunity to minimize the immersion of clinical faculty in clinical work, and provided many internship agencies with the escape hatch from any real commitment to research." [Schneider, 1992]. I think the coherence of the academic and field aspects of training for psychological wellness is, if anything, greater and much more difficult. There is no organized collectivity of field training sites. Programs will have to create their own sites, although some of these will be in established settings, and in most of these sites, students and faculty will not be dealing with other professionals, but with members of the general community. The ideal mentor should be both faculty member and field supervisor; such a person would become a true role model for students. There are examples of this model, and in my judgment Cowen is one of them. The prevailing relationship in many field sites for psychological wellness will be one of student(s) plus supervisor, with community setting representative [e.g. elementary school teacher, pastor of a church, coach of a neighborhood team, a family, workplace representative, or member of a retirement community). However, a few settings, such as Cowen's Center for Community Study and Lerner's Institute for Children, Youth, and Families at Michigan State University would be exemplars for a portion of the experiential training program. Such settings, unfortunately, are rare.

Experiential training should include exposure to formal and informal settings and groups. If a team was working with adolescents, for example, it would be important to have contact not only with families, schools, work settings, and portions of the health and justice systems, but also with odd-job situations, gangs, "hang-out" groups, peers across the board, including within and between gender relationships, etc. Much more has been written about developmental issues in young children than in any other age group, appropriately so since it is the period of life during which the greatest and most enduring changes are possible. The prospective and then actual parents, the people and settings involved in birth and well (or not so well) baby care, the family, early peers, preschool, playground, and school settings provide us with blueprints of expected experiential components, each unique in their person-setting relationship for a given individual. These become somewhat less controlled with growth and with the increasing agency of the child. The entry to settings and institutions becomes more difficult. The adolescent years have their special qualities and opportunities, a few of which have been mentioned above. The adult years in a psychological wellness program may pose the greatest experiential challenge because the autonomy of adulthood ensures that the variety of relationships and settings, and therefore of person (or group) and setting interactions, will be at their greatest during these years. Programs should try to achieve training experience with the jobless and homeless, as well as in various workplace and home settings, in leisure time situations, and with the rich panoply of relationships, including intergenerational ones, that characterize this period of life. Possibilities shrink somewhat during the older adult years, and keep shrinking with age, but this is a growing population with choices, relational, occupational, and leisure time activities, and interactions with settings that were not evident a generation ago. The range of settings (e.g. independent living in general community, retirement community, various forms of assisted living, nursing home, etc.) should be a part of student field experience. Such experience should also include varieties of independence-dependence, impact of widowhood or widowerhood, effects of retirement and involvement in work (donated as well as paid time), relationships with children, friends, significant others, groups, effects of decline in physical health and general vigor, and so forth.

What are some of the desiderata of faculty in a psychological wellness training program? At least, they should have an understanding of a contextual developmental life course perspective; hopefully, they will also have some research experience using this perspective in real life situations. There are not many such individuals, and we shall have to be training (or retraining) faculty as we begin to train students. Their contributions to an ultimate program would be very valuable. We clearly need to "borrow" the various multidisciplinary colleagues to be utilized in the program, and the use of the term "borrow" should not indicate we do not have to pay them. It is essential to pay them for their contributions. We need to woo and welcome them, to involve them, value their contributions, and hopefully have them find out how this perspective and such a program might enhance their own work. Faculty must prize and be comfortable with collaborative work with other scientists, professionals, members of the community, and with their students. They ideally should be negotiators, advocates, and partners with people in the community. Aloof academicians would be very ill suited to such a program. The degree of control that is frequently presumed by researchers may be difficult in many aspects of their work. The ability to plan for contingencies, a large tolerance for ambiguity, and the ability to deal with improvisation will be very helpful. But all of these qualities must be directed toward the end of credible research that will inform the field and the understanding and activities of the public and policymakers.

What should we expect of students in these programs? Irwin Sandler, in a personal communication, has made the very important point that we cannot expect any person to embody all of these skills (this would be true also of faculty members). I agree that it is patently impossible for any student to master the suggested scope of psychological wellness programs. Sandler envisions specialists in one of these areas, e.g. psychological wellness in adolescence, developing programs and policies to influence well-being during that period of the life course. Using Campbell's "fish scale model of omniscience" [Campbell, 1969], Sandler sees individuals trained with expertise in specific parts of the problem, who possess skills that overlap with others working on different parts of the problem so that a collaborative team can deal with the broader problem. Sandler also asks whether we are talking about a new profession or expanded or changed roles for existing professions, such as psychologists, nurses, public health professionals, educators. He clearly favors the expanded or changed role concept for existing professions. He makes a valid distinction between what the field needs and what the realistic expectations are for students.

Sandler's expectations and examples are thoroughly realistic, and I am inclined to agree with them for the short term. Over the longer term, however, I would like to see this field develop and take on its own identity and significance. Even at this early stage, I would insist that students possess an appreciation of the life course perspective and that they have at least some experience in settings that serve or characterize the diverse periods of the life course. I would strive also to have students exposed to the bandwidth of substantive knowledge, with an appreciation of experience in real-life settings reflecting that breadth.

The history of training in biological sciences at NIMH is pertinent in this regard. The program, which began to receive support in 1957, was directed by Fred Elmadjian, who had been director of biological research at Worcester State Hospital and recruited to NIMH by members of the psychology training program. He was the only professional staff member of the biological sciences program and ran it with an uncompromising dedication to multidisciplinary training. He decreed that applicants were to have behavioral and biological departments involved in their programs. Funds were not available to applicants who did not meet this condition. A promissory note was not enough; programs were ready to apply for training support only when they could demonstrate a history of multidisciplinary collaboration. The mix in these programs contained as many as thirteen departments. Psychology and/or psychiatry were the usual behavioral departments, but the biological group was exceedingly diverse, including anatomy, physiology, endocrinology, genetics, molecular biology, biochemistry, pharmacology, cell biology, and departments that already had begun to develop into neuroanatomy and neurendocrinology. These became departments with expanded or changed roles, to use Sandler's terms. Over time, however, this enterprise developed into the field known today as neuroscience. The NIMH training program was probably responsible for the greatest contribution to the development of that rich and complex area. I do not want to rule out the possibility that over time a cohesion may take place identifying a major field devoted to enhancing psychological well-being. Collaboration is a key element in training for psychological wellness. The tendency to revert to home disciplines (where the rewards are) and the tendency to overspecialize are two potential hazards to guard against. Both are forms of fragmentation, they lead to erecting walls, and they undercut collaboration and multidisciplinary endeavors. Unfortunately, it is impossible to re-create the era or the necessary monetary support that allowed Elmadjian to do what he did.

For what roles should students be trained? There is no question that we require a strong academic cadre of psychological wellness researchers, teachers, and mentors for the future. The paucity of experience and knowledge in this new field makes it absolutely necessary, because at this time it is an area lifting itself by its own bootstraps. Necessary, but not sufficient, and we need to think beyond the usual academic situations in envisioning jobs for psychological wellness students. We have a tendency to produce students in our own image in areas like prevention. It is a constant disappointment how little effect our knowledge has had beyond limited target groups and our own in-house reward systems, although there are some encouraging signs of change. If this new field is to fulfill the promise of broader impact, graduates will have to be involved with consumers, communities, settings of various kinds, broader systems including political, judicial, and educational ones at various levels of government, and with many levels of public policy. These students will have to be trained as advocates, negotiators, coalition builders, and translators of research to everyday language, disseminators, planners, and evaluators. It is noteworthy that 91% of the students in the Fordham Applied Developmental Psychology program "are planning university-based research careers" [Fisher et al. 1993, p. 300]. This is an adventurous program that embodies several of the characteristics discussed in this chapter, although it is clearly a psychology program. I suspect this will also be the goal of many graduates of psychological wellness training, but in the future I hope a fair proportion of them opt for community and policy related positions. If they can contribute to making a difference in psychological wellness knowledge, activities, and policies in the public interest and retain connections with academia, so much the better. This outcome would confirm the bidirectionality of the enterprise.

## The Academic and Community Contexts of Training for Psychological Wellness

One of the early simple questions I asked myself was, "Psychological wellness is fine, but is it psychology?" A very quick answer was, "Yes, but it is so much more than that." In thinking and reading about some of the requirements and desirables for psychological wellness, many of which haven't been mentioned in this material, the question became a much more difficult one. Is there any academic setting in which a program so multidisciplinary can be carried out? Although multidisciplinary education is becoming more evident in universities, the power of disciplinary departments is still regnant. We have suggested the need to span the substantive distance between developmental neurobiology and political science. A fair guess is that such a program would present monumental challenges. Yet the goal is well worth trying to pursue. Psychology or an already multidisciplinary department or program, such as social ecology or human development and family studies, can take the lead. Other entities, such as public health and anthropology, have been suggested as well. I feel that psychologists are indispensable to any group attempting such a program, and I am aware of the mammoth resistance that many departments of psychology would create for such an endeavor. That is a serious issue, and I would recommend that we choose our battles judiciously; attempts should be made in the few places where they may be welcome (there's not a total wasteland out there; some material I read recently from the University of Illinois at Chicago was very impressive in its multidisciplinary cooperation). I shall address many of my remarks to the example of a psychology department. One of the first tasks is getting our own ducks in a row. The intradisciplinary span of psychology seems almost as broad as the program we envision. We should not fool ourselves about that superficial resemblance. It is necessary to involve disciplines far beyond our own in a major collaborative effort. Psychology must have sufficient will to invest in such a time-consuming and costly effort. Weissberg and Greenberg specifically mention several specialties in psychology that need stronger prevention training: clinical, community, developmental, health and social [1998, p. 924]. Psychological wellness training requires input from these, and in addition school, counseling, industrial, environmental, cognitive, personality, and psychobiology or behavioral neuroscience should be tapped, suggestions based on material for pathways to psychological wellness mentioned previously. The psychobiologists can ultimately provide links with developmental neurobiology.

The job of interesting, convincing, and involving persons from disciplines outside psychology is not an easy one. The presence of a viable research base for psychological wellness will have to be made clear to them. What stake do they have in psychological wellness? What are the incentives for their cooperation, for them to give their expertise, time, and effort to such a venture? We have a tough selling job to do. All of the usual ways of garnering support—using informal collegial relationships, especially among senior faculty; soliciting the interest and active support of higher echelons of the university; gaining some allies in the medical school or school of public health—will need to be explored. Given the scope and anticipated problems, however, outside funding may be required. A long-term goal would be the creation of some doctoral level programs with the richness and breadth of contributions mentioned previously. This field, despite its name, should not be restricted to psychology majors. In order to attract other fields to such a program, we should agree to cross-train each other's students, which means that psychologists will be training, and supporting, cultural anthropologists and economists, for example. In order to maximize possibilities, postdoctoral training and mid-career shifts should be entertained. It is likely that simultaneous activities at the doctoral, postdoctoral, and mid-career levels will be needed in an effort to launch this new area. The use of postdoctorals and mid-career shift "students" in the double role as instructors for doctoral students should be considered. Consortial postdoctoral training programs, involving individuals and faculty from several universities, have been federally funded and might be models to explore for psychological wellness training. Private foundation support should also be solicited.

It is clear from what has been presented to this point that a fourth requirement indispensable to a psychological wellness training program is leadership. The qualities, motivation, experience, and time necessary to construct a program of this complexity prompt the question of whether a single individual is able to carry this off. My guess is no. Although I have qualms about programs run by committee, this sort of endeavor needs many proponents and would benefit especially from senior, respected backers who will participate. This is by no means a problem without some potential benefit, for if the necessary cooperation and involvement can be obtained from colleagues within a discipline or within a behavioral and social sciences group, the possibility of enlisting contributions from more distant disciplines is improved. Even within such a group or committee, there is usually one person who should be a leader among leaders. I am reminded of recent examples of consortial postdoctoral training programs, prevention training programs, and centers where the complexity and breadth is comparable to that envisioned in psychological wellness programs. The consortial training programs in family process and in emotion research involved contributors from ten or more universities. Mavis Hetherington directed the family process program, and Paul Ekman crafted the emotion program. In prevention research training, Roger Weissberg and Irwin Sandler come to mind as directors of complex, state-of-the-art programs, and the AIDS research center in San Francisco, directed by Thomas Coates, boasts not only a domestic but an international training program, as well as exemplary connections with the local, state, national, and international communities. If I were to try to think of a few simple terms that characterized the leaders of these programs, they would include vision, energy, and complete dedication to the task.

I have assiduously avoided providing a curriculum because I think that the major general principles governing training, i.e. the conceptual framework, the substantive scope, the recommended coherence of academic and field experience, and the qualities of leadership, are most important in guiding the development of programs. Curricula will, as always, vary from place to place, and experimentation and risk taking are encouraged. We will all need to see what works. However, I would add one recommendation based upon the provocative suggestion made by Richard Price, who served as a discussant for a symposium on training for prevention at the 1998 annual meeting of the American Psychological Association. Price advised doing away with the requirement for a dissertation. For training programs in psychological wellness, such an inherently collaborative program, that strikes me as a sterling idea. In its place, I would recommend a required collaborative study, preferably in a real life setting, of a problem of relevance to psychological wellness.

Perhaps the major changes needed in the academic context to provide a favorable environment for psychological wellness training have to do with internal revisions in the prevailing "rules of the game" in most academic departments, including those in psychology. Lerner and Miller [1993] in the attempt to "build faculty enthusiasm for, and strength in, the approach to research and outreach associated with a developmental contextual view of human ecology and development" have addressed this issue in language as clear as I have seen:

> First, we need to engage high-quality faculty in revising the way they envision their scholarly and research careers. Second, we need to alter what has been the normative connection between faculty research and the community that is served by our university. Third, then, faculty members need to see outreach not as an activity that is separate from their research but, to the contrary, as a key component in their attempts to do ecologically valid research, within specific communities, about the nature of life in these settings. A final challenge involves the need to effect changes in the reward system within institutions of higher education. In order for scholars to begin to reorient their own work, university tenure and promotion committees evaluating scientists studying development must be urged to begin to value multidisciplinary collaborative, and hence multiauthored, publications—even more than publications from individual scholars writing within their own disciplines. [p. 362]

The experiential components of psychological wellness training involving contact with individuals, families, groups, settings, communities and aspects of the legal and the political process may prove equally problematic. Many years ago, in discussing the ethical dilemmas in mental health prevention, I remarked that the community might respond to proposed interventions with the question, "Who asked you to do anything?" This is not an irrational response of healthy populations, who like to get on with their lives, science notwithstanding, and suggests that ethical questions may be even more of an issue in psychological wellness. Several interventions are mentioned by Cowen [1994] and by Weissberg and Greenberg [1998]. They predominantly involve children, and many are carried out on disadvantaged populations. Would advantaged populations, especially advantaged adults, serve as research subjects or provide openings for psychological wellness students' experiential needs? We need to be concerned that psychological wellness students have experience with people from a broad socioeconomic spectrum.

The research and experiential needs of psychological wellness students in the community bring us back once again to the relationship between psychological wellness and primary prevention. Cowen [1994] clearly states that wellness enhancement "includes, but is not limited to, primary prevention approaches. Otherwise put, although most primary prevention goals and activities fit neatly within a wellness enhancement framework, they do not exhaust that framework. Within the latter matrix, psychological wellness is the overarching goal and the term wellness enhancement is used to describe a family of strategies for advancing that goal" [p. 154]. Weissberg and Greenberg [1998] describe Cowen's position as a synthesis of the risk-oriented primary prevention and wellness enhancement positions, but my understanding of his position is that primacy is accorded to wellness enhancement. Weissberg and Greenberg subsequently state, "Primary prevention is a term that comfortably subsumes health promotion (i.e. general primary prevention), competence enhancement, universal prevention interventions, and selective interventions for epidemiologically at-risk groups" [p. 897]. Although Weissberg and Greenberg have done an extraordinary job in trying to untangle the conceptual and definitional morass of primary prevention, wellness enhancement (they use the term competence enhancement, which is only a part of Cowen's psychological wellness), and health promotion, I am not sure how comfortably they are subsumed under primary prevention. It seems to me that their statement is somewhat at odds with Cowen's conclusion, and that prevention must have an "of what" implicit in the term, the "what" being undesirable.

But there are added reasons for my concern, rooted in the restless uneasiness reflected in the comments at the beginning of this article and in the issue of change and continuity. I firmly believe we need to engage the broader concept of the enhancement of psychological wellness as something qualitatively different from, although related to, primary prevention as we have come to use the term in psychology. I agree with Cowen that psychological wellness leads to a different set of questions, a much different level of activity and engagement, and an opportunity for psychology to widen its collaborative pursuits and increase its potential impact on the well-being of the general population. Moreover, ultimately this approach should exert a corrective influence on the way we have traditionally understood and dealt with mental health and mental health casualties. We will find ourselves initially borrowing heavily from primary prevention sources because they have extended our reach and conceptualizations and are relevant to psychological wellness. If, however, we are bold enough to overcome our own insularity, we shall be in uncharted waters with a great deal to learn.

For the present, it seems likely that basic behavioral and social science research will provide the bedrock of scientific information regarding psychological wellness, and that psychological wellness experts, working closely with community participants, will disseminate this to settings and other community elements, larger systems, and social policy levels. For the future, we can hope for the development of a more extensive body of knowledge addressed systematically to the enhancement of psychological wellness and the training of people who will know how to use it for the public good.

## Additional Issues and Concluding Thoughts

- It isn't expected that all of those who aren't ill will be robustly healthy; this is a continuum, after all, and many may not be ill, but may lead what Thoreau aptly called lives of quiet desperation. Even in this group there is great diversity. There is a common danger in thinking about the continuum as one of normality and abnormality; value-laden terms of that sort are unwise, but psychological wellness does not exclude the probability of uniqueness and the possibility of many kinds of eccentricities. Special attention should be accorded to transitional periods in the life course and to counterintuitive findings, such as the large number of people who overcome obstacles and demonstrate remarkable resilience to stress and adversity.

• The nub of my uneasiness, which persists, has to do with the shifting complexity of what makes for psychological wellness over time. I realize I have used mainly microsystemic illustrations throughout the material on pathways to wellness. The strands of psychological wellness come from the rich interactions of biopsychosocial factors in multiple contexts at each period of the life course and across levels of the social ecology – ontogenetic development and elements of the micro-, meso-, exo-, and macrosystems [Bronfenbrenner, 1979; Weissberg and Greenberg, 1998; Cicchetti and Toth, 1998]. The question remains, is it possible for any training program to present this array of material with the necessary depth, clarity, and vision? Possible, perhaps, but not likely. The task, to be done well, would be daunting.

• A few years ago, I gave an address [Schneider 1993] entitled "If It Ain't Broke...". I completed the phrase, not with the expected "don't fix it," but rather by saying that sustained attention needed to be paid to the persistent and unglamorous task of making certain that "what ain't broke" stays that way. Treatment and cure, which are glamorous, are the linchpins of the health industry and of a great deal of biomedical and even behavioral research. Focus for a moment on the words *sustained attention, persistent, and unglamorous* because these describe much more accurately the tasks involved to ensure psychological wellness. Similar words may be used to characterize prevention. We hope people will understand and implement the pathways to psychological wellness and have the tools necessary to create settings and broader environments favorable to psychological wellness. As development proceeds, these tasks require sustained attention, persistence, and discipline. Psychological wellness for *all* the people is a task of enormous complexity, demanding uncommon perseverance. We need a real alliance with the public. I have suggested that a large number of psychology areas would have desirable participants in this undertaking. We have made significant contributions to the understanding of psychological illness. We may be able to do perhaps even more for psychological wellness. The generative possibilities of this field are truly exciting. This is a stellar opportunity to "give psychology away" [Miller, 1969].

## REFERENCES

Bronfenbrenner, U. (1979). *The ecology of human development: Experiments by nature and design.* Cambridge, MA: Harvard University Press.

Cairns, R. B. (1986). Phenomena lost: Issues in the study of development. In J. Valsiner (Ed.), *The individual subject and scientific psychology* (pp. 97–112). New York: Plenum Press.

Cairns, R. B. & Cairns, B. D. (1994). *Lifelines and risks: Pathways of youth in our time.* Cambridge, UK: Cambridge University Press.

Campbell, D. T. (1969). Ethnocentrism of disciplines and the fish scale model of omniscience. In M. Sherif & C. W. Sherif (Eds.), *Interdisciplinary relationships in the social sciences* (pp. 328–348). Chicago: Aldine.

Cicchetti, D. (1993). Developmental psychopathology: Reactions, reflections, projections. *Developmental Review, 13,* 471–502.

Cicchetti, D. (1996). Child maltreatment: Implications for developmental theory and research. *Human Development, 39,* 18–39.

Cicchetti, D. & Toth, S. (1991). The making of a developmental psychopathologist. In J. Cantor, C. Spiker, & L. Lipsitt (Eds.), *Child behavior and development: Training for diversity* (pp. 35–72). Norwood, NJ: Ablex.

Cicchetti, D. & Toth, S. L. (1998). The development of depression in children and adolescents. *American Psychologist, 53,* 221–241.

Coie, J. D., Watt, N. F., West, S. G., Hawkins, J. D., Asarnow, J. R., Markman, H. J., Ramey, S. L., Shure, M. B., & Long, B. (1993). The science of prevention: A conceptual framework and some directions for a national research program. *American Psychologist, 48,* 1013–1022.

Compas, B. E. (1993). Promoting positive mental health during adolescence. In S. G. Millstein, A. C. Petersen, & E. O. Nightingale (Eds.), *Promoting the health of adolescents: New directions for the twenty first century* (pp. 159–179). New York: Oxford University Press.

Cowen, E. L. (1994). The enhancement of psychological wellness: Challenges and opportunities. *American Journal of Community Psychology, 22,* 149–179.

Cowen, E. L. (1996). The ontogenesis of primary prevention: Lengthy strides and stubbed toes. *American Journal of Community Psychology, 24,* 238–249.

Cowen, E. L. (1997a). *In sickness and health: Primary prevention's vows revisited.* Revision of a paper presented at the Mt. Hope Family Center 1996 symposium, Rochester, NY.

Cowen, E. L. (1997b). Schools and the enhancement of children's wellness: Some opportunities and some limiting factors. In T. P. Gullota, R. P. Weissberg, R. L. Hampton, B. A. Ryan, & G. R. Adams (Eds.), *Healthy children 2010: Establishing preventive services* (pp. 87–123). Thousand Oaks, CA: Sage Publications.

Crockett, L. J. & Petersen, A. C. (1993). Adolescent development: Health risks and opportunities for health promotion. In S. G. Millstein, A. C. Petersen, & E. O. Nightingale (Eds.), *Promoting the health of adolescents: New directions for the twenty first century* (pp. 15–37). New York: Oxford University Press.

Dunn, J. (1994). Experience and understanding of emotions, relationships, and membership in a particular culture. In P. Ekman & R. J. Davidson (Eds.), *The nature of emotion: Fundamental questions* (pp. 352–355). New York: Oxford University Press.

Eddy, J. M., Smith, P., Brown, C. H., & Reid, J. B. (1998). *An internet-based survey on the training of prevention researchers.* Unpublished manuscript.

Elliott, D. S. (1993). Health-enhancing and health-compromising lifestyles. In S. G. Millstein, A. C. Petersen, & E. O Nightingale (Eds.), *Promoting the health of adolescents: New directions for the twenty first century* (pp. 119–145). New York: Oxford University Press.

Emde R. N. (1996, May). *Early emotional development: Integrative perspectives from longitudinal study.* Paper presented at conference sponsored by National Institute of Mental Health: "Advancing research on developmental plasticity: Integrating the behavioral science and neuroscience of mental health." Chantilly, VA.

Fisher, C. B., Rau, J. B., & Colapietro, E. (1993). The Fordham University doctoral specialization in applied developmental psychology. *Journal of Applied Developmental Psychology, 14,* 289–302.

Green, L. W. (1984). Health education models. In J. D. Matarazzo, S. M. Weiss, J. A. Herd, N. E. Miller, & S. M. Weiss (Eds.), *Behavioral health: A handbook of health enhancement and disease prevention* (pp. 181–208). New York: John Wiley & Sons.

Kent, D. (1995, May/June). Member profile: Interview with training advocate Stan Schneider. *APS Observer, 8,* 24–26.

Lerner, R. M. & Miller, J. R. (1993). Integrating human development research and intervention for America's children: The Michigan State University model. *Journal of Applied Developmental Psychology, 14,* 347–364.

Masten, A. S. & Coatsworth, J. D. (1998). The development of competence in favorable and unfavorable environments. *American Psychologist, 53,* 205–220.

Miller, G. A. (1969). Psychology as a means of promoting human welfare. *American Psychologist, 24,* 1063–1075.

Mrazek, P. J. & Haggerty, R. J. (Eds.). (1994). *Reducing risks for mental disorders: Frontiers for preventive intervention research.* Washington, DC: National Academy Press.

National Institute of Mental Health (1993). *The prevention of mental disorders: A national research agenda.* Rockville, MD: Author.

National Institutes of Health, National Institute of Mental Health (1995). *Basic behavioral science research for mental health: A national investment* (NIH Publication No. 95-3682). Washington, DC: Author.

National Institutes of Health, National Institute of Mental Health (1996). *A plan for prevention research for the National Institute of Mental Health* (NIH Publication No. 96-4093). Washington, DC: Author.

Perry C. L. & Jessor, R. (1985). The concept of health promotion and the prevention of adolescent drug abuse. *Health Education Quarterly, 12,* 169–184.

Price, R. H. (1983). The education of a prevention psychologist. In R. F. Felner, L. A. Jason, J. N. Moritsugu, & S. S. Farber (Eds.), *Preventive psychology: Theory, research, and practice* (pp. 290–296). New York: Pergamon Press.

Sandler, I. N. (chair), Aiken, L., Austin, D., Bond, L., Ginsberg, M., Lorion, R., McElhaney, S., Mandell, W., Morgan, J., Taylor, C., & Weissberg, R.

(1992). *Training researchers across disciplines and career levels: Building the future of prevention research.* Unpublished report of the panel on training in prevention research for the NIMH National Conference on Prevention Research, June, 1991.

Sarason, S. B. (1996). *Barometers of change: Individual, educational, and social transformation.* San Francisco: Jossey-Bass.

Schneider, S. F. (1992, April). *On reinventing psychology.* Paper presented at a summit meeting of the American Psychological Society, Chicago, IL.

Schneider, S. F. (1993, November). *If it ain't broke....* Paper presented at the 105th annual meeting of the American Association of Medical Colleges, Washington, DC.

Schneider, S. F. (1996, October). *The importance of being Emory.* Paper presented at a symposium, *The Promotion of Wellness in Children and Adolescents: A Tribute to Emory L. Cowen,* Rochester, NY.

Weisner, T. S. (1996). Why ethnography should be the most important method in the study of human development. In R. Jessor, A. Colby, & R. A. Schweder (Eds.), *Ethnography and human development: Context and meaning in social inquiry* (pp. 305–324). Chicago: University of Chicago Press.

Weissberg, R. P. & Greenberg, M. T. (1998). School and community competence enhancement programs. In W. Damon (Series Ed.), I. E. Siegel & K. Renninger (Vol. Eds.), *Handbook of child psychology, Vol. 5: Child psychology in practice* (5th ed.) (pp. 877–954). New York: John Wiley & Sons.

# 16

## Psychological Wellness: Some Hopes for the Future

*Emory L. Cowen*

## Introduction

The theme suggested to me for this chapter was to predict the future of a wellness enhancement approach. Because I have no control either in Heaven or on Earth over factors that will shape the future, I decided to put my own "spin" on the request (i.e., rather than trying guru-style to prognosticate that hazy future, I would simply identify several things I'd like to see happen in this domain). In that way, should some archivist uncover the chapter 50 years hence, s/he won't be able to say how wrong I was—only how my hopes failed to be realized.

Wish lists of this type can be drawn up at different levels of specificity. This one will be global because, in most areas, I'm incapable of providing fine-grained detail. My modest objectives are to: a) clarify the important distinction between currently dominant, "risk-driven, disease-prevention" notions of primary prevention and the enhancement of psychological wellness; b) make a case for the need to further develop a wellness enhancement approach; and c) sketch the rough contours of a life-span wellness-enhancement approach that can coexist peacefully with the less proactive strategies of reducing fallout from risk, or undoing existing psychological damage. A key assumption of the chapter is that amplification of the generative knowledge base about individual, familial, environmental, and societal factors that act to enhance or limit psychological wellness (i.e., charting pathways between antecedent conditions, situations and events, and wellness outcomes) is a necessary precondition for framing new, multilevel, coordinated steps designed to enhance wellness. The rest of the chapter is to flesh out the preceding views.

## Risk-Disease Views of Prevention Versus Enhancing Wellness

A favorite leisure-time activity of mine in the past decade has been to try to sharpen distinctions between risk-driven, disease-prevention views of primary prevention, often seen as synonymous with all of primary prevention, and enhancing psychological wellness. Although health promotion was an important element in early definitions of primary prevention [Cowen 1973, 1980; President's Commission on Mental Health 1978], it has since been somewhat neglected [Cowen 1994, 1996, 1997a, 1997b, 1999]. The articles cited develop several facets of the preceding point, i.e., that: a) the terms primary prevention, as currently used, and wellness enhancement are not synonymous; b) the two approaches are complementary, not antagonistic; and c) wellness enhancement is the broader of the two—broad enough to incorporate a disease prevention notion of primary prevention within its framework.

A more controversial point I first raised at a conference on "Preventive Intervention in Schizophrenia: Are We Ready?" is that effective enhancement of psychological wellness from the start may have as much to offer as a disease prevention strategy in forestalling serious psychological dysfunction [Cowen 1982]. In introducing the conference volume, Pardes [1982] depicted schizophrenia as "the most puzzling and, because of its chronicity, the most severe of the major mental disorders" [p. iii]. Conference talks focused on then-current research on neuropsychological and biochemical markers of vulnerability for schizophrenia. Speakers had very different views, both about the nature of prevention and the field's readiness for preventive intervention in schizophrenia. Goldstein [1982] summarized conference views on the readiness question as follows: "If the question refers to large-scale prevention programs, designed to prevent schizophrenia, the papers in this volume do not appear to justify such massive efforts" [1982, p. vii]. That was my view as well.

Although I said as much in my talk, I went on to speculate about the extent to which a portfolio shift toward early wellness-enhancing steps, with no special focus on averting schizophrenic outcomes, "might not result in a situation, 50 years hence in which there could be fewer, rather than more, people labeled schizophrenic." [Cowen

1982, p. 189]. The thinking behind that view, however ill-formulated at the time, was that early psychological wellness is a highly desirable outcome in its own right and an important resource (protective factor) for averting later, serious psychological dysfunction.

My conference talk won no awards for operational clarity. Although I suggested that it might be "more sensible, humane, pragmatic, and cost-effective to build health and/or to prevent dysfunction than to struggle, however nobly and skillfully, to contain or manage its costly, devastating residuals" [Cowen 1982, p. 183], I had little to say about how best to pursue that lofty goal, in good measure because I hadn't yet sharpened in my mind the important distinction between risk-driven, disorder-prevention, versus wellness enhancement, approaches. Today, I can say a bit more about what was only beginning to germinate at the "Are we ready?" conference, in the service of this chapter's prime goal, i.e., formulating a wellness wish list for the future.

In terms of need, I've urged major reallocations of energies and resources from the costly, frustrating business of trying to repair rooted dysfunction—mental health's past and still dominant way— toward both risk-driven primary prevention _and_ wellness enhancement approaches [Cowen 1994, 1997a]. These two approaches, collectively, now attract less than 3% of all mental health resources [Durlak 1997]. Within that framework, however, I: a) cautioned that the goals, methodologies, targeting, and optimal timings of these preventively directed strategies differed considerably; and b) expressed the hope that wellness enhancement approaches would be given reasonable consideration in the future, rather than playing second fiddle as they have in the past.

I speak of the latter as a hope because today's dominant view in prevention rhetoric and resource allocation begins with risk identification and, on that base, seeks first and foremost to forestall serious (i.e., DSM IV-type) psychological disorders. Indeed, influential current sources [Coie et al. 1993; Koretz 1991; Koretz & Moscicki 1997; Mrazek & Haggerty 1994; Mrazek & Hall 1997] tend either to equate this strategy with all of primary prevention, or at least see it as its true nerve center. Although I am hardly a solo voice in the wellness "cheering section" [Albee 1996; Durlak 1997; Durlak & Wells 1997a,

1997b; Elias 1995; Masten & Coatsworth 1998], in today's dominant, risk-disease prevention world, a wellness enhancement strategy is often, at best, only a polite afterthought [Cowen 1999]. Consistent with that perception, Dinges [1994] reported that only 2% of the cites in Trickett, Dahiyat & Selby's [1994] annotated primary prevention bibliography reflected mental health promotion, as opposed to disorder prevention activities. Given that Durlak and Wells' [1997a] meta-analysis of primary prevention studies showed wellness enhancement to be at least as effective as disorder prevention approaches, the question of why it has attracted less attention merits consideration.

Advocates of a disorder-targeted view of primary prevention have downplayed wellness enhancement on two counts. The first is that it is a qualitatively different "breed of cat" that doesn't belong with disorder prevention. That view is reflected in a quote from IOM Report *The Prevention of Mental Disorders* [Mrazek & Haggerty 1994]: "Health promotion is not driven by an emphasis on illness, but rather by a focus on the enhancement of well being" [p. 27]—a phrasing that comes close to saying that the goal of enhancing wellness, *per se*, bars an approach from being seen as primary prevention. As such, it turns attention away from the possibility suggested above—that enhancing well-being from the start and consistently thereafter may prove to be *one* effective way to prevent some forms of serious psychological dysfunction.

A second reason given by primary prevention devotees for by-passing wellness approaches is an alleged lack of consensus about "how to define, describe or measure mental health well-being" [Muñoz, Mrazek & Haggerty 1996, p. 1121]. In addressing this point earlier, although I recognized that the terms wellness and sickness reflect value judgments that can vary substantially across cultures and subgroups within a culture, I argued that there is enough agreement about their meaning in our culture, reflecting behavioral and psychological marker-variables, to permit formulation of consensually validated goals (outcomes) in such basic domains as primary prevention, psychotherapy, education, and child-rearing [Cowen 1994; 1999]. That view is not inconsistent with Muñoz et al.'s [1996] depiction of wellness as a "sense of coherence, self-efficacy, empowerment, zest, resilience, energy, flexibility, order, balance, harmony and integrity" [p. 1121]. Even though several of those descriptors are fuzzy, the sum of the ideals listed offers a reasonable start toward identifying agreed-upon, desirable wellness outcomes.

Hence, I resist the arguments that wellness enhancement approaches are dismissible either because: a) they are not (on the surface, at any rate) driven by the prime goal of reducing serious psychological disorder; or b) we lack a perfect consensus in defining wellness. Quite likely, several other realities have done more to restrict the development of this approach. One is the lack of systematic theory (and in some key areas, supporting research data) about factors that promote the early development of wellness and operate to maintain or enhance it. The latter, multistranded matters [cf. below] implicate families of shaping variables, some within mental health's purview, others well beyond its knowledge or competence bases.

A second major deterrent to the development of wellness enhancement approaches is that wellness, for many, is a shadowy concept that is hard to relate to in the here and now. Our society's preoccupations, as reflected in the media and by policymakers and budget shapers, pivot around florid failures in wellness (e.g., crime and delinquency, violence, child abuse and neglect, substance abuse, AIDS, major psychological disorder, depression, homelessness, and cult-related disasters) that affect individuals and society in dramatically negative ways [Durlak 1997]. Each of those attention-capturing, upsetting, conditions has vocal pressure groups clamoring for its obliteration. Legislators, and agencies that translate "legislative will" into policy and funding decisions, are inevitably swept into urgent crusades to wipe out social blights and the troublesome, costly problems associated with them. Necessarily, the concerns of these policy-shaping groups gravitate less to who is well than to who is sick, especially if the "sickness" rocks an ugly, societal boat.

Thus, the attention of policy shaping and funding groups mirrors today's eyesores, those of an immediate tomorrow, and loud constituent voices that create pressures to act. The idea that effective prevention today might make for a better, more cost-saving tomorrow in the vexing outcome areas noted above is too remote to attract serious support. Few people can relate to the idea of waiting 20 years to see how things will turn out. Thus, in practice, the objective of wellness enhancement has two strikes against it before it gets started.

In my view, some powerful arguments for a wellness enhancement strategy come from serendipitous discoveries, as, for example, the convergent conclusion of three recent reviews [Tolan & Guerra 1994; Yoshikawa 1994; Zigler, Taussig, & Black 1992] that the strongest delinquency prevention effects found came *not* from specifically targeted, "window-of-opportunity" programs [Reiss & Price 1996] for pre- or early adolescents, but rather as a hidden and delayed benefit of effective early, comprehensive, family-oriented competence enhancement programs for preschoolers. At the time those programs were conducted, their prime goal was to enhance poor children's readiness for school; they had little intended relevance for preventing delinquency. Yet, 15 years later, that's exactly what happened!

In seeking to understand this major unanticipated benefit, observers [Berrueta-Clement et al. 1984; Yoshikawa 1995] have hypothesized a chain of felicitous events. In that chain, preparedness for school entry paves the way for: a better educational experience [Kagan & Neuman 1997]; preparedness for life; and, ultimately, more positive outcomes on such bellwether indicators as education level attained, employment status and income, and fewer instances of welfare, delinquency, and crime [Schweinhart, Barnes, & Weikart 1993; Weikart & Schweinhart 1997]. The active early ingredient in these effective programs was the rooting of positive attitudes and school readiness skills in children and families. Solidifying educational accomplishment, in turn, paved the way to achieving key positive goals and averting many serious negative outcomes with roots in lack of preparedness for school. The latter include academic problems, getting into trouble with teachers, rejection by peers, and disengaging from normal school and peer contexts—each an outcome that augurs difficulty in the transition to adolescence [McLoyd 1998].

Although the preceding example of how significant benefit in *disorder prevention* can accrue from a sound early wellness start is compelling, it is not unique, i.e., it can be extended to negative outcomes other than delinquency. For example, although there is much evidence that marital disruption predisposes adjustment problems for children and interferes with the mastery of normal developmental tasks [Amato & Keith 1991; Hetherington 1989; Hetherington, Bridges, & Insabella 1998], it is also the case that children vary markedly in how they adapt to this stressor. In seeking to account for this variability, Hetherington et al. [1998] viewed early wellness as a crucial protective factor that helps children cope with the base-rate woes associated with disruption of their parents' marriage.

Cicchetti and Toth [1998] offer a structurally similar example with regard to childhood depression. Noting that depressotypic pre-dispositions have roots in infancy, they argue cogently that early wellness building steps such as strengthening parent-child attachment and communication bonds, and enhancing child competencies can act protectively to prevent later depression.

The preceding examples underscore two key points. Early wellness: a) gives the young child a "jump-start" in life; and b) can potentially have more protective value in forestalling diverse, maladaptive "end-states" than later, specifically targeted interventions for those same conditions. A cautionary note however: To argue, as I do, that early wellness importantly favors later wellness outcomes, falls well short of saying that it insures such outcomes. Subsequent threats to wellness can, and do, emerge not only from the vicissitudes of life, but from the different demands and challenges of different developmental periods. A comprehensive theory of wellness must pay heed to those realities.

To summarize: lack of vocal constituencies or promise for prompt elimination of social blights, make wellness enhancement remote and impalpable for many people. At the same time, evidence pointing to the approaches' potential efficacy [Albee & Gullotta 1997; Durlak 1997; Durlak & Wells 1997a; Weissberg & Greenberg 1998], including disorder prevention findings cited above, underscores the need for greater investment in such efforts both in their own right and in their potential for addressing the awesome problems that major psychological dysfunction poses for individuals and society.

## Undoing versus Forming Well

Historically, mental health's prime mandate has been to contain or reduce unfortunate psychological outcomes. Although there are some differences in how, precisely, people define the latter boundary limits, outcomes widely seen as "concerns of pertinence" include: the psychoses; personality and character disorders; depression; chronic unhappiness and ineffectuality; and specific deleterious conditions such as child and spouse abuse, drug and alcohol abuse, delinquency, and crime and violence. No one questions the formidable, non-repressible, costly nature of these problems; rather, the tactical issue at stake is how best to engage them. Although mental health's classic way— striving to undo or contain, dysfunction after it becomes evident—has logged important successes, it is at best an after-the-fact approach that does not reduce the need for future restorative efforts. Otherwise put, no matter how much success the system as articulated achieves, new, equally vexing problems that require similar attention will continue to spring up. A system so pressed at all times conjures up the image of the little Dutch boy striving valiantly to forestall inundation by putting his finger in the leaking dike.

Growing awareness of the limited efficacy and reach of a repair model has elevated the salience of both "risk detection-disorder prevention" *and* wellness-enhancement models for addressing the heavy, unresolved problems that plague the mental health fields. Reflecting this evolution, Masten and Coatsworth [1998] observed that "Prevention at its best represents both an effort to foster competence and to prevent problems" [p. 216]. These two conceptual alternatives are best seen as complementary [Cowen 1997b], i.e., they share common features but also diverge importantly. Two key assumptions they share are that: a) the insufficiencies of past, exclusively restorative approaches fuel a need for viable alternatives; and b) preventing dysfunction is one such promising alternative. However even among those who accept both these assumptions, important differences remain in beliefs about what prevention really means and how best to pursue its goals.

Around these divergencies lies a "Tale of Two Models." The first, more widely ascribed-to model, builds intervention on a base of identified risk factors, with the overarching goal of preventing serious psychological dysfunction. That model, adopted by the IOM report [Mrazek & Haggerty 1994] and the National Institute of Mental Health, heavily shapes current prevention activities and funding. It is a model with specified, sequential steps said to comprise *the* "prevention intervention cycle": 1) identify the disorder to be prevented; 2) review information on risk and protective factors relating to it; 3) conduct and analyze pilot studies of program models based on information about risk and prevention; 4) design, conduct, and evaluate large-scale trials based on effective pilot models; and 5) disseminate, i.e., promote large-scale community-level program applications [IOM Summary 1994, Muehrer 1997].

Specific features of this model are said to frame the essences of a new *"science of prevention"* [Coie et al. 1993; IOM Report 1994; Koretz 1991; Muehrer 1997]. Although more will be said about a science of prevention later, several of its underlying features are highlighted here. One is its prime targeting to specific psychological disorders of substantial magnitude. A second is its implicit assumption that disorder conditions are largely discrete, and that each has its own special "preventive pathway." A third is the belief that the model has equipotential applicability at different points in the life cycle, and a fourth is that the model best comes into play when "windows of opportunity" (i.e., prodromal risk indicators) appear [Reiss & Price 1996].

Although a wellness enhancement model accepts prevention of major disorder as one prime goal, it differs from a disease-prevention model in its assumptions about the genesis of dysfunction and the extent to which effective building from the start, rather than efforts to contain or undo damage, can both advance and go beyond the goals of disease prevention. It is thus broader and more inclusive than a risk-disease prevention model [Cowen 1997b]. Although it can readily accept and incorporate the latter's goals and methodologies, the sum of all that is but one (not necessarily the most important) of its components.

Inclinations toward risk-driven primary prevention versus wellness enhancement approaches may, in part, be shaped by the weights one attaches to the notions of *multicausality* and *multifinality* [Cicchetti & Cohen 1995; Cicchetti & Rogosch 1996; Durlak 1997]. The term multicausality, also called equifinality, refers to the fact that a given adverse outcome can come about for many reasons and via many different routes. Multifinality, by contrast, means that a given risk factor can potentiate many different adverse outcomes. The concept, however, does not assume that all risk indicators have the same "multifinality-potential." Egeland, Pianta, and Ogawa [1996], for example, found that young children's early internalizing symptoms had much broader dispersion of outcomes (i.e., greater multifinality) than early externalizing risk factors. The latter more narrowly favored antisocial outcomes. Most basically, however, Cicchetti and Rogosch [1996] argued that an "appreciation" of the concepts of multicausality and multifinality can enrich theory and research by directing attention to the complex ties and systemic interactions that operate to shape pathological and wellness outcomes.

Durlak [1997] considered the place of these two concepts in a prevention framework. After presenting evidence that specific risk factors do indeed predispose multiple adverse outcomes (i.e., multifinality), he argued: "If one negative outcome that is prevented is a risk factor for other (negative) outcomes, prevention programs should be able to simultaneously prevent multiple negative outcomes" [p. 184]. That view highlights the appeal of early, wellness-building steps that lay down essential roots such as a wholesome attachment relationship and acquiring stage salient competencies [Cowen 1994; 1999; Durlak 1997]. The absence of those nutrients creates a soil that predisposes maladaptive outcomes. Thus, in principle, early wellness building can provide the young child with resources that reduce the likelihood of many individually and socially costly outcomes. On that basis, Durlak [1997] argued that "future interventions should concentrate on those factors that may be particularly important in protecting against negative outcomes... or enhancing positive health" [p. 188]. Durlak and Wells' [1997a] meta-analysis provided evidence of the beneficial effects of such wellness enhancement programs.

The principle of multifinality helps to clarify why sound early wellness building may be an appealing way to reduce the occurrence of diverse negative outcomes. Although strengthening the host does not guarantee immunity, it holds much protective potential. By contrast, prevention programs that assume adverse outcomes to have specific risk antecedents may be limited by: a) missing those at risk for a given outcome who reach that point via risk factors other than the program's targeted one(s); b) including people for whom common identified risk factors predispose serious negative outcomes in areas other than the one(s) to which a given intervention is targeted; and c) identifying risk factors so late that a program's potential benefit is seriously restricted.

Preventive interventions built around specific risk-factors may thus be insufficiently sensitive to the fact that different risk precursors can predispose the same negative outcome, and the same risk factor may lead to different maladaptive outcomes. Organizational theory suggests that this happens because the effects on functioning of any specific system component depend on the broader context in which it is embedded [Cicchetti & Rogosch 1996]. Thus, the toll exacted by a given risk factor is likely to be a function of important interactions between it and specifics of the defining fabric of a person's life situation (e.g., basic attachment relationships, family milieu factors, peer influences, stressors encountered and "opportunities"). To the extent that such factors are important, it again points to the need for early wellness building that provides meaningful inoculation against the diverse vulnerabilities that many widely acknowledged risk factors predispose.

## Toward a More Comprehensive Wellness Enhancement Model

In arguing the need for a wellness enhancement approach, Cowen [1999] proposed a mini-structural model that focused on two sets of variables thought to favor _early_ wellness formation: a) a sound, caring parent-child attachment relationship; and b) the child's acquisition of early stage-salient competencies. That model identified four sets of input variables, some modifiable, others not, which, by promoting those two instrumental conditions, enhance early wellness: a) _caregiver_ variables, such as prior and current adjustment, sensitivity and responsivity to the child's needs, and sense of efficacy as a parent; b) _family milieu_ variables including a sound partner relationship and good relationships among family members, as seen by the caregiver;

c) *child* variables including such "givens" as attractiveness, an easy temperament, and intelligence; and d) the absence of major stressors that create ongoing concerns for the caregiver.

That earlier analysis was limited in two key respects. First, it dealt only cross-sectionally with factors thought to favor wellness formation in infancy and early childhood, not the salutogenic processes that undergird such felicitous outcomes [Antonovsky 1979]. Much remains to be learned about the roots of those processes, and pathways between those roots and later positive child outcomes. Indeed, in this context, recent theorizing and research on neural plasticity [Cicchetti & Tucker 1994; Nelson & Bloom 1997] suggests that the very process of brain differentiation, including aspects that relate to wellness outcomes, once thought to be tightly scripted genetically, is importantly shaped by positive and negative environmental experiences. One step beyond, Nelson & Bloom [1997] speculated that experientially stimulated brain modification "at the cellular, physiological and possibly microanatomic levels" [p. 983] may be the neural mechanism that accounts for the success of diverse wellness-related interventions.

Strengthening the conceptual footings of a wellness enhancement approach in the preceding directions would form more solid bedrock on which to build proactive, wellness-oriented interventions. Illustratively, the extent to which a sound, current parent-child attachment relationship evolves depends on significant experiences in the caregiver's life history, as well as her sense of efficacy and wellness as a person [Belsky 1984]. Relatedly, family milieus are likely to be shaped by the nature of the spousal relationship, the psychological environment in which each grew up, and the "mix" of interpersonal interaction patterns and conflict resolution styles that these antecedents favor. Implicit in this historical-interactional focus is the belief that certain types of early experiences are likely to have intergenerational predisposing qualities, for better or worse. If so, effective here-and-now wellness building efforts can help to break down repetitive intergenerational cycles that lead to socially and personally unfortunate outcomes.

Narrowness is a second, even more serious, limitation of my prior analysis [Cowen 1998]. The skeletal model proposed must be expanded to reflect complex determinants that significantly shape wellness outcomes over the long haul (e.g., the environmental conditions under which children develop; the nature and shaping impact of key social institutions such as schools). The latter input sources are more complex and less controllable than the two [cf. above] that govern sound early wellness starts. However, because they become more important as direct wellness-shaping forces as children grow up, they must be taken into serious account in moving from a circumscribed theory of early wellness development to a more complex lifespan framework for understanding how wellness comes about, and how it is supported or eroded over time.

Bronfenbrenner's [1977] article "Towards An Experimental Ecology of Human Development," targeted primarily to developmental research issues when it was written, provides a rich conceptual framework that reflects the complex input sources—some fully visible, others subtle—that shape wellness outcomes. Bronfenbrenner argued that "an understanding of human development" (and, in my view, the ontogenesis and maintenance of psychological wellness) "requires examination of multiperson systems of interaction, not limited to a single setting, and must take into account aspects of the environment beyond the immediate situation containing the subject" [1977, p. 514]. Achieving this goal calls for "study of the progressive mutual accommodations, throughout the life-span, between a growing human organism and the changing immediate environments in which it actually lives and grows," as this process is affected by relations within and between the "immediate settings containing the developing person... and the larger social contexts, both formal and informal, in which these settings are embedded" [1977, p. 513]. Bronfenbrenner's thesis underscores several key points, i.e., that: a) human development (and wellness) are shaped by multiple sources of influence and diverse person-environment interactions; b) these sources change in number, impact, and ways of interacting over time; and consequently, c) adaptation is susceptible to change over the course of development [Emde & Harmon 1984].

Bronfenbrenner identified four levels of input that importantly shape human development. The first and most visible, the *microsystem*, is "a complex of relations between the developing person and environment in an immediate setting (e.g., home, school, workplace) containing that person" [1977, p. 514]. Cowen's [1999] analysis of the ontogenesis of early psychological wellness was built around one important microsystem, i.e., the family context into which the child is born, particularly the nature of the caregiver-child interaction.

*Mesosystems* are a second source of influence on development. They are made up of "interrelationships among major settings (e.g., family, school), containing the developing person at a particular point in life" [1977, p. 515]. Because mesosystems involve major interactive components, they are more diffuse and difficult to assess than a microsystem. The *exosystem*, a third level of influence, is "an extension of the mesosystem embracing other specific social structures, both formal and informal, that do not themselves contain the developing person, but impinge upon [those] settings and thus influence... what goes on there" [1977, p. 515]. These sources include "major institutions of the society... as they operate at a concrete local level... e.g., the world of work, the neighborhood, the mass media, communication and transportation facilities, and informal social networks" [1977, p. 515].

Although the fourth source of influence, the *macrosystem*, differs qualitatively from all others and is the most difficult to pin down, it is a shaping force that has major impact on people's wellness. The macrosystem differs from the three prior systems in that it does not reflect specific contexts that affect people's lives, but rather "general prototypes (or blueprints)... that set the pattern for the structures and activities occurring at the concrete level" [1977, p. 515]. Although some aspects of a macrosystem are explicit, (e.g., in laws or regulations), most are "informal and carried out unwittingly;" Sarason [1971] called the latter "hidden regularities."

Specifically, Bronfenbrenner defined a macrosystem as "the overarching institutional patterns of ... economic, social, educational, legal and political systems of which micro- meso-, and eco-systems are the concrete manifestations. Macrosystems ... explicitly and implicitly endow meaning and motivation to particular agencies, social networks, roles and activities, and their interrelations. What place or priority children and those responsible for their care have in such macrosystems is of special importance in determining how a child and his or her caretakers are treated and interact with each other in different types of settings" [1977, p. 515].

Bronfenbrenner's analysis highlights the enormous complexity and changing nature of the influence sources that shape human development and wellness, at any cross-sectional point and over the lifetime course. For that reason, it is much easier to pedestalize the ideal of wellness enhancement, than it will be to bring off the many steps needed to advance that goal systematically. The latter "tall order" will at best be pursued only slowly over time, at many different levels, using diverse change strategies that rest upon different knowledge bases and expertise.

A small case in point: I have long argued that a warm, caring attachment relationship and rooting stage salient competencies is the stuff that shapes good wellness starts in infancy and early childhood. Others have said much the same [e.g., Carlson & Sroufe 1995; Masten & Coatsworth 1998]. Yet even those who have ardently championed the importance of wholesome early starts, and their protective value against, for example, the ravages of poverty [McLoyd 1990; 1998; Zigler & Styfco 1994], caution that good starts *alone* cannot wipe out the disastrous effects of such massive and widespread stressors.

The preceding is just another way of saying that enhancing wellness systematically calls for complex, not simple, solutions. Although rooting early wellness in the child is a giant step in the right direction, it wins only one battle in a major, ongoing war. A cohesive, lifespan-oriented effort to enhance psychological wellness will require inputs from diverse specialists working in concert, in different ways and at different levels, to advance a set of shared (wellness-related) goals. It is a challenge that calls for multiple approaches, multiple solutions, multiple sources of expertise, new modes of communication and interaction, and much dedication, patience, and tenacity. Like Bronfenbrenner's overarching model, and this chapter's broad wellness enhancement framework, Cicchetti and Lynch's [1993] more focused, ecological/transactional model for preventing community violence and child maltreatment also rests on the view that any serious approach to such goals would "need to be carried out at different levels of the ecology" [p. 114].

## Science of Prevention Revisited

Bronfenbrenner's framework provides a helpful backdrop against which to revisit the concept of science of prevention—a term used increasingly in the 1990s, often in a haloed way. Although those who introduced it and advocated its adoption [e.g., Coie et al. 1993; IOM

Report 1994] have defined it clearly, some users have strayed from that definition and capitalized on the term's "in" status to legitimize what they are doing—however removed that may be from the concept's intended usage. Although such misuse, of course, is not the responsibility of those who introduced the term, it is nevertheless a bothersome, counterproductive reality. More relevant for this chapter, however, are several of the good and limiting aspects of a *correct* (i.e., as intended) usage of the term "science of prevention," as the latter relates to wellness enhancement goals.

One good thing is the reminder it offers that prevention's early development and credibility were seriously hampered by a porous scientific substrate. Like a bright, flashing neon sign, the term advertises the need for sound documenting research in this area and serves as a rallying cry to do such research. Although prevention's weak research base posed serious problems early on [Price, Cowen, Lorion & McKay 1988], several recent comprehensive reviews [Albee & Gullotta 1997; Durlak 1997; Durlak & Wells 1997a; Weissberg & Greenberg 1998] highlight the field's solidly growing empirical base and confirm that this early shortcoming is being overcome.

Before considering the down side of current use of the term "science of prevention," an oversimplified statement about shared goals for adaptive outcomes may help to put key terminological issues in perspective. The essence of such a statement is that most of us would welcome a world filled with happy, healthy, effective people, free of debilitating psychological problems. The real question is not whether that is a desirable goal but rather how it can best be approached. It is around this latter issue that the term science of prevention, properly used, may have unintended constraining features.

To address the challenging, "how-best-realized" question in the light of the full complexity of Bronfenbrenner's analysis calls for the use of many different investigative and programmatic strategies, with different foci, goals and methodologies. Good science, including a good science of prevention, must necessarily come in different forms to reflect particular issues being studied and the diverse contexts in which such studies must unfold. What establishes good science in the prevention-wellness sphere is neither the specific substantive problem being studied, nor the particular model being used to study it, but rather the extent to which a range of sound methodologies succeed in identifying diverse pathways to wellness enhancement and problem reduction, and thus set the stage for change/intervention to advance those shared objectives

Unfortunately, the currently dominant use of the term science of prevention is confined to a particular *one* of those multipathways, i.e., the specific goal of preventing serious psychological disorder in those at risk, following the lock-step sequence in program development, evaluation, and dissemination described above [IOM 1994; Muehrer 1997]. Although this is a legitimate, appropriate usage in its own sphere of application, it scarcely scratches the surface of the broad range of approaches needed to advance wellness-promotion objectives and, if taken as gospel, rivets on a part-strategy that can, at best, address only a fraction of the complex, challenging issues that must be resolved to advance both the goals of preventing disorder and promoting wellness. In so doing, it constrains, or at least directs attention away from, other promising forms of a "science of wellness enhancement."

An earlier article [Cowen 1994] provides a base for concretizing this point. In that paper, I described five qualitatively different approaches to wellness enhancement: a) promoting wholesome early attachments; b) rooting early core competencies; c) engineering wellness-enhancing settings; d) acquiring effective stress coping skills; and e) empowerment. These strands were depicted as "mutually enhancing elements, in an elaborate system, not elements in competition with each other" [p. 159]. Whereas none fits cozily into the current, narrowly defined science of prevention-mould, each is integral to a life-span wellness enhancement model and must be carried out in different contexts and settings, using different "scientific" methodologies.

Illustratively, although steps taken to promote a wholesome attachment relationship and to root stage salient competencies seem, phenotypically, to be 180° removed from empowerment promotion steps, those on-the-surface disparate worlds come together meaningfully when seen as exemplars of a cohesive genotype of wellness enhancement. That is to say that they differ not in the ultimate goals that link them, but in their qualitatively different defining methods.

The latter differences are as they must be because the strategies in question approach the centrally shared goal of wellness enhancement at very different levels of Bronfenbrenner's framework. Thus, whereas early attachment is a microsystem issue, empowerment steps implicate complex changes in exosystems and the macrosystem.

A further complicating factor is that a given wellness issue can take on different forms at different times and under different circumstances. Steps taken to enhance wellness must necessarily fit such developmental and contextual realities. This point can be illustrated with the concept of empowerment. The natural roots of this notion lie in the soil of social inequity and *dis*empowerment [Rappaport 1981; 1987]. In the broadest sense, empowerment efforts are intended to promote opportunity and justice, and to enable people to control their own lives—each seen as instrumental to wellness. Many long-term empowerment efforts must thus be targeted to complex, difficult to change levels within Bronfenbrenner's framework, i.e., to exo- and macrosystems.

Although the justification of that thrust is self-evident, empowerment issues come up in contexts quite removed from the construct's original and most salient sphere of relevance. There is, for example, an intriguing *structural* parallel between classic empowerment issues and the promotion of autonomy support in young children [Deci & Ryan 1985]. Justification for this parallel can be drawn from Ryan and Stiller's [1991] report of consistent relationships between autonomy supportive conditions and a range of positive educational and behavioral outcomes in children. Although the technologies of classic empowerment and autonomy support in children are worlds apart, reflecting major developmental and contextual differences in their application, they share the wellness-related goals of strengthening people's sense of efficacy, and beliefs in their ability to master life situations and control their fate. For young children, a wholesome attachment relationship and success in acquiring stage salient competencies may, *ipso facto*, be "empowering." Put another way, because the wellness related ideal of empowerment can come up in very different forms, advancing that generic goal systematically requires a range of technologies calibrated to different stages, contexts, and realities.

The point to highlight in this discussion is that the diverse approaches described above, each central to wellness theory, are *not* readily incorporable into the framework of a "science of prevention" as that term is now narrowly defined and used. Without questioning the need for, or legitimacy of, that concept, it can be a source of confusion bordering on imperialism when put forth as the only way to "prevent." Moreover, should it turn out that some types of disorder reduction can better be realized by a wellness enhancement than by a risk-disease prevention approach, exclusive emphasis on the latter will act to obscure the former's potential for cutting down the flow of the very adverse conditions that a frontal disease-prevention strategy seeks to eradicate.

## Some Implications for Research

Establishing a sound generative base [Cowen 1980] for a wellness enhancement approach calls for: a) different research and program development activities than a risk-detection, disease-prevention strategy; and b) more diverse research methodologies that differ qualitatively from those said to define a "science of prevention" [Coie et al. 1993; IOM Report 1994; Muehrer 1997]. The first point is neatly illustrated by current research on childhood resilience [Cicchetti & Garmezy 1993; Masten & Coatsworth 1998; Werner & Smith 1982, 1992]. Resilience has been defined as "manifested competence in the context of significant challenges to adaptation or development" [Masten & Coatsworth 1998, p. 206]. When Garmezy [1982] depicted resilient children as "keepers of a dream" [p. xix], he meant to suggest that society (and wellness enhancement theory) could profit greatly from an understanding of the forces that moved profoundly stressed children to wholesome adaptation.

The odds-defying phenomenon of resilient child outcomes fits hand-in-glove with a wellness orientation. Generative findings about the pathways to wholesome adaptation among vulnerable, high-risk children form a base on which interventions to promote early wellness and avert later serious adaptive problems can rest. In this vein, Cowen, Wyman, Work and Parker [1990] spoke of resilience in the context of a shifting emphasis "away from the past dominant question of 'how can psychological malfunction best be undone', toward the potentially more fruitful questions of 'how wellness comes about in the first place and what can be done to promote it?'" [p. 195]. Thus the broad paradigmatic question being proposed is: what makes people healthy [Antonovsky 1979], rather than what makes them sick? A special appeal of the notion of child resilience is that it speaks directly to that question [Masten & Coatsworth 1998].

Several other thrusts that also reflect the emerging wellness paradigm include: a) the development of early, effective Head-Start programs [Ramey & Ramey 1998; Zigler & Styfco 1994], designed to promote child and family competencies that enhance both short- and long-term wellness [Masten & Coatsworth 1998; McLoyd 1998; Yoshikawa 1994]; b) conceptualizing early childhood problems as competence deficits and structuring change efforts around competence building [Strayhorn 1988]; and c) articulating and refining ongoing, school-based, wellness-oriented programs, from kindergarten through high school, to promote development of a broad range of essential social competencies [Elias & Tobias 1996; Weissberg & Elias 1993; Weissberg & Greenberg 1998]. An even more sweeping approach, in this same tradition, is the development of comprehensive, enduring school structures and programs built around the core goal of systematic enhancement of children's wellness [Battistich et al. 1995; Battistich et al. 1989; Dryfoos 1994; Iscoe & Keir 1997; Keir & Millea 1997]. This development places wellness enhancement in one key natural habitat, i.e., the school.

Without downplaying the importance of the above examples for a wellness enhancement framework, it is clear that they illustrate the strategy at its simplest, most accessible levels. Far more challenging in all likelihood will be the complex issues posed for this approach at the crucial, but difficult to access, levels of the exosystem and macrosystem.

## Concluding Remarks

Several recurrent themes of this chapter bear underscoring: a) my prior analysis of factors that promote wellness in the first years of life [Cowen 1999] reflects but one limited aspect of a broad array of wellness issues that must be addressed; b) different settings, systems, and sources of input, individually and interactively, affect wellness outcomes, as people develop; c) these sources vary both in their accessibility to study and potential for manipulation, control, and change; d) the full challenge of wellness enhancement will entail tortuously slow, pebble-piling steps that call for many different types of expertise and levels of study, and diverse change efforts; and e) these steps range from the individual to the societal level, and involve both visible and hidden regularities.

Although I cannot offer a detailed blueprint for navigating all the many byways (known and unknown) of this labyrinth, it is a labyrinth that must ultimately be negotiated to create a solid generative base for a comprehensive wellness enhancement thrust. Sudden cataclysmic breakthroughs in this quest are unlikely. But even if systematic wellness enhancement is no more than an ideal that will never *fully* be realized—and that is likely to be the case—it offers a fruitful, forward-looking framework for guiding conceptual formulations, program development, and research in mental health and other fields.

## Acknowledgments

My boundless gratitude to editors and authors for their Congressional Medal contributions to this tome, built around a notion and a vision (i.e., the enhancement of psychological wellness) that has been central to my professional being for several decades. Special thanks to Dante Cicchetti for his careful and caring edits and on-target suggestions for improving the chapter. I reserve exclusive claim, however, to the chapter's multisplendored sins.

## References

Albee, G. W. (1996). Revolutions and counterrevolutions in prevention. *American Psychologist, 51*, 1130–1133.

Albee, G. W. & Gullotta, T. P. (1997). *Primary prevention works*. Thousand Oaks, CA: Sage Publications.

Amato, P. R. & Keith, B. (1991). Parental divorce and the well being of children. *Psychological Bulletin, 110*, 26–46.

Antonovsky, A. (1979). *Health, stress and coping.* San Francisco: Jossey-Bass.

Battistich, V., Schaps, E., Watson, M., & Solomon, D. S. (1995). Prevention effects of the Child Development Project: Early findings from an ongoing multisite demonstration trial. *Journal of Adolescent Research, 11,* 12–35.

Battistich, V., Solomon, D. S., Watson, M., Solomon, J., & Schaps, E. (1989). Effects of an elementary school program to enhance prosocial behavior and children's cognitive social problem solving skills and strategies. *Journal of Applied Developmental Psychology, 10,* 147–169.

Belsky, J. (1984). The determinants of parenting: A process model. *Child Development, 55,* 83–96.

Berrueta-Clement, J. R., Schweinhart, L. J., Barnett, M. W., Epstein, A. S., & Weikart, D. P. (1984). *Changed lives: The effects of the Perry Preschool Project on youths through age 19.* Ypsilanti, MI: High/Scope Press.

Bronfenbrenner, U. (1977). Toward an experimental ecology of human development. *American Psychologist, 32,* 513–531.

Carlson, E. A. & Sroufe, L. A. (1995). Contributions of attachment theory to developmental psychopathology. In D. Cicchetti & D. J. Cohen (Eds.), *Developmental psychopathology: Vol. 1. Theory and methods* (pp. 581–617). New York: John Wiley & Sons.

Cicchetti, D. & Cohen, D. J. (1995). Perspectives on developmental psychopathology. In D. Cicchetti & D. J. Cohen (Eds.), *Developmental psychopathology: Vol. 1. Theory and methods* (pp. 3–20). New York: Wiley-Interscience.

Cicchetti, D. & Garmezy, N. (1993). Milestones in the development of resilience. *Development and Psychopathology, 4,* 497–783.

Cicchetti, D. & Lynch, M. (1993). Toward an ecological/transactional model of community violence and child maltreatment: Consequences for children's development. *Psychiatry, 56,* 96–118.

Cicchetti, D. & Rogosch, F. A. (1996). Equifinality and multifinality in developmental psychopathology. *Development and Psychopathology, 8,* 597–600.

Cicchetti, D. & Toth, S. L. (1998). The development of depression in children. *American Psychologist, 53,* 221–241.

Cicchetti, D. & Tucker, D. (1994). Development and self-regulatory structures of the mind. *Development and Psychopathology, 6,* 533–549.

Coie, J. D., Watt, N. F., West, S. G., Hawkins, J. D., Asarnow, J. R., Markman, H. J., Ramey, S. L., Shure, M. B., & Long, B. (1993). The science of prevention: A conceptual framework and some directions for a national research program. *American Psychologist, 48*, 1013–1022.

Cowen, E. L. (1973). Social and community interventions. In P. Mussen & M. Rosenzweig (Eds.), *Annual Review of Psychology* (Vol. 24) (pp. 423–472).

Cowen, E. L. (1980). The wooing of primary prevention. *American Journal of Community Psychology, 8*, 258–284.

Cowen, E. L. (1982). Choices and alternatives for primary prevention in mental health. In M. P. Goldstein (Ed.), *Preventive intervention in schizophrenia: Are we ready?* (pp. 178–191). Washington, DC: NIMH Primary Prevention Series, Government Printing Office.

Cowen, E. L. (1994). The enhancement of psychological wellness: Challenges and opportunities. *American Journal of Community Psychology, 22*, 149–179.

Cowen, E. L. (1996). The ontogenesis of primary prevention: Lengthy strides and stubbed toes. *American Journal of Community Psychology, 24*, 235–249.

Cowen, E. L. (1997a). The coming of age of primary prevention: Comments on Durlak and Wells' meta-analysis. *American Journal of Community Psychology, 25*, 153–167.

Cowen, E. L. (1997b). On the semantics and operations of primary prevention and wellness enhancement: Or, will the real primary prevention please stand up? *American Journal of Community Psychology, 25*, 245–255.

Cowen, E. L. (1999). In sickness and in health: Primary prevention's vows revisited. In D. Cicchetti & S. L. Toth (Eds.), *Rochester Symposium on Developmental Psychopathology: Vol 9. Developmental approaches to prevention and intervention* (pp. 1–24). Rochester, NY: University of Rochester Press.

Cowen, E. L., Wyman, P. A., Work, W. C., & Parker, G. R. (1990). The Rochester Child Resilience Project (RCRP): Overview and summary of first year findings. *Development and Psychopathology, 2*, 193–212.

Deci, E. L. & Ryan, R. M. (1985). *Intrinsic motivation and self-determination in human behavior*. New York: Plenum Press.

Dinges, N. (1994). Mental health promotion. In P. J. Mrazek & R. J. Haggerty (Eds.), *Reducing risks for mental disorders: Frontiers for preventive intervention* (pp. 333–355). Washington, DC: National Academy Press.

Dryfoos, J. G. (1994). *Full-service schools: A revolution in health and social services for children, youth, and families*. San Francisco: Jossey-Bass.

Durlak, J. A. (1997). *Successful prevention programs for children and adolescents*. New York: Plenum.

Durlak, J. A. & Wells, A. M. (1997a). Primary prevention programs for children and adolescents: A meta-analytic review. *American Journal of Community Psychology, 25,* 115–152.

Durlak, J. A. & Wells, A. M. (1997b). Primary prevention programs: The future is exciting. *American Journal of Community Psychology, 25,* 233–243.

Egeland, B., Pianta, R., & Ogawa, J. (1996). Early behavior problems: Pathways to mental disorders in adolescence. *Development and Psychopathology, 8,* 725–750.

Elias, M. J. (1995). Primary prevention as health and social competence promotion. *Journal of Primary Prevention, 16,* 5–24.

Elias, M. J. & Tobias, S. E. (1996). *Social problem solving: Interventions in the schools.* New York: Guilford.

Emde, R. N. & Harmon, R. J. (1984). *Continuities and discontinuities in behavior.* New York: Plenum.

Garmezy, N. (1982). Foreword. In E. E. Werner & R. S. Smith, *Vulnerable but invincible: A study of resilient children* (pp. xiii–xix). New York: McGraw-Hill.

Goldstein, M. P. (1982). Preface. In M. P. Goldstein (Ed.), *Preventive intervention in schizophrenia: Are we ready?* (pp. v–vii). Washington, DC: NIMH Primary Prevention Series, Government Printing Office.

Hetherington, E. M. (1989). Coping with family transitions: Winners, losers and survivors. *Child Development, 60,* 1–14.

Hetherington, E. M., Bridges, M., & Insabella, G. M. (1998). What matters? What does not? Five perspectives on the association between marital transition and children's adjustment. *American Psychologist, 53,* 167–184.

Institute of Medicine Report. (1994). *Reducing risks for mental disorders: Summary.* Washington, DC: National Academy Press.

Iscoe, L. K. & Keir, S. S. (1997). *Revisiting the school of the future: The evolution of a school based services project.* Austin, TX: Hogg Foundation for Mental Health.

Kagan, S. L. & Neuman, M. J. (1997). Defining and implementing school readiness: Challenges for families, early care and education, and schools. In R. P. Weissberg, T. P. Gullota, R. L. Hampton, B. A. Ryan, & G. R. Adams (Eds.), *Establishing preventive services: Issues in children's and families' lives* (Vol. 9) (pp. 61–96). Thousands Oaks, CA: Sage Publications.

Keir, S. S. & Millea, S. (1997). *Challenges and realities: Evaluating a school based service project*. Austin, TX: Hogg Foundation for Mental Health.

Koretz, D. S. (1991). Prevention-centered science in mental health. *American Journal of Community Psychology, 19*, 453–458.

Koretz, D. S. & Moscicki, E. K. (1997). An ounce of prevention: What is it worth? *American Journal of Community Psychology, 25*, 189–196.

Masten, A. S. & Coatsworth, J. D. (1998). The development of competence in favorable and unfavorable environments: Lessons from research on successful children. *American Psychologist, 53*, 205–220.

McLoyd, V. C. (1990). The impact of economic hardship on Black families and children: Psychological stress, parenting and socioemotional development. *Child Development, 61*, 311–346.

McLoyd, V. C. (1998). Socioeconomic disadvantage and child development. *American Psychologist, 53*, 185–204.

Mrazek, P. J. & Haggerty, R. J. (Eds.). (1994). *Reducing risks for mental disorders: Frontiers for preventive intervention*. Washington, DC: National Academy Press.

Mrazek, P. J. & Hall, M. (1997). A policy perspective on prevention. *American Journal of Community Psychology, 25*, 221–226.

Muehrer, P. (1997). Introduction to the special issue: Mental health prevention science in rural communities and contexts. *American Journal of Community Psychology, 25*, 421–424.

Muñoz, R. F., Mrazek, P. J., & Haggerty, R. J. (1996). Institute of Medicine report on prevention of mental disorders: Summary and commentary. *American Psychologist, 51*, 1116–1122.

Nelson, C. A. & Bloom, F. E. (1997). Child development and neuroscience. *Child Development, 68*, 970–987.

Pardes, H. (1982). Foreword. In M. P. Goldstein (Ed.), *Preventive intervention in schizophrenia: Are we ready?* (pp. iii–v). Washington, DC: NIMH Primary Prevention Series, Government Printing Office.

President's Commission on Mental Health. (1978). *Report to the President*. (Stock No. 040-000-00390-8). Washington, DC: U.S. Government Printing Office.

Ramey, C. T. & Ramey, S. L. (1998). Early intervention and early experience. *American Psychologist, 53*, 109–120.

Rappaport, J. (1981). In praise of paradox: A social policy of empowerment over prevention. *American Journal of Community Psychology, 9*, 1–25.

Rappaport, J. (1987). Terms of empowerment/exemplars of prevention: Toward a theory of community psychology. *American Journal of Community Psychology, 15*, 121–148.

Reiss, D. & Price, R. H. (1996). National research agenda for prevention research: The National Institute of Mental Health Report. *American Psychologist, 51*, 1109–1115.

Ryan, R. M. & Stiller, J. (1991). The social contexts of internalization: Parent and teacher influences on autonomy, motivation, and learning. In R. P. Pintrich & M. L. Maehr (Eds.), *Advances in motivation and achievement: Goals and self-regulatory processes* (Vol. 7) (pp. 115–149). Greenwich, CT: JAI.

Sarason, S. B. (1971). *The culture of the school and the problem of change*. Boston: Allyn Bacon.

Schweinhart, L. J., Barnes, H. V., & Weikart, D. P. (1993). *Significant benefits: The High/Scope Perry Preschool Project through age 27*. Ypsilanti, MI: High Scope Press.

Strayhorn, J. M. (1988). *The competent child: An approach to psychotherapy and preventive mental health*. New York: Guilford.

Tolan, P. H. & Guerra, N. G. (1994). Prevention of delinquency: Current status and issues. *Applied and Preventive Psychology, 3*, 251–273.

Trickett, E. J., Dahiyat, C., & Selby, P. (1994). *Primary prevention in mental health: An annotated bibliography, 1983–1991*. Rockville, MD: U.S. Department of Health and Human Services.

Weikart, D. P. & Schweinhart, L. J. (1997). High/Scope Perry Preschool Program. In G. W. Albee & T. P. Gullotta (Eds.), *Primary prevention works: Issues in children's and families lives, Vol. 6* (pp. 146–166). Thousand Oaks, CA: Sage Publications.

Weissberg, R. P. & Elias, M. J. (1993). Enhancing young children's social competence and health behavior: An important challenge for educators, scientists, policy makers and funders. *Applied and Preventive Psychology, 2*, 179–190.

Weissberg, R. P. & Greenberg, M. T. (1998). School and community competence-enhancement and prevention programs. In W. Damon (Series Ed.), I. E. Siegel & K. A. Renninger (Vol. Eds.), *Handbook of child psychology: Vol. 4. Child psychology in practice* (5th ed.) (pp. 877–954). New York: John Wiley & Sons.

Werner, E. E. & Smith, R. S. (1982). *Vulnerable but invincible: A study of resilient children*. New York: McGraw-Hill.

Werner, E. E. & Smith, R. S. (1992). *Overcoming the odds: High risk children from birth to adulthood*. Ithaca, NY: Cornell University Press.

Yoshikawa, H. (1994). Prevention as cumulative protection: Effects of early family support and education on chronic delinquency and its risks. *Psychological Bulletin, 115*, 28–54.

Yoshikawa, H. (1995). Long-term effects of early childhood programs on social outcomes and delinquency. *The Future of Children, 5*, 51–75.

Zigler, E. & Styfco, S. J. (1994). Head Start: Criticisms in a constructive context. *American Psychologist, 49*, 127–132.

Zigler, E., Taussig, C., & Black, K. (1992). A promising preventative for juvenile delinquency. *American Psychologist, 47*, 997–1006.

Zigler, E. F. & Finn-Stevenson, M. (1997). Policy efforts to enhance child and family life: Goals for 2010. In R. P. Weissberg, T. P. Gullotta, R. L. Hampton, B. A. Ryan, & G. R. Adams (Eds.), *Establishing preventive services: Issues in children's and families' lives* (Vol. 9) (pp. 27–60). Thousand Oaks, CA: Sage Publications.

# About the Authors

## Editors

**Dante Cicchetti, Ph.D.,** is professor of clinical and social sciences in psychology, and professor of psychiatry and pediatrics at the University of Rochester. Dr. Cicchetti received his Ph.D. in clinical psychology and child development from the University of Minnesota. Subsequently, he was an assistant professor and the Norman Tishman associate professor of psychology and social relations at Harvard University. Since 1985, Dr. Cicchetti has served as the director of Mt. Hope Family Center. He has published extensively in the areas of emotional development, Down Syndrome, child maltreatment, childhood depression, and developmental psychopathology, and has edited and contributed to many books, including *Attachment in the Preschool Years; Child Maltreatment,: Risk and Protective Factors in the Development of Psychopathology; The Self in Transition; Child Abuse, Child Development and Social Policy,* and *Developmental Psychopathology.* Included among Dr. Cicchetti's awards and honors are the 1983 Boyd McCandless Award (for early career contributions to developmental psychology) from the American Psychological Association, the 1997 Research Career Achievement Award from the American Professional Society on the Abuse of Children, the 1999 Distinguished Scientific Contribution to Child Clinical Psychology Award, and the 1999 Nicholas Hobbs Award for contributions to social policy and child development (both from the American Psychological Association). Dr. Cicchetti is the founding editor of *Development and Psychopathology* as well as on the editorial board of the *Psychological Bulletin.*

**Julian Rappaport, Ph.D.,** is professor of psychology at the University of Illinois at Urbana-Champaign and a faculty member in the programs in clinical/community psychology and personality and social ecology. He is a recipient of the American Psychological Association's (Division 27) Career Award for Distinguished Contributions to Theory and Research, a past president of the Society for Community Research and Action, and Editor-Emeritus of the *American Journal of Community Psychology.*

**Irwin Sandler, Ph.D.,** is a professor in the Department of Psychology at Arizona State University and is the director of an NIMH-funded Prevention Research Center. He has been the president of the Society for Community Research and Action and chair of the Council of Community Psychology Program Directors. He is the 1999 recipient of the Distinguished Contributions to Theory and Research award from the Society for Community Research and Action. He has also been a member of several task forces and advisory committees on prevention and promotion for the American Psychological Association and the National Institute of Mental Health. He has written over 100 scholarly articles, chapters, books, and intervention manuals concerning stress and coping and prevention for children. His research focuses on understanding children's adaptation to highly stressful situations such as parental divorce, parental death, and economic strain in the family and on the development of preventive programs for children in high stress situations. Among his publications are the coedited *Handbook of Children's Coping* (Plenum), and recent scholarly publications on children's coping and coping efficacy.

**Roger P. Weissberg, Ph.D.,** is a professor of psychology and education at the University of Illinois at Chicago (UIC). He is the chair of UIC's Community and Prevention Research Division, and directs an NIMH-funded, multidisciplinary predoctoral and postdoctoral prevention research training program in urban children's mental health and AIDS prevention. Dr. Weissberg is a senior research associate for the Mid-Atlantic Regional Laboratory for Student Success. He also is executive director of the Collaborative to Advance Social and Emotional Learning (CASEL). Dr. Weissberg has written more than 100 publications focusing on preventive interventions with children, and has coauthored nine school-based, competence-promotion curricula to prevent problem behaviors including drug use, high-risk sexual behaviors, and aggression. Three recent coedited books include: *Enhancing Children's Wellness* [Sage 1997], *Establishing Preventive Services*, [Sage 1997], and *Promoting Positive Outcomes* [CWLA Press 1999]. He also coauthored *Promoting Social and Emotional Learning: Guidelines for Educators* [Association for Supervision and Curriculum Development 1997]. He has been the president of the American Psychological

Association's Society for Community Research and Action and co-chaired an APA Task Force on "Prevention: Promoting Strength, Resilience, and Health in Young People." He has received the William T. Grant Foundation's 5-year Faculty Scholars Award in Children's Mental Health, and the National Mental Health Association's Lela Rowland Prevention Award.

## Contributors

**Mark Aber, Ph.D.,** is associate professor of psychology at the University of Illinois at Urbana-Champaign and a faculty member in the programs in Clinical/Community Psychology and Personality and Social Ecology. His primary research interests concern neighborhoods, community organization, and community development. He is a member, Council of Community Psychology Program Directors, Society for Community Research and Action, and chair of the Children and Youth Interest Group, Society for Community Research and Action.

**Manuel Barrera, Jr., Ph.D.,** is professor of psychology at Arizona State University and adjunct research scientist at Oregon Research Institute. He received his Ph.D. in clinical psychology from the University of Oregon. For the past 20 years he has studied social support, including its conceptualization, measurement, and relations to the mental health of adolescents. Currently he is involved in research to evaluate the efficacy of social support interventions.

**Dina Birman, Ph.D.,** is a research fellow at Georgetown University Medical Center in Washington, D.C. Her professional interests involve understanding adaptation and acculturation experiences of immigrants, refugees, and ethnic minorities. Prior to coming to Georgetown University, she was working at the National Institute of Mental Health, as chief of minority institutions programs. She had also worked for the Refugee Mental Health Program, at the National Institute of Mental Health, and later at the Center for Mental Health Services in the Substance Abuse and Mental Health Services Administration. While there, she provided technical assistance and consultation to domestic refugee resettlement programs on psychological adjustment of refugees, and the development of refugee mental health services and preventive interventions.

**Jacob A. Burack, Ph.D.,** received his Ph.D. in developmental psychology from Yale University. He is an associate professor of school/applied developmental psychology in the Department of Educational Psychology at McGill University and is the founder and director of the McGill Youth Study Team (MYST). Jake's scholarly interests include the study of the development of cognition, attention and perception among persons with autism and mental retardation, and theoretical writings about the developmental course of autism and related disorders. A secondary area is focused on the study of cultural attitudes and beliefs of First Nations' children in relation to academic, emotional, and social well-being. In addition to their academic work, Jake and his students work with school administrators, teachers, aides, families, at-risk students, and students with special needs on the development of educational services for children in Quebec and elsewhere in Canada.

**Emory L. Cowen, Ph.D.,** is professor of psychology and director of the University of Rochester Center for Community Study. He was a founder of the Primary Mental Health Project (PMHP) and directed the project for its first 34 years. Cowen is past president of Division 27 of the American Psychological Association (APA) and the recipient of its Distinguished Contributions and Seymour B. Sarason awards. He also received the APA Award for Distinguished Contributions to Psychology in the Public Interest. He has authored 300+ articles, chapters and books in the professional literature, focusing on the areas of primary prevention, wellness enhancement, school-based early detection and prevention programs, and resilient adaptation among highly stressed children.

**Joseph A. Durlak, Ph.D.,** is a professor of psychology at Loyola University Chicago. After receiving his Ph.D. from Vanderbilt University in 1972, he served in the U.S. Army as a clinical psychologist and began work in school-based prevention. He has written two books on prevention and coedited a third, *School-based prevention programs for children and adolescents* published by Sage, *Successful prevention programs for children and adolescents*, published by Plenum, and *Program imple-*

*mentation in preventive trials* coedited with Joseph Ferrari and published by Haworth Press. His major interests, in addition to prevention, include community psychology, child clinical psychology, meta-analysis, and the use of paraprofessionals.

**Maurice J. Elias, Ph.D.,** is a professor in the Department of Psychology at Rutgers University. He is co-developer of the Improving Social Awareness-Social Problem Solving Project. This project received the 1988 Lela Rowland Prevention Award from the National Mental Health Association, is approved by the Program Effectiveness Panel of the National Diffusion Network as a federally validated prevention program, and most recently, has been named as a Model Program by the National Educational Goals Panel. In 1990, he was awarded the National Psychological Consultants to Management Award by the American Psychological Association. In 1993, he received the Distinguished Contribution to Practice of Community Psychology Award from the Society for Community Research and Action (APA Division 27). Dr. Elias is a member of the Leadership Team of the Collaborative to Advance Social and Emotional Learning (CASEL). His books include: *Social Decision Making Skills: A Curriculum Guide for Elementary Grades, Building Social Problem Solving Skills: Guidelines from a School-Based Program, Social Decision Making Skills: Guidelines for Middle School Educators, Promoting Student Success Through Group Intervention, Social Problem Solving Interventions in Schools, Promoting Social and Emotional Learning: Guidelines for Educators,* and *Emotionally Intelligent Parenting.*

**John W. Fantuzzo, Ph.D.,** is the Diana Riklis Professor in the School, Community, and Clinical Child Psychology Program in the Graduate School of Education at University of Pennsylvania. His research interests and grant activity primarily involve the design, implementation, and evaluation of school- and community-based assessment and prevention strategies for vulnerable, low-income children and families in high-risk environments. Research related to enhancing Head Start services for urban preschool children and their families is a major interest at this time.

**Robert D. Felner, Ph.D.,** received his doctorate in clinical and community psychology from the University of Rochester, where he had the good fortune to have Emory L. Cowen as his master's and dissertation advisor. He also spent a year on internship at the Center for Community Studies under Cowen's supervision and, throughout his graduate career, worked there as a graduate research assistant.

Currently, Felner is director of the School of Education and the National Center on Public Education and Social Policy at the University of Rhode Island. He is also the director of the project on High Performance Learning Communities at the University of Illinois, which includes evaluation research on a number of major school reform initiatives, including those funded by the Carnegie Corporation, the Lilly Endowment, and the Kellogg foundation.

Previously, Felner was founding director of the Center for Prevention Research and Development in the Institute for Government and Public Affairs at the University of Illinois, where he was also professor of public policy, education, and social welfare. Prior to that he served as professor of psychology and director of the graduate programs in clinical and community psychology at both the University of Illinois and Auburn University. He began his academic career as an assistant professor in clinical and community psychology at Yale University in 1976.

**James G. Kelly, Ph.D.,** has been the professor of psychology and public health at the University of Illinois at Chicago since 1982. Previous academic appointments have been at the University of Oregon, University of Michigan, and Ohio State University. He was also on the staff of the National Institute of Mental Health. Two postdoctoral years were spent at the Department of Psychiatry of Massach us etts General Hospital and the Harvard School of Public Health where he received a Master's Degree in public health. His Ph.D. degree is from the University of Texas in clinical psychology.

He is an author or coauthor of seven books and numerous journal articles and book chapters. He is recognized for his ecological thesis to conduct community based research and to design preventive interventions. During the past eight years he has been documenting the development of African American community leaders. This work has been collaborative with the host community organization in the selection of topics, research methods, and ways to implement the findings from this work.

He is a fellow of four divisions of the American Psychological Association, as well as fellow of the American Association for the

Advancement of Science. He was first elected president of the Society for Community Research and Action and has received the award for Distinguished Contributions to Theory and Research from the Society. In August 1988 he received the Senior Career award for Distinguished Contributions to Psychology in the Public Interest from the American Psychological Association.

**Raymond P. Lorion, Ph.D.,** received his doctorate in clinical psychology from the University of Rochester in 1972 under the direction of Emory Cowen and served as a research coordinator for the Primary Mental Health Project from 1972–1974. Dr. Lorion is currently professor and chair of psychology at Ohio University and editor of the *Journal of Community Psychology*. From 1982–1984, he served as visiting scientist to the National Institute of Mental Health and acting associate administrator for Prevention of the Alcohol, Drug Abuse and Mental Health Administration. In those capacities, he assisted in the development and implementation of the Prevention Research Centers program. Throughout his career, he has worked on the identification of risk and protective factors for child and adolescent emotional and behavioral disorders and on the design, implementation and evaluation of interventions to reduce the incidence and prevalence of those disorders. He is the author/editor of 10 books and approximately 120 chapters and scientific papers.

**Suniya S. Luthar, Ph.D.,** is associate professor of psychology and education at Teachers College, Columbia University, and director of child and family research at the APT Foundation, New Haven. She received a Ph.D. in developmental/clinical psychology from Yale University. Her interests are in developmental psychopathology, and current studies involve adjustment processes among inner-city and suburban youth; vulnerability and resilience among substance abusers' children; and group psychotherapy for at-risk mothers. Professional honors include a dissertation award from the American Psychological Association's Division 37 and a Boyd McCandless Young Scientist Award from APA's Division 7.

**Wanda K. Mohr, Ph.D., R.N., F.A.A.N.,** is an assistant professor and director of psychiatric mental health nursing in the School of Nursing at the University of Pennsylvania. Her research interests focus specifically on children exposed to family violence and more generally on issue related to child mental health service delivery models. She is national chairperson for research and education for the Association of Child and Adolescent Psychiatric Nursing and recipient of numerous awards for research and child advocacy.

**Kathleen Nelson** is a doctoral student in the clinical psychology program at Arizona State University. Her primary interest is in the area of stress and coping among families facing adversity. Kathleen's master's degree research focused on identification of families who benefit from participation in parenting programs for newly divorced mothers. Currently, her research is focused upon environmental and interpersonal risk and resiliency factors among families coping with poverty. Clinically, Kathleen works with low-income families in which children are at high-risk for out-of-home placement.

**Martin Nieto, M.A.,** is a Ph.D. candidate in the Clinical/Community Program at the Department of Psychology, University of Illinois, Urbana-Champaign. He is also visiting research specialist for the Children and Family Research Center at the University of Illinois, Urbana-Champaign. Main research interests concern the theoretical and empirical understanding of neighborhood and community influences on child and adolescent development and adjustment.

**Hazel Prelow, Ph.D.,** is an assistant professor of psychology at the State University of New York at Albany. After receiving her Ph.D. in clinical psychology from the University of North Texas, she completed a postdoctoral fellowship in child mental health/primary prevention at Arizona State University. Her current research seeks to understand how the sociocultural context influences risk and protective factors for minority adolescents. She is also interested in cross-cultural and measurement equivalence.

**Fred A. Rogosch, Ph.D.,** is associate professor in clinical and social sciences in psychology at the University of Rochester and a researcher at the Mt. Hope Family Center. He has published papers and chapters in the areas of child maltreatment, offspring of parents with mental disorders, substance abuse, prevention, resilience, and social development.

**Seymour B. Sarason, Ph.D.,** received his B.A. in 1939 from the University of Newark (now the Newark Campus of Rutgers, The State University of New Jersey). He did his graduate work at Clark University where he received his Ph.D. in 1942. He was the

1996 recipient of the Gold Medal Award for Life Contribution by a Psychologist in the Public Interest, as well as other awards from the American Association on Mental Deficiency and the American Psychological Association.

In 1962 he founded and directed the Yale Psycho-Educational Clinic, one of the first research and training sites in community psychology. He has contributed to a number of areas of psychology, including mental retardation, culture and personality, projective techniques, teacher training, anxiety in children, and school reform. He has published numerous books, chapters, and articles that reflect his broad interests in the field.

Seymour is professor of Psychology Emeritus in the Department of Psychology and at the Institution for Social and Policy Studies of Yale University. He retired in 1989 from Yale University after two decades of directing the clinical training program. Seymour continues to be an active and productive scholar, having published over 10 books since his retirement.

**Stanley F. Schneider, Ph.D.**, received his doctorate in psychology from the University of Michigan in 1953, where he remained on the faculty of the Departments of Psychology and Psychiatry until 1962, teaching and supervising internship training of graduate students in clinical psychology. He joined the National Institute of Mental Health (NIMH) in 1963. In his long career there he was chief of the Psychology Education Branch, the program that supported the training of research and clinical psychologists at universities and other training centers throughout the nation. He championed the development of community psychology, health psychology, social ecology, environmental psychology, programs to broaden methodology, training for prevention, and increased attention to the inclusion of women and ethnic minorities in all aspects of psychology. He became Associate Director for Research Training and Resource Development in the Division of Neuroscience and Behavioral Science in 1985. His interests and activities were articulated in a growing commitment to life course development as a cohering paradigm for psychology. He was an early contributor to the institute's AIDS program and saw this disease as a vivid example of the need to link research with the community and with social policy. He also stimulated interest in emotion as a neglected area of NIMH research and training, and was active in promoting the development of research centers in AIDS and in behavioral sciences. He retired from NIMH in 1995, and in some valedictory remarks underlined the importance of increased attention to the enhancement of psychological wellness as an urgent matter of health economics.

**Sheree L. Toth, Ph.D.,** is associate professor of psychology at the University of Rochester and associate director of the Mt. Hope Family Center. She has published in the areas of child maltreatment, parental depression, and prevention and intervention and has contributed chapters to many books, including *Developmental Psychopathology, Handbook of Developmental Psychology,* and *Handbook of Psychotherapies with Children and Families.* Toth also has coedited eight volumes for the *Rochester Symposium on Developmental Psychopathology.*

**Edison J. Trickett, Ph.D.,** is professor of psychology at the University of Maryland, College Park. He is a past president of Division 27 of the American Psychological Association, past editor of the *American Journal of Community Psychology,* and recipient of Division 27's award for Distinguished Contribution to Theory and Research in Community Psychology. He has written extensively on the development of an ecological perspective on community research and intervention and is currently conducting research with Dina Birman on the adaptation of adolescents from the former Soviet Union to life in the United States. His most recent book, coedited with Dina Birman and Roderick Watts, is entitled *Human Diversity: Perspectives on People in Context.*

**Angela Wiley, Ph.D.,** is assistant professor of human and community development and a family life extension specialist at the University of Illinois at Urbana-Champaign. She received her Ph.D. in developmental psychology from Clark University and has been a postdoctoral student at the University of Illinois at Urbana-Champaign.

**Sharlene Wolchik, Ph.D.,** is a professor in the Department of Psychology at Arizona State University. She is head of the Divorce Core in the Prevention Research Center at Arizona State University. She has been secretary of the Society for Community Research and Action and editor of the *Community Psychologist.* She has authored four books and over sixty chapters and journal articles. She has developed the New Beginnings Program, a parenting program for divorced mothers that has demonstrated efficacy in two randomized experimental trials and is currently conducting a six-year follow-up study on these families as the children move into late adolescence. Among her publications are the coedited *Handbook of Children's Coping* (Plenum), and recent scholarly publications on parenting in highly stressed families.

**Peter A. Wyman, Ph.D.,** is codirector of the Rochester Child Resilience Project, an ongoing program investigating resilience in children and families and seeking to apply this knowledge to promote children's adaptation. Dr. Wyman has authored numerous articles on the topics of children's resilience and development in adverse environments and preventive interventions. He is coauthor of School-Based Prevention for Children at Risk, published in 1996 by the American Psychological Association. Dr. Wyman is also director of research at the Primary Mental Health Project, and associate professor in clinical and social sciences in psychology at the University of Rochester. Dr. Wyman also is a clinical associate professor of psychiatry at the University of Rochester School of Medicine, where he teaches in the clinical training program.